Trends in Drug Discovery in Diabetes and Obesity

Further Volumes of the Series "*Trends in Drug Discovery*"

Szabo, G. T. and Pardi, N. (eds.)

Trends in mRNA Vaccine Research

2025

Print ISBN: 9783527350582

Doller, D. and Hodgetts, K. J. (eds.)

Trends in CNS Drug Discovery

2026

Print ISBN: 9783527352807

Sofia, M. J. and Wang, Z. (eds.)

Trends in Antiviral Drug Development

2025

Print ISBN: 9783527353019

Trends in Drug Discovery in Diabetes and Obesity

Edited by Lars Linderoth and Søren Østergaard

WILEY-VCH

Editors

Dr. Lars Linderoth
Novo Nordisk
Novo Nordisk Park
Building H5.s.39
Måløv
Denmark

Dr. Søren Østergaard
Novo Nordisk
Novo Nordisk Park
Building H5.1.11
Måløv
Denmark

Series Editors

Dr. János Fischer
Richter Co., Ltd.
Budapest
Hungary

Dr. Christian Klein
Roche Innovation Center Zürich
Roche Pharma, Research & Early Development, pRED, Wagistrasse 10
8952, Schlieren
Switzerland

Dr. Wayne E Childers
Moulder Center for Drug Discovery Research
School of Pharmacy, Temple University
3307 N Broad Street
Philadelphia, PA
USA

Dr. David P Rotella
Department of Chemistry and Biochemistry
Montclair State University
Montclair, NJ
USA

Cover Images: © Søren Østergaard

Typesetting: Straive, Chennai, India

Library of Congress Card No.: applied for

British Library Cataloguing-in-Publication Data A catalogue record for this book is available from the British Library.

Bibliographic information published by the Deutsche Nationalbibliothek
The Deutsche Nationalbibliothek lists this publication in the Deutsche Nationalbibliografie; detailed bibliographic data are available on the Internet at <http://dnb.d-nb.de>.

Print ISBN: 978-3-527-35330-9
ePDF ISBN: 978-3-527-84542-2
ePub ISBN: 978-3-527-84541-5
oBook ISBN: 978-3-527-84540-8

Printed and bound by
CPI Group (UK) Ltd, Croydon, CR0 4YY

C9783527353309_290726

Contents

Series Editors Preface *xi*
Preface *xiii*

1 **The Role of Gut Peptides in the Regulation of Body Weight** *1*
Jens J. Holst and Sten Madsbad
Introduction and Methodological Considerations *1*
Mimicry *2*
Hormone Antagonists *3*
Activation and Inactivation *3*
Somatostatin as a Tool *4*
Gut Hormones with a Possible Role in Food Intake *5*
Cholecystokinin *5*
GLP-1 *7*
Role of Endogenous GLP-1 in Food Intake Regulation *8*
Mechanism of Action of Exogenous GLP-1 Receptor Agonists *9*
Development of GLP-1 Receptor Agonists for Obesity Therapy *9*
Oxyntomodulin and Glucagon-GLP-1 Coagonists *10*
PYY *11*
GIP *13*
Ghrelin *16*
Conclusion *18*
References *19*

2 **Agonists and Antagonists of the Human GIP Receptor** *33*
Hüsün S. Kizilkaya, Lærke S. Gasbjerg, Jens J. Holst, and Mette M. Rosenkilde
Introduction *33*
Objective of the Chapter *34*
Background *35*
Glucose-Dependent Insulinotropic Polypeptide – Rationale for Initial Therapeutic Interest *35*
GIP – Posttranslational Processing, Secretion, and Degradation *36*
Glucose-Dependent Insulinotropic Polypeptide Receptor (GIPR) *37*
Receptor Activation and Signaling *37*

Desensitization, Internalization, and Receptor Trafficking *40*
Expression in Humans and Animals *45*
Important Species Differences in the GIP System *45*
Physiological Actions of GIP *46*
GIP's Effect on the Pancreas of Healthy Individuals *46*
GIP's Effect on the Pancreas of Individuals with Type 2 Diabetes *47*
GIP's Effect on the Pancreas of Individuals with Obesity *48*
Extrapancreatic Physiological Effects of GIP *49*
Adipose Tissue *49*
Body Weight *50*
Energy Expenditure *51*
Cardiovascular System *51*
Bones *52*
Central Nervous System *53*
Pharmacological GIPR Agonism *54*
Animal Studies *54*
Human Studies *55*
Pharmacological GIPR Antagonism *60*
Animal Studies *60*
Human Studies *61*
Theories Bridging GIPR Agonism and Antagonism *62*
Conclusion *63*
References *64*

3 Amylin – Biological Aspects *87*
Thomas A. Lutz
Introduction *87*
Amylin Synthesis and Secretion *87*
Different Molecular Forms of Amylin *88*
Amylin Signaling at the Amylin Receptor *88*
Amylin Receptor Activation and Intracellular Signaling *88*
Amylin's Effect on Energy Homeostasis *89*
Amylin Effects on Eating; Induction of Satiation *89*
Amylin Effects on Energy Expenditure *90*
Sex Differences in Amylin Action *91*
Brain Sites of Amylin Action *91*
Caudal Hindbrain with the AP and the NTS *91*
Projections from the AP – Role of the Lateral Parabrachial Nucleus *92*
Single Cell Studies to Define the Phenotype of Caudal Hindbrain Neurons Involved in Amylin Action *93*
Other Brain Areas Mediating the Actions of Amylin *94*
Direct Amylin Action in the Hypothalamus *94*

Central Reward Processing of Amylin in the Ventral Tegmental Area (VTA), the Nucleus Accumbens (NAc), the Dorsal Tegmental Area, and the Medial Prefrontal Cortex *95*
Amylin–Leptin Interactions in the Regulation of Energy Homeostasis *96*
Amylin–Leptin Interactions in the AP and NTS *97*
Amylin–Leptin Interactions in the VMH (ARC + VMN) *98*
Amylin–Leptin Interactions in the VTA *98*
Other Molecular Forms of Amylin and Their Potential Role in Physiology and Pathophysiology *99*
Amylin Forms *99*
Amylin Analogs Mimic Amylin's Effects on Eating *100*
Amyloid Formation in Pancreatic Islets *102*
Mechanisms of Amyloid Genesis *102*
Pathological Effects of Amylin Deposits on Pancreatic β-Cells *103*
Therapeutic Approach to Reduce Amylin-Derived Fibrillogenic *103*
Conclusion *104*
Acknowledgments and Disclosures *104*
References *105*

4 Peptide-Based GLP-1 Receptor Agonists for the Treatment of Type 2 Diabetes and Obesity *121*
János T. Kodra, Lars Linderoth, Steffen Reedtz-Runge, Thomas Kruse, and Jacob C. Kofoed
Introduction *121*
GLP-1 Biology *122*
GLP-1 Receptor Binding and Activation *123*
Clinical Relevant Peptide GLP-1 Receptor Agonists *124*
Exendin-4-Based Analogs *124*
Exenatide *124*
Exenatide Long-Acting Release (LAR) *125*
Lixisenatide *126*
Efpeglenatide *126*
Loxenatide *127*
Noiiglutide *127*
Visepegenatide *128*
GLP-1-Based Analogs *128*
Liraglutide *128*
Semaglutide *129*
Taspoglutide *129*
Albiglutide and Albenatide *130*
Dulaglutide *131*
Ecnoglutide *131*

Utreglutide 132
HyGlutide 132
ZT002 133
Bofanglutide 133
Summary and Outlook 134
References 134

5 Oral Agents Used to Treat Type 2 Diabetes and Obesity 141
John Liddle, Ekaterina Ratkova, Cátia A. Bonito, Christopher J. Rhodes, and Sarah Will
Introduction 141
Type 2 Diabetes Oral Agents 141
Sulfonylureas 145
Biguanides 146
Alpha-Glucosidase Inhibitors 147
Meglitinides (Glinides) 147
Thiazolidinediones 148
Dipeptidyl Peptidase-4 (DPP4) Inhibitors 150
Bile Acid Sequestrants 150
Dopamine-2 Agonists 152
Sodium-Glucose Transporter-2 (SGLT2) Inhibitors 153
Glimins 154
Other (Non-Approved) Small Molecule T2D Treatments 154
Obesity Oral Agents 154
Nicotine 155
Thyroxine 155
Dinitrophenol 158
Amphetamines 159
Centrally-Acting Combinations 159
Lorcaserin 161
Orlistat 162
Cannabinoid Receptor Antagonists 162
β3-Adrenoreceptor Agonists 163
Melanocortin 4 Receptor (MC4R) Agonist 163
A Current Perspective for Oral Diabetes and Obesity Small Molecules 164
Small Molecule Glucagon-Like Peptide 1 Receptor (GLP-1R) Agonists 164
Introduction 164
The First Reported Small Molecule GLP-1R Agonists 165
GLP-1R Agonists and Positive Allosteric Modulators 168
Small Molecule GLP-1R Agonists in Clinical Development 173
TTP273 from vTv Therapeutics 173
Danuglipron and Lotiglipron 173
Orforglipron 176

Summary of the GLP-1R Small Molecule Agonist Landscape *179*
Outlook for GLP-1R Small Molecule Agonists and Beyond *180*
References *180*

6 **Trends in the Field of Insulin Drug Design** *197*
Thomas Hoeg-Jensen
Introduction *197*
Native Insulin *198*
Meal Insulin Designs and Formulations *199*
Once-Daily Basal Insulin Designs *199*
Once-Weekly Insulin Designs *201*
Tissue Selective and Functionally Selective Insulin *203*
Oral and Pulmonary Insulin *204*
Glucose-Sensitive Insulin *204*
Insulin Pumps and Cell-Based Therapy *206*
Conclusions *206*
Abbreviations *207*
Biography *207*
References *207*

7 **Neuropeptide Y Receptor Ligands and Opportunities Within Diabetes and Obesity** *215*
Søren Østergaard
The Neuropeptide Y (NPY) Peptide and Receptor Family *215*
Neuropeptides NPY, PYY, and PP *215*
NPY Receptors and Distribution *217*
Knockout Studies in Rodents *218*
Y_1R/Y_5R Agonism *219*
Y_1R/Y_5R Antagonists for Diabetes or Obesity Treatment *220*
PP and Y_4R Interaction *222*
PYY and Y_2R Interaction *223*
Regulator of Food Energy Homeostasis *223*
Regulator of Glucose Homeostasis *224*
Lessons from Bariatric Surgery Support the Critical Role of PYY *224*
SAR and Y_2R Selective Agonists *225*
Half-Life Extension of PYY Analogs *226*
Y_2R Agonism and Combinations with Other Peptide Agonists *227*
Human Studies and Trials with PYY and Analogs *229*
Prospects of Obesity and Diabetes Treatment with PYY *231*
References *232*

8 **PrRP-GPR10 Signaling and Metabolism** *243*
Claire H. Feetham, Amy A. Worth, Sam Groom, and Simon M. Luckman
Modified PrRP Peptides as a New Pharmacological Tool *243*

The Discovery of GPR10 and PrRP 244
Prolactin-Releasing Hormone – A Misnomer? 244
Central Metabolic Effects of PrRP 246
Receptor Coupling and Distribution 246
Prlh and *Prlhr* Knockout Mouse Models 248
Natural Polymorphisms in the *PRLHR* Gene 248
Genetic Mutations Affecting NPFF Signaling Related to Metabolism 249
Brainstem $PrRP^{NTS}$ Neurons 250
Hypothalamic $PrRP^{DMH}$ Neurons 252
Systemically Administered PrRP Analogs 252
Conclusions 253
References 254

9 The Becoming of Dasiglucagon 263
Ditte Riber, Jesper M. Mathiesen, Lise Giehm, Francesca Macchi, Mikael Elander, and Jesper S. Villadsen
The Becoming of Dasiglucagon 263
The Discovery of Glucagon and Its Physiological Effects 263
Medical Use of Glucagon as a Rescue Treatment for Insulin Induced Hypoglycemia in Diabetes Mellitus 264
Rational Design of Dasiglucagon 265
Basis for the Chemical and Physical Instability of Native Glucagon 265
Design Strategy and Assays 267
1st Design: Exploring Substitution of Residues Susceptible for Isomerization, Cleavage, and Oxidation 268
2nd Design: Exploring Substitution of Potential Deamidation Sites and Disruption of an Aggregation Prone Hydrophobic Region 268
3rd Design: Combining the Learnings from Previous SAR Rounds 270
4th Design 272
5th Design 274
Characterization of Dasiglucagon 279
Physical and Chemical Stability of Dasiglucagon 279
Rotation Study – Simulating Real Use by Patients 279
Structural Characterization by Circular Dichroism 281
Pharmacological Effect of Dasiglucagon in Humans 282
Conclusion 283
Amino Acid Abbreviations 283
References 284

Index 287

Series Editors Preface

The **Trends in Drug Discovery** book series focuses on recent drug discoveries, including preclinical studies and successful drug development leading to newly approved drugs in major therapeutic fields. The scope of this series includes both small-molecule and large-molecule drugs including biologics.

Each volume gives an overview of a specific therapeutic field, discusses concepts and technologies, and describes the discoveries of recently approved drugs.

The **series editors** are introduced as follows:

János Fischer (Emeritus Fellow of IUPAC, research advisor at Richter, Hungary) participated in the editing of two book series of Wiley-VCH: Analogue-based Drug Discovery (Vols. 1–3, 2006–2011) and Successful Drug Discovery (Vols. 1–5, 2015–2021).

David Rotella (Sokol Professor of Chemistry, Montclair State University, United States) was a co-editor for Analogue-based Drug Discovery (Vol. 3) and Successful Drug Discovery (Vol. 1).

Christian Klein (former Department Head Cancer Immunotherapy and Site Head at the Roche Innovation Center, Zurich, Switzerland) was a co-editor for Successful Drug Discovery (Vols. 3–5).

Wayne E. Childers (Professor of Pharmaceutical Sciences at Temple University School of Pharmacy, Philadelphia, Pennsylvania, United States) was a co-editor for Successful Drug Discovery (Vols. 2–5).

The goals of this book series are to provide the drug discovery community with reference books and to support teaching in the field of drug discovery.

The fourth volume has the title: **Trends in Drug Discovery in Diabetes and Obesity.** GLP-1 receptor agonists represent a revolutionary class of medications for the treatment of diabetes and obesity. In the last 20 years, a great development could be observed in this drug class affording very successful, long-lasting pharmaceutical products. Editors of this volume, Lars Linderoth and Søren Østergaard (Novo Nordisk), focus on new research trends in this field.

Preface

Obesity is one of the most urgent health issues of the 21st century. Once seen mainly as a result of lifestyle and personal choices, obesity is now understood as a complex, multifactorial disease with significant effects on both individual and public health. It is a well-known risk factor for many chronic diseases, including type 2 diabetes, cardiovascular disease, MASH, and certain cancers. Perhaps most concerning, obesity has reached pandemic levels, impacting over almost 1 billion adults worldwide, with no indication that this trend will slow down.

The scientific understanding of obesity has improved significantly over the past few decades. Where it was once viewed as a simple calculation of calorie intake versus expenditure, it is now recognized as a disorder caused by complex biochemical, genetic, environmental, and psychosocial interactions. This deeper knowledge of the physiological factors driving obesity, especially the role of neuroendocrine signaling and metabolic pathways, has laid the groundwork for developing more effective treatments to address this urgent need.

At the forefront of this therapeutic revolution are innovations in the design and delivery of engineered endogenous peptides, such as glucagon-like peptide-1 (GLP-1), glucose-dependent insulinotropic polypeptide (GIP), glucagon (Gcg), amylin (Amy), prolactin-releasing peptide (PrRP), and peptide YY (PYY), as they represent key components of the body's intricate network of hormonal signals that regulate food intake, glycemic control, and metabolism.

In this context, the long-acting GLP-1 analog, semaglutide, and the long-acting dual receptor agonist GLP-1/GIP, tirzepatide, have demonstrated unprecedented weight loss in overweight or obese individuals, with or without type 2 diabetes mellitus (T2DM). Additionally, we also observe extra health benefits that are not necessarily related to weight loss alone. Lowering the risk of cardiovascular diseases (CVD), slowing the progression of chronic kidney disease (CKD), and improving MASH are among some of the benefits seen after longer-term treatment. Leveraging these peptides in new innovative ways therefore holds the promise of addressing not only obesity but also its related disorders, with the hope of eliminating the surge, particularly in type 2 diabetes, and even reducing it.

Through contributions from some of the world's leading scientists, the chapters provide an in-depth examination of the mode of action and of how peptide design is transforming the treatment of obesity and diabetes. The book covers the discovery of

GLP-1, including its mechanisms of action and the pharmacological effects of GLP-1 receptor agonists. It also discusses GIP, amylin, glucagon, PrRP, and PYY, along with their implications for clinical practice. Additionally, it explores cutting-edge approaches like dual- and multiagonist strategies, which combine multiple peptides for synergistic weight-loss effects. Furthermore, next-generation glucose-sensitive insulins mark a paradigm shift in insulin therapy.

One fascinating area discussed is the emergence of small-molecule GLP-1 receptor agonists. These compounds have the potential to disrupt the field by offering the benefits of peptide therapies in an oral form that is easier to produce, store, and administer. This breakthrough has important implications for making modern obesity treatments more accessible and scalable, providing hope for meeting the increasing demand for effective therapies in resource-limited settings.

The journey from scientific insight to clinical application is rarely straightforward, and the development of peptide-based medicines for obesity is no exception. This book highlights the many challenges researchers face in improving the efficacy, stability, and safety of these therapies while navigating strict regulatory and translational hurdles. It also captures the remarkable progress made, providing analogs with improved properties such as dual or triple functions or ultra-long half-lives.

By combining cutting-edge research with expert analysis, this book aims to serve as both a reference and a source of inspiration for a broad audience of scientists, clinicians, and healthcare professionals. We hope these chapters will not only inform but also motivate further advancements in designing safer, more effective medicines to combat obesity and diabetes.

We extend our deepest gratitude to the distinguished contributors whose expertise and pioneering efforts lay the groundwork for this book. Their insights and dedication to pushing the boundaries of peptide science have greatly enriched this work. As you continue reading the upcoming chapters, we encourage you to see the innovations discussed here not as the final achievement but as the starting point for the next wave of scientific breakthroughs in obesity and diabetes. The journey to address the immense complexities of obesity and its effects persists, but the advances highlighted in this book mark a step forward in new molecular treatment options. Together, we move closer to a future where the burden of obesity and related diseases is not only eased but ultimately prevented.

December 2025

Lars Linderoth and Søren Østergaard
Maalov, Copenhagen

1

The Role of Gut Peptides in the Regulation of Body Weight

Jens J. Holst[1] and Sten Madsbad[2]

[1] University of Copenhagen, The Panum Institute, NovoNordisk Foundation Center for Basic Metabolic Research and Department of Biomedical Sciences, Blegdamsvej 3, DK-2200 Copenhagen N, Denmark
[2] University of Copenhagen, Hvidovre Hospital, Department of Endocrinology, Kettegaard Alle 36, DK-2650 Hvidovre, Denmark

Introduction and Methodological Considerations

The recent success of therapeutics based on gut hormones, in particular the insulin-stimulating incretin hormones (glucose-dependent insulinotropic polypeptide [GIP] and glucagon-like peptide-1 [GLP-1]), has drawn attention to the gut as an organ involved in the regulation of food intake and body weight. In this review, we will discuss the specific role of gut hormones in the overall regulation of body weight. The fundamental assumption is that body weight is tightly regulated; indeed, overfeeding and starvation experiments, also in humans, have provided ample evidence that weight changes elicited by overfeeding as well as starvation elicit counterregulatory responses that eventually restore body weight [1, 2]. The adjustment of food intake to correspond to the energy expended (due to basic metabolism as well as the individual's physical activity level), thereby ensuring energy balance, is referred to as *homeostatic* regulation of food intake. However, the homeostatic regulation can be overridden by *hedonic* processes that reflect the rewarding, palatable, and pleasurable properties of food. Hedonic feeding has been increasingly invoked to explain how obesity may develop despite the presence of adaptive, homeostatic mechanisms that should protect against overeating. Immediately, one would anticipate that both the hedonic and the homeostatic regulation were matters for the central nervous system, as indicated by numerous studies of the importance of hypothalamic nuclei, including for instance the arcuate nucleus and its interactions with the paraventricular nucleus and other nuclei [3]. However, since the original description by Gibbs et al. that injections of (impure) cholecystokinin (CCK) reduced short-term food intake in a dose-related manner in rats [4], there has been an interest in understanding the role of the gut in the regulation. Gibbs et al. suggested a set of criteria for evaluation of hormones like CCK as physiological regulators: (1) the hormonal signal should be activated by feeding; (2) the hormone, administered exogenously, should significantly decrease meal size; (3) it should have a rapid onset and a brief duration of action (if it were to be involved in meal termination or meal frequency); (4) its effect should not be due to illness (e.g., evaluated by conditioned taste aversion); and (5) the proposed signal should be effective in physiological doses. The last criterion would be consistent with an endocrine mode of action, i.e., that the signal was transmitted to the brain via the circulation. Subsequent research has shown that this may not be relevant for all gastrointestinal hormones. Furthermore, such criteria, designed for evaluation of the physiological role of the gut hormones, are not necessarily relevant when it comes to the evaluation of the pharmacological potential of the hormones. In early experimental studies, emphasis was often put on effects on meal size versus meal frequency, which again would be physiologically relevant, but may be less important for the therapeutic exploitation of a hormone. The number of gut hormones (which are mainly peptides) evaluated for effect on food intake has been growing steadily over the years; for many years these peptides were thought of as signals released to the bloodstream to act on distant targets (in this case the brain), but many of the newer peptides identified in the gut were eventually localized to nerve cells and fibers of the enteric nervous system, suggestive of nonendocrine mechanisms of action. For many of these *neuropeptides* of the gut, it is currently not possible to estimate their role in food intake because too little is known about their projections, the localization of the receptors, and their mechanisms of activation; for some of them, it seems evident that they have local actions as parts of the enteric nervous system. Many of the peptides are also expressed in the central nervous system where they may serve additional regulatory functions. This makes evaluations very complex. A good example is CCK itself, which probably mainly acts as a classical hormone when it comes to regulation of gall bladder emptying and pancreatic enzyme secretion, but for which other actions depend on interaction with vagal sensory fibers expressing the CCK receptors [5]. Such receptors are also expressed in numerous cortical and noncortical neurons of the brain, and CCK is also produced in numerous CNS neurons where it appears to have a transmitter function, the nature of which and possible role in feeding are still unclear.

CCK will be discussed further below, but otherwise focus will be on the hormones ghrelin, GLP-1, and peptide YY (PYY), while also the potential of glucose-dependent insulinotropic polypeptide (GIP) and oxyntomodulin will be discussed. All these hormones have the actions with which they were originally associated, such as regulation of insulin secretion (GIP and GLP-1), gastrointestinal motility and secretion (GlP-1, ghrelin, and PYY), and stimulation of growth hormone (GH) secretion (ghrelin), but in addition they have all been reported to inhibit food intake (in the case of ghrelin, increase food intake). But what is the evidence that they take part in the physiological regulation of food intake? The fact that they under certain circumstances can inhibit food intake does not necessarily mean that they are important for normal regulation.

Mimicry

Traditionally, in gastrointestinal hormone research, physiological relevance is initially established using the mimicry approach, whereby the assumed actions of the endogenous hormones are mimicked by administration (infusion) of an exogenous hormone. This requires that the release of the hormone, e.g., during meal intake, is measured (the availability of an accurate assay is therefore essential), followed by infusion of the hormone in question to concentrations similar to those observed during the meal. A positive response (reduction of food intake) supports a physiological function for the peptide, but, of course, only represents a necessary, not a sufficient, condition for this. Indeed, to establish a positive mimicry experiment is often sufficiently difficult to render fulfillment of this criterion problematic – for instance, measurements of the actual hormone concentrations (particularly in rodents) have often been unreliable.

Hormone Antagonists

A much better way of establishing the importance of a new peptide is to acutely block the activities of the peptide with a receptor antagonist. This, of course, requires knowledge about the responsible receptor and, furthermore, requires access to reliable (specific, potent) antagonists, which is clearly a limiting factor. Genetic manipulations may be very useful but also have serious limitations; a knock-in experiment is useless since hyper-expression/-secretion will always be unphysiological. Global knockout, although sometimes informative, very often leads to compensatory changes, which may completely perturb the picture, and acute targeted knockout experiments are difficult to produce and most often involve mice, which are difficult to study and not always relevant for human physiology. A good example is the hormone GLP-1 and its analogs, some of which are among the most powerful appetite and food intake suppressors we know, but where a global knockout of the receptor does not lead to changes in body weight or food intake [6]. Does this mean that endogenous GLP-1 does not participate in the regulation of food intake? Probably not, but a global knockout experiment is not the way to demonstrate this.

Activation and Inactivation

Is there a reliable way to demonstrate unequivocally that the gut hormones contribute to the regulation of food intake under physiological conditions? As already discussed, the most reliable tool we have is blockade with hormone receptor antagonists, since it is a fundamental dogma that these peptides act on (a) specific receptor(s); therefore, acute blockade of these should remove the effect they are responsible for. The use of receptor antagonists has one more very important advantage: if we are talking *small molecule* antagonists (and most are at least as small as the hormones themselves), they are likely to access the same tissues and compartments as the hormones. This means that it will also be possible for the antagonists to interfere with paracrine interactions and activations of neural mechanisms that might be involved, provided the effects depend on interaction with the receptors. In line with this, there are other approaches that may yield similarly specific and relevant results. Thus, if the hormones can somehow be deactivated or their activation prevented, this may have a similar effect as antagonism.

An illustrative example is the use of dipeptidyl peptidase 4 (DPP-4) inhibitors to prevent the conversion of the orexigenic primary secretion product of PYY, PYY 1–36, to PYY 3–36, which is generated by cleavage of the peptide by the enzyme DPP-4 [7]. Conversely, the DPP-4 inhibitors prevent the DPP-4 mediated inactivation of GLP-1 and GIP (and several other substrates), and the plasma concentration of the active forms of these hormones will therefore increase, leading, for instance, to increased insulin secretion [8]. For ghrelin, its biological activity depends on the octanoylation of the serine residue in position no. 2, and inhibitors of the enzyme, ghrelin O-acyl transferase (GOAT) that catalyzes this modification, will inactivate the hormone [9].

Somatostatin as a Tool

There is another approach, which might be described as a physiological sledgehammer: the use of somatostatin. Somatostatin acts via its five different receptors [10], and virtually all gut endocrine cells express one or more of these receptors, which typically inhibit adenylate cyclase via a Gi protein subunit. Administration of somatostatin therefore inhibits the secretion of most (all?) gut hormones [11]. Some of the more long-acting somatostatin analogs developed for clinical use differentially activate the various receptor subtypes (e.g., lanreotide has greater affinity for peripheral rather than central receptors). Somatostatin, however, has actions on many tissues and cells and is an important regulator of pituitary secretion, for instance of growth hormone. In addition, it regulates gastrointestinal function via presynaptic inhibition of neurons of the enteric nervous system. Even more problematic, somatostatin also inhibits the secretion of pancreatic islet hormones [12], which have all been suspected of influencing appetite and food intake. Thus, an effect observed after somatostatin infusion (or injection) is not necessarily due to specific inhibition of (a) gut hormone(s), but might, of course, be compatible with such an effect. Indeed, in experiments with octreotide, a long-acting somatostatin agonist, an increase in food intake was *not* observed in healthy controls, whereas in patients after esophagectomy and with elevated secretion of gut hormones, a positive response, i.e., an increase in food intake, was observed [13].

An even more dramatic experimental approach is to study patients with short bowel syndrome. These individuals have a natural drive to eat since insufficient energy intake in their situation would be deleterious. Fortunately, the patients show a ferocious appetite and hyperphagia [14], but, of course, have a clear homeostatic problem to solve. Complicating matters further, a discordance between secretion of gut-derived appetite hormones and energy intake in humans was recently reported [15]. In these studies, volunteers ingested a low-fat (LF) or a low-carbohydrate (LC) diet in a crossover design. The LC meal increased plasma concentrations of GLP-1, GIP, and PYY but lowered ghrelin levels compared to the isocaloric LF meal, while energy intake was 550 kcal greater on the LC meal. Thus, the effects of gut-derived appetite hormones on ad libitum energy intake can be overridden by other diet-related factors, at least in the short-term [15].

In conclusion, in spite of 50 years of research, there is no clear answer to the question of the role of the gut hormones in the regulation of appetite and food intake under physiological conditions. It appears that the closest we can get is to evaluate, for each hormone, the evidence derived from mimicry and other experiments with exogenous hormone administration and studies with whatever antagonists have been available. In the following, we will discuss some of the evidence for the contribution of the most important gut hormone candidates for regulation of food intake.

Gut Hormones with a Possible Role in Food Intake

An overview of the gut hormones and their main actions discussed in this chapter are presented next.

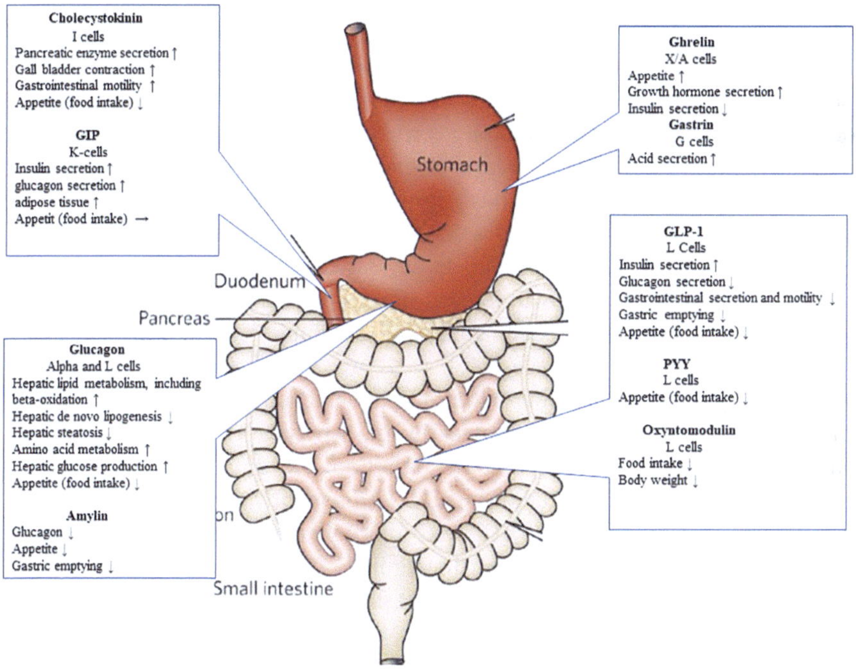

Cholecystokinin

CCK was discovered in 1929 by Ivy and Oldberg as a physiological principle (endocrine regulation of gall bladder emptying), but it took another 40 years before the chemical nature of the hormone was revealed: a peptide of 33 amino acids [16]. During the purification of CCK, it became clear that the specific bioactivity of the compound in terms of gall bladder motility and stimulation of pancreatic enzyme secretion increased in parallel; eventually, the pure (and subsequently synthetic) peptide exhibited similar dual bioactivity and it was concluded that CCK and pancreozymin were one and the same peptide [16]. The peptide is produced in the endocrine I-cells of the upper small intestinal mucosa and, upon development of radioimmunoassays for CCK, it could be demonstrated to be released in response to protein and lipid ingestion [17]. Like other peptides, CCK is produced as a larger precursor molecule (95 amino acids), which undergoes posttranslational cleavage and modification including sulfation and amidation of the C-terminus, both of which are essential for its bioactivity, but it has been difficult to reach an agreement regarding the chain length of "cholecystokinin." As mentioned, the structure was originally determined to comprise 33 amino acids, but incomplete cleavage of the precursor and metabolism of the various cleavage fragments results in the formation of several molecular forms, among which the 33-amino acid peptide is only one. A C-terminal (amidated and sulfated) fragment of 8 amino acids (CCK-8) has apparently full biological activity, and several other components, including a 22- and a 58-amino acid component, have been described [18]. The various components have different potencies and different half-lives in the circulation, and these factors complicate interpretation and determination of the physiological functions of "CCK." Furthermore, CCK has two receptors, the CCK 1 and 2 (or A and B) receptors, for which CCK-8 has about the same affinity and potency, whereas the related stomach hormone, gastrin (their C-terminal structures are very similar), also has affinity for the B-form (which is therefore commonly referred to as the gastrin receptor although it has affinity for both), and there is a differential expression of the two receptors [19]. Complicating matters even further, CCK and the CCK receptors are also expressed in several regions of the central nervous system [20] where CCK seems to exert a transmitter function (typically exerted by CCK-8). Obviously, experiments consisting of simple infusions of "CCK" are difficult to interpret.

However, with the advent of specific receptor antagonists (loxiglumid, proglumide), it became possible to analyze at least some aspects of CCK physiology. Smith et al. were again the first to show that the inhibition of feeding with CCK depended on intact afferent fibers of the vagus [21]. Subsequently, Smith and coworkers could demonstrate that a specific CCK1 receptor antagonist resulted in significant increases in meal size, strongly supporting a role for CCK in the regulation of food intake at least in rats [22]. Furthermore, a rat strain with inactive CCK-A receptors (Olefsky rats) showed disordered food intake and obesity [23]. It should be noted that CCK also importantly influences gastric emptying, apparently involving a vago-vagal reflex activity, and it has been suspected that this effect could explain some of the anorexic effects. The CCK receptors are found in numerous locations in the brain [24], but they hardly serve as targets for peripheral CCK, but rather for CCK released from local CCK-containing neurons. Importantly, CCK receptors can also be demonstrated to be expressed on vagal afferent neurons with cell bodies in the nodose ganglion, and there is substantial evidence for the importance of this pathway for the actions of CCK on food intake [25]. Given the solid status of CCK in feeding regulation in rodents, one would expect CCK/CCK receptors to be an attractive target for therapy of humans. However, the role of the CCK system in humans is not nearly as clear as it is in rodents, and long-acting CCK-A receptor agonists did not result in weight loss in overweight or obese individuals [25, 26]. In addition,

CCK-1 receptor agonists may induce pathological findings, including pancreatitis and pancreatic neoplasia, and a long-acting agonist was demonstrated to cause increased pancreas weight and neoplasia at the expected therapeutic exposure levels in monkeys [27]. Indeed, the agonists would also be expected to increase the risk of bile system complications including gallstones and gallstone-related pancreatitis [27]. As discussed earlier, investigations in patients subjected to bariatric surgery, in particular gastric bypass surgery, generally reveal elevations of gut hormones, secondary to accelerated intestinal exposure of nutrients, and these elevations are thought to contribute importantly to the weight loss observed. CCK concentrations are mildly elevated after gastric bypass surgery [28, 29], which may be surprising since the operation bypasses the site of most dense localization of I-cells, but apparently more distally located I-cells are sufficient to explain the elevation. The other operation, sleeve gastrectomy (SG), is also associated with increased intestinal nutrient exposure and shows exaggerated release of several gut hormones, but here the increase in CCK secretion is nevertheless minor [29]. In conclusion, while the evidence for an important role in the regulation of food intake in rodents is extensive, the situation in humans is less clear, and utilization of CCK agonism for therapeutic purposes seems far away.

GLP-1

GLP-1 is a 30-amino acid peptide product of intestinal expression of the gene encoding proglucagon (PG), the precursor of glucagon [30]. When produced in the gut, the 160-amino acid prohormone is cleaved to produce glicentin (corresponding to amino acids no. 1–69 of PG, a fraction of which [about a third] may be cleaved to oxyntomodulin [PG 33–69]), GLP-1 (PG 78–107), and GLP-2 (PG 126–158). In the pancreas, the major products are glucagon (PG 33–61) and the Major Proglucagon Fragment (PG 72–158) [31]. Because GLP-1 was originally thought to correspond to PG 72–107 (which is formed in small amounts in the pancreas and is inactive), the naturally occurring form is often designated GLP-1 7–37 or, since it is often amidated C-terminally (a process that involves the C-terminal Gly residue), GLP-1 (7–36) amide. The cellular origin is the endocrine L-cell [32], one of the most abundant gut endocrine cells, a cell type that also gives rise to the gut hormone PYY (see below). The L-cells are found in increasing numbers along the intestine with a majority in the colon, even in the distal colon and the rectum [33]. The proglucagon products are secreted in response to ingestion of all the major macronutrients, because the L-cells are equipped with both apical and basolateral proteins [34] that either sense G-protein coupled receptors (GPCRs) or transport digested nutrients (like SGLT-1). For instance, for lipids, the cells express the GPCR, GPR 119, reacting with 2-monoacyl glycerols, a major digestive product of nutritional triglycerides [35]. And for protein breakdown products, several apical and basolateral membrane-bound proteins (GPCRs and transporters) are known to react to amino acids and stimulate secretion [36]. Immediately after its release, and already in the capillaries draining the mucosa of the gut, GLP-1 is broken down by the enzyme DPP-4, which is expressed by the endothelial cells of the capillaries [37]. DPP-4 cleaves off the two N-terminal amino acids, and the metabolite GLP-1 9–39 is inactive. The half-life in the circulation is one to two minutes. Thus, very little GLP-1 reaches the liver in the intact form and even less reaches the peripheral circulation [38]. This creates a problem regarding relevant measurements. It is possible to measure the intact hormone with sandwich ELISA targeting the terminals of the peptide. But the concentrations are very low and do not reflect the secretion of the peptide. Instead, it is possible in humans to measure the metabolite GLP-1 9–36 amide, the concentration of which will reflect secretion [31]. However, it is now believed that GLP-1 mainly signals by activating afferent sensory pathways, a process that may take place in the lamina propria before the entry of the hormone into the mucosal capillaries and degradation by DPP-4 [39, 40]. Measurement of the metabolite may therefore also reflect the actions of the hormone. In mice, measurements are even more difficult because of the actions of the enzyme neprilysin, which destroys the metabolite [41, 42].

Role of Endogenous GLP-1 in Food Intake Regulation

Although discovered on the basis of its insulin releasing properties, GLP-1 is also considered one of the ileal brake hormones, i.e., an enterogastrone hormone, released from the ileal mucosa in response to remaining nutrients, with inhibitory effect on upper gastrointestinal secretion and motility ([43, 44]). This hormonal axis also involves inhibition of appetite and food intake. GLP-1 was shown in 1996 to inhibit food intake, when administered intra-cerebro-ventricularly (ICV) [45], but it is doubtful whether this mode of administration is relevant for peripherally secreted GLP-1 or for subcutaneously injected GLP-1 receptor agonists. Rather, the numerous cerebral receptors are targets for GLP-1 produced by a small group of neurons in the nucleus of the solitary tract of the brain stem [46]. These neurons appear to receive excitatory input from peripheral stimuli, e.g., gastric distension [47], but they are not activated by peripherally administered GLP-1. Appetite suppression and food intake inhibition by peripheral GLP-1 were first demonstrated in 1998 by Flint et al. [48], and soon confirmed by many other groups, and in 2001 it was determined in a meta-analysis that the effect was dose dependent, i.e., the more GLP-1 infused the more food intake would be inhibited [49]. In spite of this, mice with deletion of the GLP-1 receptor do not become obese. Similarly, the antagonist of the GLP-1 receptor, exendin 9–39, only variably and weakly influences food intake and appetite sensations [50] in humans although it apparently did block CNS responses to palatable food consumption as determined by functional Magnetic Resonance Imaging (fMRI) [51]. The antagonist is probably doing its job, since it blocks the food intake inhibiting actions of exogenous GLP-1 receptor agonists. Because the lack of effect of the antagonist contrasts to the powerful inhibition of food intake with GLP-1 receptor agonists, one may ask whether exendin 9–39 elicits other effects that may counteract the effects of the GLP-1 blockade on appetite and food intake. Thus, in humans, Ex9 invariably increases plasma concentrations of glucagon and glucose, which may both dampen appetite. It may be that effects of GLP-1 are mainly seen during conditions of strong stimulation of secretion as in conditions with accelerated gastric emptying [31]. Attempting to identify the roles of the exaggerated secretion of both GLP-1 and PYY (see below) for the weight loss after gastric bypass surgery, Svane et al. [7] studied ad libitum food intake after blockade of either or both of these hormones. For GLP-1 receptor blockade, they used the GLP-1 receptor antagonist exendin 9–39. For PYY, there is no antagonist for human use, but the conversion of PYY 1–36 to PYY 3–36, which is required for activation (see below), can be prevented by inhibitors of the responsible enzyme, DPP-4. Svane et al. also studied the secretion of the two hormones in response to a test meal. Importantly, blockade of the GLP-1 receptor led to greatly augmented PYY 3–36 responses (caused by a negative feedback mechanism regulating L-cell activity), and DPP-4 inhibition greatly increased intact GLP-1 responses; thus, as the effects of one hormone were prevented, secretion of the other hormones increased, presumably negating the effect of the inhibition and vice versa. Consistent with this, combined blockade resulted in a 20% increase in ad libitum intake, providing strong support for the importance of these two hormones for weight loss after gastric bypass surgery.

Mechanism of Action of Exogenous GLP-1 Receptor Agonists

As mentioned earlier, the injected agonists of the GLP-1 receptor powerfully inhibit food intake, and it has been demonstrated that their activity depends on interaction with cerebral receptors [52]. Fluorescent or radioactive GLP-1 agonists can be shown to access several of the circumventricular organs, where the blood-brain barrier is leaky, including the median eminence, the area postrema, and the subfornical organ [53, 54]. Notably, no binding is observed in animals with a deletion of the GLP-1 receptor gene, suggesting that GLP-1 and its analogs do need to enter the brain to exert activity. A subsequent activation (as determined by c-Fos staining) can be demonstrated in the nucleus of the solitary tract, in several nuclei of the hypothalamus, in the amygdala, and in the parabrachial nucleus [53]. These, therefore, should be considered the initially engaged pathways.

Development of GLP-1 Receptor Agonists for Obesity Therapy

In the earliest studies, GLP-1 was infused to mimic high physiological increases in plasma concentration and did result in significant inhibition of food intake and appetite sensations, consistent with a physiological effect on food intake [48], and, as already mentioned, the response could also be demonstrated to be dose-dependent. However, side effects consisting of nausea, vomiting, and stomach pain, observed during sudden increases in plasma levels of GLP-1, prevented investigations of higher doses [55]. With the advent of GLP-1 receptor agonists, developed for diabetes therapy, similar problems were observed [56], but further studies showed that a slow up-titration of dosing to some extent could mitigate the side effects [57], and in a study where liraglutide was given in a fixed combination with the long-acting insulin analog, insulin degludec, and where the up-titration was done according to the insulin component (fasting blood glucose) and thus took place over a 14-week period, there were virtually no gastrointestinal side effects [58]. Subsequent careful dose-response studies with increasing doses of liraglutide revealed that higher doses of this once-daily agonist resulted in weight losses up to 7–8 kg over a 20-week period [59]. This led to the SCALE trials, phase 3 trials [60] of 3 mg liraglutide daily for obesity therapy. The large SCALE 1 trial, which was extended over three years, showed persistent weight loss and an 80% reduction in the risk of developing diabetes during the trial [61]. The SCALE trials led to approval of liraglutide 3 mg for obesity therapy, under the name of Saxenda. This marked the opening of the therapy of obesity with the GLP-1 agonists. A second generation agonist, semaglutide, developed for improved actions on both food intake and insulin secretion and for a longer half-life (weekly) [62] was also tested in a dose-response study (with daily doses to avoid side effects of the larger weekly doses) [63]. The trial showed that 0.4 mg daily over a year would result in a weight loss of 14%. A series of phase 3 trials, the STEP trials [64], with semaglutide at 2.4 mg per week given to people with obesity but no diabetes were then initiated. In these studies, weight losses of up to 18% were observed, and the compound was approved for therapy of obesity under the trade name of Wegovy. In March 2026, a higher dose of semaglutide was approved for chronic weight management.

It has been discussed whether the side effects of high doses of GlP-1 receptor agonists are inseparably associated with the appetite reducing effect and involve the same cerebral pathways [65]. However, the fact that it is possible to develop some insensitivity to the effect, while the effect on food intake is preserved, suggests that separate mechanisms are involved. This raises the possibility that agonists without these side effects could be developed. Recently, it has been proposed that co-administration of GIP with GLP-1 reduces the side effects of GLP-1 [66], and this might explain why the GLP-1-GIP coagonist tirzepatide can be administered in higher doses and therefore may have an even greater effect on body weight (up to 25%). Proof for this hypothesis is still lacking, however.

Oxyntomodulin and Glucagon-GLP-1 Coagonists

Oxyntomodulin is a 37-amino acid product of proglucagon, corresponding to residues no. 33–69 of proglucagon [67]. The peptide was known to exist as a glucagon-related peptide in gut extracts by size exclusion chromatography of "gut glucagon" (enteroglucagon) [68], and its definitive structure was determined in 1982 [69, 70]. Dominique Bataille felt that it had special effects on oxyntic gland secretion (gastric glands) in experimental models and therefore suggested the catchy name oxyntomodulin. In extracts of human intestinal mucosa, it constitutes about a third of the glucagon-containing products of proglucagon (with glicentin [PG 1–69] responsible for the remaining 2/3), and it is released from the L-cells in about the same proportion [68]. This also means that its concentration is rather low under most circumstances and that its secretion follows the secretion patterns of glicentin and GLP-1. Subsequent studies revealed that it binds to the glucagon receptor and the GLP-1 receptor but with about 1/100 of the affinity of the cognate ligands [71]. Thus, it is difficult to see that it plays a major physiological role under normal circumstances. However, under conditions with severely increased secretion of the proglucagon-derived intestinal products, the levels may rise sufficiently to influence these receptors [72]. Such conditions are almost all associated with accelerated gastric emptying, and the secretion is particularly pronounced after gastric bypass operations [72], where secretion and, therefore, the levels of glicentin and oxyntomodulin may increase up to 30-fold.

The current interest in oxyntomodulin relates to the discovery that it is a natural glucagon-GLP-1 coagonist. Two groups showed in 2009, based on studies with oxyntomodulin, that stabilized and long-acting analogs might have a particularly pronounced effect on food intake and body weight, as expected because of the anorexic properties of both GLP-1 and glucagon. It was also found that the combination with GLP-1 ensured that the hyperglycemic effects of their glucagon agonism did not predominate [73, 74]. Thus, glucagon-GLP-1 coagonists appeared to have treatment potential. Since then, several companies have engaged in the production of glucagon-GLP-1 coagonists. This development is surprising in view of the efforts previously made to produce glucagon *antagonists* for diabetes therapy in recognition of the importance of glucagon for diabetic hyperglycemia [75]. Although the glucose-lowering effects of such antagonists were confirmed with several compounds, they also had unwanted effects on lipid metabolism, with aggravation of hepatic steatosis and hyperlipidemia [76]. Glucagon *agonism*, on the other hand, importantly affects hepatic lipid metabolism, including increased beta-oxidation, lipolysis, and inhibition of de novo lipogenesis [77]. GLP-1 was of course already effective in antidiabetic treatment; thus, by combining glucagon and GLP-1 action, one would further augment the anorexic effect and improve the metabolism-associated steatosis of most patients with obesity and type 2 diabetes. This assumption seems to be correct. Several published studies with various GLP-1/glucagon coagonists have shown important reductions in hepatic steatosis and weight loss in patients both with and without type 2 diabetes [78]. So far, only a single compound (Mazdutide) has reached the market (in China), and there may be outstanding issues with adverse effects – both GLP-1 and glucagon may cause nausea and vomiting and both increase heart rate. In addition, the powerful effects of glucagon on amino acid metabolism may be associated with unwanted increases in protein turnover.

PYY

PYY is a peptide of 36 amino acids with tyrosine residues (one letter code: Y) at both terminals (hence the name) and a member of a family of peptides that also comprises the very similar 36-amino acid peptides, pancreatic polypeptide (PP) and neuropeptide Y (NPY). It was discovered by Kazuhiko Tatemoto who, working with Victor Mutt in Stockholm, isolated the peptide from pig intestinal extracts using an original assay for amidated peptides [79]. Thus, it was isolated without any notions about biological activity [79]. Early studies suggested that it would inhibit pancreatic and gastric secretion. It is produced in the endocrine L-cells of the intestinal mucosa, most of which also produce proglucagon and the proglucagon-derived peptides (GLP-1 and oxyntomodulin); indeed, PYY is even localized to the same granules as these hormones [79, 80]. However, not all L-cells contain both hormones; most of the proximal L-cells of the small intestine do not contain PYY [81], whereas some of the distal cells do not secrete proglucagon-derived peptides [82]. The density of L-cells increases distally and is highest in the colon [83]. This family of peptides is also called the PP-fold peptides, because of a definite secondary structure: the peptides make a turn around the middle so that the two termini come close together in a hairpin-like shape. The proximity of the termini is essential for the receptor interaction [84]. The PP-fold family of peptides binds to the so-called Y or NPY receptors [85], comprising five subtypes; thus, the type and proximity of the terminals of the peptides determine the interaction with the extracellular compartment of the Y receptors. In the gut, PYY is produced as PYY 1–36, which has a high affinity for the Y1 receptor, which transmits increased appetite, and initially PYY was also found to stimulate food intake, undoubtedly because of its Y1 receptor activation in the models investigated, for instance intracerebroventricular injection. Even in 2002, PYY was designated "a key mediator of orexigenic behavior" [86]. However, a truncated form, produced by cleavage mediated by the enzyme dipeptidyl peptidase-4 (DPP-4), was also identified [87]. The product, PYY 3–36, no longer binds to Y1 but instead to the Y2 receptor [88]. Batterham et al. demonstrated inhibition of food intake by exogenous PYY 3–36 in both rats and humans acting via the Y2 receptor [89] and showed that PYY 3–36 was effective also in obese individuals (unlike leptin) [90]. These reports gave rise to considerable controversies [91, 92]. However, Boey et al. studied mice with knockout of PYY and found that they were prone to the development of obesity and glucose intolerance [93], and today there seems to be agreement regarding the inhibitory effects of PYY on food intake [94]. Batterham et al. also reported lower levels of PYY in plasma, suggesting that PYY might be involved in the pathogenesis of obesity. The effect is thought to be exerted by interaction of the peptide with Y2 receptor containing neurons in the arcuate nucleus, suggesting that circulating PYY 3–36 reaches these regions of the brain, possibly via the median eminence (one of the circumventricular organs with a leaky blood-brain barrier). This hypothesis is supported by the finding that peripheral PYY can cross the blood-brain barrier by a nonsaturable mechanism [95]. However, other data point toward a vagal route of PYY signaling since the food intake-reducing effect of PYY following intraperitoneal injection was found to be blocked by vagotomy in rats. Moreover, vagotomy also greatly decreased the PYY-induced expression of Fos in the arcuate nucleus (ARC) [96, 97]. Therefore, peripheral PYY is likely to signal to the brain via the vagus nerve and via direct interaction with hypothalamic nuclei after crossing the blood-brain barrier.

Measurements of PYY in plasma are by no means simple. First, the close structural relationship between the members of this family of peptides (also including the neuropeptide NPY and the islet peptide, pancreatic polypeptide) poses great demands on the specificity of the antibodies employed for immunoassays; second, to be interpretable in terms of metabolic consequences of secretion, it is necessary to distinguish between the 1–36 and the 3–36 forms. In addition, it turns out that the peptide is also degraded rapidly from the C-terminus, where plasma enzymes are responsible for sequential cleavage of the 36 and 35 residues, rendering PYY

3–34 a significant metabolite [98]. Importantly, both PYY 3–34 and the intermediate, PYY 3–35, are biologically inactive. Thus, there are no immunoassays currently available that can accurately measure active PYY 3–36, and predictions on the biological impact of changes in its plasma concentrations cannot be made. However, perhaps with recent mass spectrometry methods, this might now be possible [99].

Side effects (nausea and vomiting) during infusion into humans were also a concern, and in a series of studies, Sloth et al. attempted to identify conditions that would result in robust inhibition of food intake with both PYY 1–36 and 3–36 in humans, while minimizing the side effects [100, 101]. However, the effects of both hormones were disappointing after subcutaneous injections, and inhibition of appetite was invariably associated with adverse effects and signs of sympathoadrenal activation during intravenous infusions of PYY 3–36, whereas PYY 1–36 was without effect. Support for a role for PYY in appetite regulation in humans came from studies of gastric bypass surgery, where the bypass was associated with greatly elevated levels of PYY and GLP-1 [102, 103] (see above).

In further studies, Neary et al. [104] found additive effects of infusions of PYY and GLP-1 on appetite and food intake, and Schmidt et al., who studied very low doses of the two hormones, were able to identify a clearly potentiating interaction between the two, meaning that the inhibition of food intake after combined infusion was greater than the sum of the inhibitory effects of the separate infusions [105]. Attempting to identify the roles of the exaggerated secretion of both PYY and GLP-1 in the weight loss after gastric bypass surgery, Svane et al. studied ad libitum food intake after blockade of either or both hormones using the GLP-1 receptor antagonist exendin 9–39 and inhibiting conversion of PYY 1–36 to PYY 3–36 with an inhibitor of the enzyme DPP-4, as described earlier [7]. Combined blockade resulted in a 20% increase in ad libitum intake, supporting an important interaction between the two hormones and providing strong support for the importance of these two hormones for the weight loss after gastric bypass surgery.

So far there are no reports of a suitable PYY agonist for human use in the treatment of obesity, but a dual agonist with efficacy for both GLP-1 and Y2 receptors has been described [106]. Furthermore, coadministration of PYY, GLP-1, and oxyntomodulin, mimicking the pattern observed after gastric bypass operations in humans, by subcutaneous infusions for four weeks, has been effective in providing weight loss in healthy humans [107] as well as individuals with prediabetes and obesity.

GIP

The 42-amino acid hormone, glucose-dependent insulinotropic polypeptide, GIP, was discovered by John Brown, working with Victor Mutt in Stockholm, on the basis of its inhibitory effects on acid secretion in denervated gastric pouches in dogs – hence its original name: gastric inhibitory polypeptide[108]. After the discovery that it also stimulated insulin secretion in humans [109] (whereas its role in gastric inhibition in humans was less clear), it got its new name, retaining the acronym, and a series of mimicry experiments indicated that the new hormone was likely to be one of the long-sought incretin hormones [110], hormones from the gut that would enhance insulin secretion during oral intake of glucose (and perhaps other nutrients). In 2017, a GIP receptor antagonist suitable for human use was discovered [111], and in experiments with antagonists against the GIP and the GLP-1 receptor, it could be demonstrated that GIP was an important incretin hormone in humans, responsible for almost half of the incretin effect [112].

GIP is secreted from the endocrine K-cells of the duodenal and the proximal jejunal epithelium in response to carbohydrate and fat ingestions [113]. Like GLP-1 and PYY, it is degraded by the enzyme DPP-4, and the metabolite of GIP is inactive [114, 115]. The half-life of GIP is about 7 minutes in humans, and that of the metabolite about 30 minutes, compatible with renal elimination by glomerular filtration [116]. GIP is processed from a 92-amino acid precursor molecule, which is not known to produce alternative molecular forms of GIP or additional bioactive molecules [117]. A shorter form, GIP 1–30 amide, which is fully biologically active on the GIP receptor, may be formed in very small amounts, but does not seem to play a specific role [118, 119]. As for the other substrates of DPP-4, the hormone circulates in an intact form (GIP 1–42), representing about 50%, and as the truncated metabolite, GIP 3–42, but the ratio between the two molecular forms does not seem to change much. Regarding its circulating concentrations, measurements of the intact form would of course be preferable, but in qualitative terms more or less similar results are obtained with total GIP assays [120]. Assays employed in the older literature showed cross reactions with poorly characterized substances, among these is the so-called GIP 8000, with little or no relationship to GIP secretion [121]. Current assays seem to be more specific. The GIP receptor is expressed in the beta cells of the pancreatic islets in agreement with the activity on insulin secretion (but also in the other islet cell types) [122]. There is also a somewhat diffuse expression in numerous other tissues, including the adipose tissues, where the receptor may be expressed on both adipocytes and nonadipocyte cell types [123, 124]. The glucose-dependent insulinotropic polypeptide receptor (GIPR) is apparently also expressed in the brain [125], but currently the more precise localization is uncertain [126], and in particular expression in the human brain is unclear. Interestingly, the effect of GIP on insulin secretion in people with type 2 diabetes is lost or nearly absent [127]. The reason for this is unknown, but it may be related to defective glucose-induced insulin secretion.

The current interest in GIP and its effects in food intake derives from the remarkable effects of the GIP-GLP-1 coagonist, tirzepatide [128]. In the phase 3 trials for the obesity indication, treatment with this compound resulted in up to 25% weight loss in the course of 72–88 weeks [129], seemingly greater than those obtained with semaglutide, which is a monoagonist of the GLP-1 receptor. Also, the effect on glucose control in people with T2DM seems to be greater than that of semaglutide, with more than 50% of treated individuals reaching hemoglobin A1c values below 5.7% [130].

These findings are surprising indeed, since GIP has been thought to *promote* obesity based on numerous experimental observations. The early literature was summarized by Vincent Marks in 1988 in his paper "GIP – The Obesity Hormone"

[131], and a detailed follow-up was provided by Yip and Wolfe in 2000 [132]. The notion of a role of GIP in promoting obesity was supported by several findings including the following: it appears to stimulate fatty acid synthesis in the adipose tissues; it enhances insulin-stimulated incorporation of fatty acids into triglycerides and may increase insulin receptor affinity and insulin-stimulated glucose transport; and it was also reported to enhance postprandial lipid clearance from the circulation. A lipolytic activity has also been demonstrated, and it has been proposed that insulin may act as a switch between lipolysis and lipogenesis. Importantly, mice with knockout of GIP or the GIP receptor are resistant to diet-induced obesity [133]. Furthermore, the GIP receptor antagonist was demonstrated to block the effects of GIP on adipose tissue blood flow and lipid uptake, and the antagonist also impairs GIP-induced increases in splanchnic blood flow and nutrient uptake [134]. In genetic studies, inactivating variants of the GIP receptor are associated with leanness [135]. The lack of activity of GIP on glucose control in patients with type 2 diabetes has been confirmed in many studies, but its effects on food intake are more important for the current discussion. The development of tirzepatide was preceded by rodent studies carried out in Munich, where a GIP-GLP-1 coagonist was demonstrated to have good effects in experimental animals in 2013 [136]. In 2019, in a paper summarizing the effects of GIP on food intake and body weight in rodents, it was shown that while GIP mono-agonism did not have impressive effects on body weight, combinations with GLP-1 were remarkably effective [137]. Paradoxically, in other laboratories, GIP antagonists, developed on the basis of assumptions of its role to promote obesity, showed similar results [124], and indeed currently a GIP antagonist (a monoclonal antibody directed against the GIP receptor to which is attached a GLP-1 moiety) has shown remarkable weight-reducing and glycemia-improving effects [138] and is currently in phase 3 clinical trials.

Isolated experiments, designed to demonstrate effects of GIP on food intake in humans, have so far not been able to reveal any effects [139]. Addition of GIP to GLP-1 administrations has had only negative effects on plasma glucose and lipids, on liver fat, and has shown no effect on food intake [140]. Development of a long-acting GIP mono-agonist produced by NovoNordisk was terminated in 2023 due to lack of additional activity when combined with semaglutide (press release April 2023). A long-acting GIP agonist was presented by Eli Lilly at diabetes conferences in 2023 but showed very moderate and barely significant effects on blood glucose levels and body weight, and similar findings have been presented by NovoNordisk.

Two interesting hypotheses have been presented to explain the apparent superiority of tirzepatide. Tirzepatide has been demonstrated to be a “wild-type” agonist for the GIP receptor but a biased agonist on the GLP-1 receptor with preference for the cAMP pathway compared to the beta-arrestin pathway, which is responsible for receptor internalization and termination of activity [141]. Presumably a biased agonist may therefore have prolonged activity. The other proposal is that coadministration of GIP decreases the gastrointestinal side effect of GLP-1 administration [66]. With a GIP-GLP-1 coagonist, it may, therefore, be possible to use higher doses of the coagonist without running into the limiting side effects of GLP-1 agonism.

In conclusion, the effects of GIP on the control of food intake, particularly with regard to humans, are uncertain. However, the GIP/GLP-1 coagonist, tirzepatide, no doubt represents an remarkable advancement in the treatment of both diabetes and obesity.

Ghrelin

Ghrelin was discovered in 1999 as a ligand for the secretagogue receptor of the growth hormone-producing somatotrophs in the pituitary (the GHSR-1A receptor) [142]. Surprisingly, its natural ligand, ghrelin, turned out to be produced and secreted from endocrine cells of the gastric mucosa, until then designated A-like or X-cells. Expression of the gene gives rise to a preproghrelin of 117 amino acids [143], which is homologous to promotilin. Ghrelin is a 28-amino acid peptide carrying an unusual posttranslational modification, octanoylation of the serine residue in position 3, catalyzed by the enzyme GOAT (ghrelin O-acyl-transferase) [9]. The octanoylation (other fatty acids may also be used) may be lost after release in the circulation, and the deacylated molecule loses some of its actions. In agreement with its receptor localization, ghrelin stimulates GH secretion, but measurements of its secretion revealed an unusual pattern, with increasing concentrations in the interprandial periods, followed after initiation of food intake by decreases proportional to the size of the meal [144, 145]. In agreement with this pattern, ghrelin is thought to increase appetite and contribute to meal initiation. The most important receptors for this activity appear to be localized on the food intake-promoting NPY and agouti-related protein (AGRP) cells of the arcuate nucleus of the hypothalamus [146]. It is not clear how peripheral ghrelin gets there, and a hypothalamic source of ghrelin has been proposed, but remains controversial. Alternatively, ghrelin seems to engage afferent vagal fibers [5], and the growth hormone secretagogue receptor (GHSR) also appears to be expressed in gastrointestinal sensory neurons emanating from spinal dorsal root ganglia; thus, sensory neuron GHSR deletion attenuated diet-induced obesity [147]. Furthermore, viral tracing suggested crosstalk between gut non-vagal sensory afferents and adipose sympathetic outflow, pointing to alternative pathways for regulation of energy homeostasis [147]. Interestingly, ghrelin and GLP-1 may have opposing effects on behavioral patterns related to obtaining and consuming palatable foods. While meal anticipation is largely driven by endogenous ghrelin, GLP-1 has opposing effects. Preference for high-fat/sugar foods is also heightened by ghrelin and reduced by GLP-1 signaling [148].

Peripheral administration of ghrelin has been reported to lead to increased food intake in both rats and humans [149, 150], but endogenous ghrelin levels are lower in obesity, suggesting that the hormone is not directly responsible for the increased food intake [144, 151]. On the other hand, ghrelin levels increase in response to weight loss and may contribute to the difficulties of maintaining weight loss. Ghrelin appears to be involved also in glucose regulation, perhaps in particular the ghrelin produced locally in the epsilon cells of the pancreatic islets. Here, ghrelin increases somatostatin secretion and inhibits insulin secretion with resulting impairments of glucose tolerance [152]. Interestingly, ghrelin levels have been found to be elevated in individuals with the Prader-Willi syndrome, a syndrome of obesity associated with chromosomal deletions and associated with "ferocious appetite," which may be partly due to the high ghrelin levels [153]. The biology of ghrelin has been extensively studied in rodents and the number of publications is overwhelming (see Muller et al. [154] for comprehensive review [154]). Stimulation of food intake in humans was found already in 2001 [149] and has been confirmed in several subsequent studies, also including obese subjects [155]. The studies have generally included few individuals, and in some studies, for instance, in vagotomized individuals [156], there was no effect of the infusion. Also in gastrectomized subjects, there were no effects [157]. These results would be compatible with an essential role of the stomach and/or the vagus for the effects of ghrelin. The studies generally used high doses (5 pmol/kg × minutes) that give rise to supraphysiological plasma concentrations, and one group concluded that circulating ghrelin was unlikely to function as a physiological regulator of food intake since more physiological doses had no effects on food intake [158]. Such experiments obviously depend on the accuracy of the assays employed, but with a peptide the size of ghrelin, infusion rates of 5 pmol/kg × minutes would be expected to result in very high levels compared to those usually reported for peptides in human studies.

Knockout studies have not been entirely conclusive; ghrelin knockout mice (ghrelin−/−) have a normal body size, body composition, bone density, growth rate, gastric emptying, food intake, reproduction, gross behavior, and tissue pathology [159, 160]; and *Ghsr*-null mice are not dwarfs; their appetite and body composition are comparable to that of wild-type littermates [161]. Other investigators using another knockout model concluded that ghrelin signaling is required for the development of the full phenotype of diet-induced obesity, but also in those studies, the spontaneous effects of the knockout were inconspicuous [162] and a clear role in the development of obesity could not be identified [163].

Antagonist studies have so far not led to compounds with a clear therapeutic potential in obesity, and small molecule agonists and inverse agonists have not yet reached clinical development [164].

An interesting pharmacological approach is the application of inhibitors of the GOAT enzyme, preventing the octanoylation and thereby inactivating the circulating ghrelin, but this approach has so far not been clinically successful [9].

Measurements of ghrelin after bariatric surgery are generally consistent with a contribution of ghrelin to the weight loss observed since plasma levels fall considerably after surgery as might have been suspected [165]. In a study where the patients were especially selected to be comparable regarding both preoperative weight and weight loss, it was possible to evaluate the importance for the weight loss of differences regarding hormonal changes [7]. In this study (the results of which differ markedly from those obtained in consecutive patient groups without weight matching ([166])), postoperative levels of PYY and GLP-1 were much less elevated after gastric sleeve compared to gastric bypass, and ghrelin levels were much lower (in agreement with the removal of a large part of the stomach). This pointed to a particularly important role for ghrelin changes after SG. A follow-up study was therefore performed to evaluate the importance of the ghrelin changes by substitution. Twelve participants scheduled for SG were included. Before and three months after surgery, a mixed-meal test followed by an ad libitum meal test were performed with concomitant infusions of acyl-ghrelin (1 pmol/kg/minutes) or placebo. Infusions began 60 minutes prior to meal intake to reach a steady state before the mixed-meal and were continued throughout the study day. Two additional experimental days with 0.25 pmol/kg × minutes and 10 pmol/kg × minutes and acyl-ghrelin infusions were conducted three months after surgery. Both before and after SG, postprandial glucose concentrations increased dose-dependently during ghrelin infusions compared with placebo infusions (notably, complete substitution to preoperative levels was obtained with the 0.25 pmol/kg × minutes dose). Ghrelin infusion inhibited basal and postprandial insulin secretion rates, resulting in lowered measures of β-cell function. Ad libitum meal intake did not differ during ghrelin administration compared with placebo. It was concluded that the permanently lower concentration of ghrelin following SG surgery may contribute to the improved glycemic control after SG, but apparently had no influence on food intake [167].

LEAP2 is a liver-produced antimicrobial peptide that was demonstrated to act as a specific antagonist of the ghrelin receptor [168, 169]. Infusions of LEAP2 were recently found to decrease appetite and food intake [169]. The release of LEAP2 from the liver (and intestine) is not yet well defined, but the findings so far suggest that ghrelin levels should be compared with circulating levels of LEAP2 to estimate the impact of the ghrelin system on, e.g., food intake.

Conclusion

It is clear from the aforementioned presentation that the gut harbors several peptides with powerful effects on food intake. The results of bariatric surgery, where in particular Roux-en-Y gastric bypass is associated with grossly elevated plasma levels of several of these gut hormones, indicate that this endogenous appetite-regulating system is sufficiently powerful to cause weight losses that correspond to the aspirations of many obese individuals. It is also sufficient to cause great improvements in the health status of the patients with reductions in the risk of development of the complications of obesity and extension of life expectancies, by five years in patients with normal glucose tolerance and nine years in those with diabetes. Fortunately, it seems that several of the hormones, when applied in forms with extended half-lives in the circulation, are capable of producing weight losses approaching those of bariatric surgery, with for instance tirzepatide, the GIP-GLP-1 coagonist, causing weight losses of 25% after 88 weeks of treatment. If one assumes – and admittedly, it remains an assumption, although well supported by experimental and observational data – that the results of the surgery are mainly due to these hormonal changes, then it follows that similar results may be obtained after long-term treatment with the exogenous agonists. If true, this is greatly encouraging and raises hopes of much improved future therapy for many more people living with obesity and elevated risk of complications. Conversely, the results also support the notions about the importance of the gut hormones for appetite and food intake regulation in healthy individuals, although the evidence for their role is weaker. Thus, the normal regulation of food intake undoubtedly involves many more factors than merely the release of gut hormones.

References

1 Leibel, R.L., Rosenbaum, M., and Hirsch, J. (1995). Changes in energy expenditure resulting from altered body weight. *N. Engl. J. Med.* 332 (10): 621–628. https://doi.org/10.1056/NEJM199503093321001.

2 Lund, J. and Clemmensen, C. (2023). Physiological protection against weight gain: evidence from overfeeding studies and future directions. *Philos. Trans. R. Soc. Lond. Ser. B Biol. Sci.* 378 (1885): 20220229. https://doi.org/10.1098/rstb.2022.0229.

3 Schwartz, M.W., Woods, S.C., Porte, D. Jr., et al. (2000). Central nervous system control of food intake. *Nature* 404 (6778): 661–671. http://www.ncbi.nlm.nih.gov/pubmed/10766253.

4 Gibbs, J., Young, R.C., and Smith, G.P. (1973). Cholecystokinin decreases food intake in rats. *J. Comp. Physiol. Psychol.* 84 (3): 488–495. https://doi.org/10.1037/h0034870.

5 Dockray, G.J. (2013). Enteroendocrine cell signalling via the vagus nerve. *Curr. Opin. Pharmacol.* 13 (6): 954–958. https://doi.org/10.1016/j.coph.2013.09.007.

6 Scrocchi, L.A., Brown, T.J., MaClusky, N. et al. (1996). Glucose intolerance but normal satiety in mice with a null mutation in the glucagon-like peptide 1 receptor gene. *Nat. Med.* 2 (11): 1254–1258.

7 Svane, M.S., Jorgensen, N.B., Bojsen-Moller, K.N. et al. (2016). Peptide YY and glucagon-like peptide-1 contribute to decreased food intake after Roux-en-Y gastric bypass surgery. *Int. J. Obes.* 40 (11): 1699–1706. https://doi.org/10.1038/ijo.2016.121.

8 Holst, J.J. and Deacon, C.F. (1998). Inhibition of the activity of dipeptidyl-peptidase IV as a treatment for type 2 diabetes. *Diabetes* 47 (11): 1663–1670.

9 Iyer, M.R., Wood, C.M., and Kunos, G. (2020). Recent progress in the discovery of ghrelin O-acyltransferase (GOAT) inhibitors. *RSC Med. Chem.* 11 (10): 1136–1144. https://doi.org/10.1039/d0md00210k.

10 Moller, L.N., Stidsen, C.E., Hartmann, B., and Holst, J.J. (2003). Somatostatin receptors. *Biochim. Biophys. Acta* 1616 (1): 1–84. https://doi.org/10.1016/s0005-2736(03)00235-9.

11 Le Roux, C.W., Welbourn, R., Werling, M. et al. (2007). Gut hormones as mediators of appetite and weight loss after Roux-en-Y gastric bypass. *Ann. Surg.* 246 (5): 780–785. http://www.ncbi.nlm.nih.gov/pubmed/17968169.

12 Weir, G.C., Samols, E., Loo, S. et al. (1979). Somatostatin and pancreatic polypeptide secretion: effects of glucagon, insulin, and arginine. *Diabetes* 28 (1): 35–40.

13 Elliott, J.A., Jackson, S., King, S. et al. (2015). Gut hormone suppression increases food intake after esophagectomy with gastric conduit reconstruction. *Ann. Surg.* 262 (5): 824–829; discussion 829–830. https://doi.org/10.1097/SLA.0000000000001465.

14 Fourati, S., de Dreuille, B., Bettolo, J. et al. (2023). Hyperphagia is prominent in adult patients with short bowel syndrome: a role for the colon? *Clin. Nutr.* 42 (11): 2109–2115. https://doi.org/10.1016/j.clnu.2023.09.003.

15 Hengist, A., Sciarrillo, C.M., Guo, J. et al. (2023). Discordance between gut-derived appetite hormones and energy intake in humans. *medRxiv*. https://doi.org/10.1101/2023.05.10.23289718

16 Mutt, V. (1980). Chemistry, isolation and purification of gastrointestinal hormones. *Biochem. Soc. Trans.* 8 (1): 11–14. https://doi.org/10.1042/bst0080011.

17 Rehfeld, J.F., Friis-Hansen, L., Goetze, J.P., and Hansen, T.V. (2007). The biology of cholecystokinin and gastrin peptides. *Curr. Top. Med. Chem.* 7 (12): 1154–1165. https://doi.org/10.2174/156802607780960483.

18 Rehfeld, J.F. and Bundgaard, J.R. (2010). Cell-specific precursor processing. *Results Probl. Cell Differ.* 50: 45–62. https://doi.org/10.1007/400_2009_32.

19 Monstein, H.J., Nylander, A.G., Salehi, A. et al. (1996). Cholecystokinin-A and cholecystokinin-B/gastrin receptor mRNA expression in the gastrointestinal tract and pancreas of the rat and man. A polymerase chain reaction study. *Scand. J. Gastroenterol.* 31 (4): 383–390. http://www.ncbi.nlm.nih.gov/pubmed/8726308.

20 Sanders, D.J., Zahedi-Asl, S., and Marr, A.P. (1982). Glucagon and CCK in human brain: controls and patients with senile dementia of Alzheimer type. *Prog. Brain Res.* 55: 465–471.

21 Smith, G.P., Jerome, C., and Norgren, R. (1985). Afferent axons in abdominal vagus mediate satiety effect of cholecystokinin in rats. *Am. J. Phys.* 249 (5 Pt 2): R638–R641. https://doi.org/10.1152/ajpregu.1985.249.5.R638.

22 Weller, A., Smith, G.P., and Gibbs, J. (1990). Endogenous cholecystokinin reduces feeding in young rats. *Science* 247 (4950): 1589–1591. https://doi.org/10.1126/science.2321020.

23 Moran, T.H., Katz, L.F., Plata-Salaman, C.R., and Schwartz, G.J. (1998). Disordered food intake and obesity in rats lacking cholecystokinin A receptors. *Am. J. Phys.* 274 (3): R618–R625. https://doi.org/10.1152/ajpregu.1998.274.3.R618.

24 Ding, Y., Zhang, H., Liao, Y.Y. et al. (2022). Structural insights into human brain-gut peptide cholecystokinin receptors. *Cell Discov.* 8 (1): 55. https://doi.org/10.1038/s41421-022-00420-3.

25 Cawthon, C.R. and de La Serre, C.B. (2021). The critical role of CCK in the regulation of food intake and diet-induced obesity. *Peptides* 138: 170492. https://doi.org/10.1016/j.peptides.2020.170492.

26 Jordan, J., Greenway, F.L., Leiter, L.A. et al. (2008). Stimulation of cholecystokinin-A receptors with GI181771X does not cause weight loss in overweight or obese patients. *Clin. Pharmacol. Ther.* 83 (2): 281–287. https://doi.org/10.1038/sj.clpt.6100272.

27 Nyborg, N.C.B., Kirk, R.K., de Boer, A.S. et al. (2020). Cholecystokinin-1 receptor agonist induced pathological findings in the exocrine pancreas of non-human primates. *Toxicol. Appl. Pharmacol.* 399: 115035. https://doi.org/10.1016/j.taap.2020.115035.

28 Jacobsen, S.H., Olesen, S.C., Dirksen, C. et al. (2012). Changes in gastrointestinal hormone responses, insulin sensitivity, and beta-cell function within 2 weeks after gastric bypass in non-diabetic subjects. *Obes. Surg.* 22 (7): 1084–1096. https://doi.org/10.1007/s11695-012-0621-4.

29 Svane, M.S., Bojsen-Moller, K.N., Martinussen, C. et al. (2019). Postprandial nutrient handling and gastrointestinal hormone secretion after Roux-en-Y gastric bypass vs sleeve gastrectomy. *Gastroenterology* 156 (6): 1627–1641.e1. https://doi.org/10.1053/j.gastro.2019.01.262.

30 Muller, T.D., Finan, B., Bloom, S.R. et al. (2019). Glucagon-like peptide 1 (GLP-1). *Mol. Metab* 30: 72–130. https://doi.org/10.1016/j.molmet.2019.09.010.

31 Holst, J.J., Albrechtsen, N.J.W., Rosenkilde, M.M., and Deacon, C.F. (2019). Physiology of the incretin hormones, GIP and GLP-1-regulation of release and posttranslational modifications. *Compr. Physiol.* 9 (4): 1339–1381. https://doi.org/10.1002/cphy.c180013.

32 Eissele, R., Goke, R., Willemer, S. et al. (1992). Glucagon-like peptide-1 cells in the gastrointestinal tract and pancreas of rat, pig and man. *Eur. J. Clin. Investig.* 22 (4): 283–291.

33 Knudsen, J.B., Holst, J.J., Asnaes, S., and Johansen, A. (1975). Identification of cells with pancreatic-type and gut-type glucagon immunoreactivity in the human colon. *Acta Pathol. Microbiol. Scand. A* 83 (6): 741–743.

34 Gribble, F.M. and Reimann, F. (2016). Enteroendocrine cells: chemosensors in the intestinal epithelium. *Annu. Rev. Physiol.* 78: 277–299. https://doi.org/10.1146/annurev-physiol-021115-105439.

35 Hansen, H.S., Rosenkilde, M.M., Holst, J.J., and Schwartz, T.W. (2012). GPR119 as a fat sensor. *Trends Pharmacol. Sci.* 33 (7): 374–381. https://doi.org/10.1016/j.tips.2012.03.014.

36 Modvig, I.M., Kuhre, R.E., Jepsen, S.L. et al. (2021). Amino acids differ in their capacity to stimulate GLP-1 release from the perfused rat small intestine and stimulate secretion by different sensing mechanisms. *Am. J. Physiol. Endocrinol. Metab.* 320 (5): E874–E885. https://doi.org/10.1152/ajpendo.00026.2021.

37 Hansen, L., Deacon, C.F., Orskov, C., and Holst, J.J. (1999). Glucagon-like peptide-1-(7–36)amide is transformed to glucagon-like peptide-1-(9–36)amide by dipeptidyl peptidase IV in the capillaries supplying the L cells of the porcine intestine. *Endocrinology* 140 (11): 5356–5363. http://www.ncbi.nlm.nih.gov/pubmed/0010537167.

38 Hjollund, K.R., Deacon, C.F., and Holst, J.J. (2011). Dipeptidyl peptidase-4 inhibition increases portal concentrations of intact glucagon-like peptide-1

(GLP-1) to a greater extent than peripheral concentrations in anaesthetised pigs. *Diabetologia* 54 (8): 2206–2208. https://doi.org/10.1007/s00125-011-2168-7.

39 Brierley, D.I., Holt, M.K., Singh, A. et al. (2021). Central and peripheral GLP-1 systems independently suppress eating. *Nat. Metab.* 3 (2): 258–273. https://doi.org/10.1038/s42255-021-00344-4.

40 Holst, J.J. and Deacon, C.F. (2005). Glucagon-like peptide-1 mediates the therapeutic actions of DPP-IV inhibitors. *Diabetologia* 48 (4): 612–615. http://www.ncbi.nlm.nih.gov/pubmed/15759106.

41 Smits, M.M., Galsgaard, K.D., Jepsen, S.L. et al. (2024). in vivo inhibition of dipeptidyl peptidase 4 allows measurement of GLP-1 secretion in mice. *Diabetes* 73 (5): 671–681. https://doi.org/10.2337/db23-0848.

42 Windelov, J.A., Wewer Albrechtsen, N.J., Kuhre, R.E. et al. (2017). Why is it so difficult to measure glucagon-like peptide-1 in a mouse? *Diabetologia* 60 (10, 10): 2066–2075. https://doi.org/10.1007/s00125-017-4347-7.

43 Holst, J.J. (1999). Glucagon-like peptide 1(GLP-1): an intestinal hormone signalling nutritional abundance, with an unusual therapeutic potential. *Trends Endocrinol. Metab.* 10 (6): 229–234.

44 Schirra, J. and Goke, B. (2005). The physiological role of GLP-1 in human: incretin, ileal brake or more? *Regul. Pept.* 128 (2): 109–115. http://www.ncbi.nlm.nih.gov/pubmed/15780430.

45 Turton, M.D., O'Shea, D., Gunn, I. et al. (1996). A role for glucagon-like peptide-1 in the central regulation of feeding. *Nature* 379 (6560): 69–72.

46 Larsen, P.J., Tang-Christensen, M., Holst, J.J., and Orskov, C. (1997). Distribution of glucagon-like peptide-1 and other preproglucagon- derived peptides in the rat hypothalamus and brainstem. *Neuroscience* 77 (1): 257–270.

47 Vrang, N., Phifer, C.B., Corkern, M.M., and Berthoud, H.R. (2003). Gastric distension induces c-Fos in medullary GLP-1/2-containing neurons. *Am. J. Physiol. Regul. Integr. Comp. Physiol.* 285 (2): R470–R478. http://www.ncbi.nlm.nih.gov/pubmed/12714357.

48 Flint, A., Raben, A., Astrup, A., and Holst, J.J. (1998). Glucagon-like peptide 1 promotes satiety and suppresses energy intake in humans. *J. Clin. Invest.* 101 (3): 515–520.

49 Verdich, C., Flint, A., Gutzwiller, J.P. et al. (2001). A meta-analysis of the effect of glucagon-like peptide-1 (7–36) amide on ad libitum energy intake in humans. *J. Clin. Endocrinol. Metab.* 86 (9): 4382–4389. http://www.ncbi.nlm.nih.gov/pubmed/11549680.

50 Gasbjerg, L.S., Bari, E.J., Christensen, M., and Knop, F.K. (2021). Exendin (9–39) NH (2): recommendations for clinical use based on a systematic literature review. *Diabetes. Obes. Metab.* 23 (11): 2419–2436. https://doi.org/10.1111/dom.14507.

51 Ten Kulve, J.S., Veltman, D.J., van, B.L. et al. (2015). Endogenous GLP-1 mediates postprandial reductions in activation in central reward and satiety areas in patients with type 2 diabetes. *Diabetologia* 58 (12): 2688–2698. https://doi.org/10.1007/s00125-015-3754-x.

52 Sisley, S., Gutierrez-Aguilar, R., Scott, M. et al. (2014). Neuronal GLP1R mediates liraglutide's anorectic but not glucose-lowering effect. *J. Clin. Invest.* 124 (6): 2456–2463. https://doi.org/10.1172/JCI72434.

53 Gabery, S., Salinas, C.G., Paulsen, S.J. et al. (2020). Semaglutide lowers body weight in rodents via distributed neural pathways. *JCI Insight* 5 (6): https://doi.org/10.1172/jci.insight.133429.

54 Orskov, C., Poulsen, S.S., Moller, M., and Holst, J.J. (1996). Glucagon-like peptide I receptors in the subfornical organ and the area postrema are accessible to circulating glucagon-like peptide I. *Diabetes* 45 (6): 832–835.

55 Ritzel, R., Orskov, C., Holst, J.J., and Nauck, M.A. (1995). Pharmacokinetic, insulinotropic, and glucagonostatic properties of GLP-1 [7–36 amide] after subcutaneous injection in healthy volunteers. Dose–response-relationships. *Diabetologia* 38 (6): 720–725.

56 Larsen, J., Hylleberg, B., Ng, K., and Damsbo, P. (2001). Glucagon-like peptide-1 infusion must be maintained for 24 h/day to obtain acceptable glycemia in type 2 diabetic patients who are poorly controlled on sulphonylurea treatment. *Diabetes Care* 24 (8): 1416–1421. http://www.ncbi.nlm.nih.gov/pubmed/11473079.

57 Fineman, M.S., Shen, L.Z., Taylor, K. et al. (2004). Effectiveness of progressive dose-escalation of exenatide (exendin-4) in reducing dose-limiting side effects in subjects with type 2 diabetes. *Diabetes Metab. Res. Rev.* 20 (5): 411–417. http://www.ncbi.nlm.nih.gov/pubmed/15343588.

58 Ostergaard, L., Frandsen, C.S., Dejgaard, T.F., and Madsbad, S. (2017). Fixed-ratio combination therapy with GLP-1 receptor agonist liraglutide and insulin degludec in people with type 2 diabetes. *Expert. Rev. Clin. Pharmacol.* 10 (6): 621–632. https://doi.org/10.1080/17512433.2017.1313109.

59 Astrup, A., Rossner, S., Van, G.L. et al. (2009). Effects of liraglutide in the treatment of obesity: a randomised, double-blind, placebo-controlled study. *Lancet* 374 (9701): 1606–1616. https://doi.org/10.1016/S0140-6736(09)61375-1.

60 Pi-Sunyer, X., Astrup, A., Fujioka, K. et al. (2015). A randomized, controlled trial of 3.0 mg of liraglutide in weight management. *N. Engl. J. Med.* 373 (1): 11–22. https://doi.org/10.1056/NEJMoa1411892.

61 Le Roux, C.W., Astrup, A., Fujioka, K. et al. (2017). 3 years of liraglutide versus placebo for type 2 diabetes risk reduction and weight management in individuals with prediabetes: a randomised, double-blind trial. *Lancet* 389 (10077): 1399–1409. https://doi.org/10.1016/S0140-6736(17)30069-7.

62 Knudsen, L.B. and Lau, J. (2019). The discovery and development of liraglutide and semaglutide. *Front. Endocrinol. (Lausanne)* 10: 155. https://doi.org/10.3389/fendo.2019.00155.

63 O'Neil, P.M., Birkenfeld, A.L., McGowan, B. et al. (2018). Efficacy and safety of semaglutide compared with liraglutide and placebo for weight loss in patients with obesity: a randomised, double-blind, placebo and active controlled, dose-ranging, phase 2 trial. *Lancet* 392 (10148): 637–649. https://doi.org/10.1016/S0140-6736(18)31773-2.

64 Wilding, J.P.H., Batterham, R.L., Calanna, S. et al. (2021). Once-weekly semaglutide in adults with overweight or obesity. *N. Engl. J. Med.* 384 (11): 989. https://doi.org/10.1056/NEJMoa2032183.

65 Geisler, C.E. and Hayes, M.R. (2023). Metabolic hormone action in the VTA: reward-directed behavior and mechanistic insights. *Physiol. Behav.* 268: 114236. https://doi.org/10.1016/j.physbeh.2023.114236.

66 Samms, R.J., Cosgrove, R., Snider, B.M. et al. (2022). GIPR agonism inhibits PYY-induced nausea-like behavior. *Diabetes* 71 (7): 1410–1423. https://doi.org/10.2337/db21-0848.

67 Holst, J.J., Albrechtsen, N.J.W., Gabe, M.B.N., and Rosenkilde, M.M. (2018). Oxyntomodulin: actions and role in diabetes. *Peptides* 100: 48–53. https://doi.org/10.1016/j.peptides.2017.09.018.

68 Baldissera, F.G. and Holst, J.J. (1984). Glucagon-related peptides in the human gastrointestinal mucosa. *Diabetologia* 26 (3): 223–228.

69 Bataille, D., Tatemoto, K., Gespach, C. et al. (1982). Isolation of glucagon-37 (bioactive enteroglucagon/oxyntomodulin) from porcine jejuno-ileum. Characterization of the peptide. *FEBS Lett.* 146 (1): 79–86.

70 Holst, J.J. (1982). Evidence that enteroglucagon (II) is identical with the C-terminal sequence (residues 33–69) of glicentin. *Biochem. J.* 207 (3): 381–388.

71 Baldissera, F.G., Holst, J.J., Knuhtsen, S. et al. (1988). Oxyntomodulin (glicentin-[33–69]): pharmacokinetics, binding to liver cell membranes, effects on isolated perfused pig pancreas, and secretion from isolated perfused lower small intestine of pigs. *Regul. Pept.* 21 (1–2): 151–166.

72 Nielsen, M.S., Ritz, C., Wewer Albrechtsen, N.J. et al. (2020). Oxyntomodulin and glicentin may predict the effect of bariatric surgery on food preferences and weight loss. *J. Clin. Endocrinol. Metab.* 105 (4): https://doi.org/10.1210/clinem/dgaa061.

73 Day, J.W., Ottaway, N., Patterson, J.T. et al. (2009). A new glucagon and GLP-1 co-agonist eliminates obesity in rodents. *Nat. Chem. Biol.* 5 (10): 749–757. https://doi.org/10.1038/nchembio.209.

74 Pocai, A., Carrington, P.E., Adams, J.R. et al. (2009). Glucagon-like peptide 1/glucagon receptor dual agonism reverses obesity in mice. *Diabetes* 58 (10): 2258–2266. https://doi.org/10.2337/db09-0278.

75 Bagger, J.I., Knop, F.K., Holst, J.J., and Vilsboll, T. (2011). Glucagon receptor antagonism for the treatment of type 2 diabetes. *Diabetes. Obes. Metab.* 13: 965–971.

76 Guzman, C.B., Zhang, X.M., Liu, R. et al. (2017). Treatment with LY2409021, a glucagon receptor antagonist, increases liver fat in patients with type 2 diabetes. *Diabetes. Obes. Metab.* 19 (11): 1521–1528. https://doi.org/10.1111/dom.12958.

77 Galsgaard, K.D., Pedersen, J., Knop, F.K. et al. (2019). Glucagon receptor signaling and lipid metabolism. *Front. Physiol.* 10: 413. https://doi.org/10.3389/fphys.2019.00413.

78 Haedersdal, S., Andersen, A., Knop, F.K., and Vilsboll, T. (2023). Revisiting the role of glucagon in health, diabetes mellitus and other metabolic diseases. *Nat. Rev. Endocrinol.* 19 (6): 321–335. https://doi.org/10.1038/s41574-023-00817-4.

79 Tatemoto, K. and Mutt, V. (1980). Isolation of two novel candidate hormones using a chemical method for finding naturally occurring polypeptides. *Nature* 285 (5764): 417–418. http://www.ncbi.nlm.nih.gov/pubmed/6892950.

80 Bottcher, G., Alumets, J., Hakanson, R., and Sundler, F. (1986). Co-existence of glicentin and peptide YY in colorectal L-cells in cat and man. An electron microscopic study. *Regul. Pept.* 13 (3–4): 283–291. http://www.ncbi.nlm.nih.gov/pubmed/3754646.

81 Svendsen, B., Pedersen, J., Jacob Wewer, A.N. et al. (2014). An analysis of co-secretion and co-expression of gut hormones from male rat proximal and distal small intestine. *Endocrinology* 156 (3): 847–857. https://doi.org/10.1210/en.2014-1710.

82 van der Beek, C.M., Canfora, E.E., Lenaerts, K. et al. (2016). Distal, not proximal, colonic acetate infusions promote fat oxidation and improve metabolic markers in overweight/obese men. *Clin. Sci. (Lond.)* 130 (22): 2073–2082. https://doi.org/10.1042/CS20160263.

83 Sjolund, K., Sanden, G., Hakanson, R., and Sundler, F. (1983). Endocrine cells in human intestine: an immunocytochemical study. *Gastroenterology* 85 (5): 1120–1130. https://doi.org/10.1016/S0016-5085(83)80080-8.

84 Fuhlendorff, J., Johansen, N.L., Melberg, S.G. et al. (1990). The antiparallel pancreatic polypeptide fold in the binding of neuropeptide Y to Y1 and Y2 receptors. *J. Biol. Chem.* 265 (20): 11706–11712. https://www.ncbi.nlm.nih.gov/pubmed/2164012.

85 Blomqvist, A.G. and Herzog, H. (1997). Y-receptor subtypes – how many more? *Trends Neurosci.* 20 (7): 294–298. https://doi.org/10.1016/s0166-2236(96)01057-0.

86 Lecklin, A., Lundell, I., Paananen, L. et al. (2002). Receptor subtypes Y1 and Y5 mediate neuropeptide Y induced feeding in the guinea-pig. *Br. J. Pharmacol.* 135 (8): 2029–2037. https://doi.org/10.1038/sj.bjp.0704667.

87 Eberlein, G.A., Eysselein, V.E., Schaeffer, M. et al. (1989). A new molecular form of PYY: structural characterization of human PYY (3–36) and PYY (1–36). *Peptides* 10 (4): 797–803. https://doi.org/10.1016/0196-9781(89)90116-2.

88 Grandt, D., Dahms, P., Schimiczek, M. et al. (1993). Proteolytic processing by dipeptidyl aminopeptidase IV generates receptor selectivity for peptide YY (PYY). *Med. Klin. (Munich)* 88 (3): 143–145. https://www.ncbi.nlm.nih.gov/pubmed/8097274.

89 Batterham, R.L., Cowley, M.A., Small, C.J. et al. (2002). Gut hormone PYY(3–36) physiologically inhibits food intake. *Nature* 418 (6898): 650–654. http://www.ncbi.nlm.nih.gov/pubmed/12167864.

90 Batterham, R.L., Cohen, M.A., Ellis, S.M. et al. (2003). Inhibition of food intake in obese subjects by peptide YY3–36. *N. Engl. J. Med.* 349 (10): 941–948. http://www.ncbi.nlm.nih.gov/pubmed/12954742.

91 Boggiano, M.M., Chandler, P.C., Oswald, K.D. et al. (2005). PYY3–36 as an anti-obesity drug target. *Obes. Rev.* 6 (4): 307–322. https://doi.org/10.1111/j.1467-789X.2005.00218.x.

92 Tschop, M., Castaneda, T.R., Joost, H.G. et al. (2004). Physiology: does gut hormone PYY3–36 decrease food intake in rodents? *Nature* 430 (6996), 1 p following 165; discussion 162 p following 165. https://doi.org/10.1038/nature02665.

93 Boey, D., Lin, S., Karl, T. et al. (2006). Peptide YY ablation in mice leads to the development of hyperinsulinaemia and obesity. *Diabetologia* 49 (6): 1360–1370. https://doi.org/10.1007/s00125-006-0237-0.

94 Manning, S. and Batterham, R.L. (2014). The role of gut hormone peptide YY in energy and glucose homeostasis: twelve years on. *Annu. Rev. Physiol.* 76: 585–608. https://doi.org/10.1146/annurev-physiol-021113-170404.

95 Nonaka, N., Shioda, S., Niehoff, M.L., and Banks, W.A. (2003). Characterization of blood–brain barrier permeability to PYY3–36 in the mouse. *J. Pharmacol. Exp. Ther.* 306 (3): 948–953. https://doi.org/10.1124/jpet.103.051821.

96 Abbott, C.R., Monteiro, M., Small, C.J. et al. (2005). The inhibitory effects of peripheral administration of peptide YY (3–36) and glucagon-like peptide-1 on food intake are attenuated by ablation of the vagal-brainstem-hypothalamic pathway. *Brain Res.* 1044 (1): 127–131. http://www.ncbi.nlm.nih.gov/pubmed/15862798.

97 Koda, S., Date, Y., Murakami, N. et al. (2005). The role of the vagal nerve in peripheral PYY3–36-induced feeding reduction in rats. *Endocrinology* 146 (5): 2369–2375. https://doi.org/10.1210/en.2004-1266.

98 Torang, S., Bojsen-Moller, K.N., Svane, M.S. et al. (2016). in vivo and in vitro degradation of peptide YY3–36 to inactive peptide YY3–34 in humans. *Am. J. Physiol. Regul. Integr. Comp. Physiol.* 310 (9): R866–R874. https://doi.org/10.1152/ajpregu.00394.2015.

99 Kowalka, A.M., Alexiadou, K., Cuenco, J. et al. (2023). The postprandial secretion of peptide YY (1–36) and (3–36) in obesity is differentially increased after gastric bypass versus sleeve gastrectomy. *Clin. Endocrinol.* 99 (3): 272–284. https://doi.org/10.1111/cen.14846.

100 Sloth, B., Davidsen, L., Holst, J.J. et al. (2007). Effect of subcutaneous injections of PYY1–36 and PYY3–36 on appetite, ad libitum energy intake, and plasma free fatty acid concentration in obese males. *Am. J. Physiol. Endocrinol. Metab.* 293 (2): E604–E609. http://www.ncbi.nlm.nih.gov/pubmed/17566112.

101 Sloth, B., Holst, J.J., Flint, A. et al. (2007). Effects of PYY1–36 and PYY3–36 on appetite, energy intake, energy expenditure, glucose and fat metabolism in obese and lean subjects. *Am. J. Physiol. Endocrinol. Metab.* 292 (4): E1062–E1068. http://www.ncbi.nlm.nih.gov/pubmed/17148749.

102 Korner, J., Bessler, M., Cirilo, L.J. et al. (2005). Effects of Roux-en-Y gastric bypass surgery on fasting and postprandial concentrations of plasma ghrelin, peptide YY, and insulin. *J. Clin. Endocrinol. Metab.* 90 (1): 359–365. https://doi.org/10.1210/jc.2004-1076.

103 Korner, J., Bessler, M., Inabnet, W. et al. (2007). Exaggerated glucagon-like peptide-1 and blunted glucose-dependent insulinotropic peptide secretion are associated with Roux-en-Y gastric bypass but not adjustable gastric banding. *Surg. Obes. Relat. Dis.* 3 (6): 597–601. http://www.ncbi.nlm.nih.gov/pubmed/17936091.

104 Neary, N.M., Small, C.J., Druce, M.R. et al. (2005). Peptide YY3–36 and glucagon-like peptide-17–36 inhibit food intake additively. *Endocrinology* 146 (12): 5120–5127. https://doi.org/10.1210/en.2005-0237.

105 Schmidt, J.B., Gregersen, N.T., Pedersen, S.D. et al. (2014). Effects of PYY3–36 and GLP-1 on energy intake, energy expenditure, and appetite in overweight men. *Am. J. Physiol. Endocrinol. Metab.* 306 (11): E1248–E1256. https://doi.org/10.1152/ajpendo.00569.2013.

106 Ostergaard, S., Paulsson, J.F., Kjaergaard Gerstenberg, M., and Wulff, B.S. (2021). The design of a GLP-1/PYY dual acting agonist. *Angew. Chem. Int. Ed. Engl.* 60 (15): 8268–8275. https://doi.org/10.1002/anie.202016464.

107 Behary, P., Tharakan, G., Alexiadou, K. et al. (2019). Combined GLP-1, oxyntomodulin, and peptide YY improves body weight and glycemia in obesity and prediabetes/type 2 diabetes: a randomized, single-blinded, placebo-controlled study. *Diabetes Care* 42 (8): 1446–1453. https://doi.org/10.2337/dc19-0449.

108 Brown, J.C. (1982). Gastric inhibitory polypeptide. *Monogr. Endocrinol.* 24 (III-XI): 1–88.

109 Dupre, J., Ross, S.A., Watson, D., and Brown, J.C. (1973). Stimulation of insulin secretion by gastric inhibitory polypeptide in man. *J. Clin. Endocrinol. Metab.* 37: 826–828.

110 Nauck, M., Schmidt, W.E., Ebert, R. et al. (1989). Insulinotropic properties of synthetic human gastric inhibitory polypeptide in man: interactions with glucose, phenylalanine, and cholecystokinin-8. *J. Clin. Endocrinol. Metab.* 69 (3): 654–662. http://www.ncbi.nlm.nih.gov/pubmed/2668324.

111 Sparre-Ulrich, A.H., Gabe, M.N., Gasbjerg, L.S. et al. (2017). GIP (3–30) NH2 is a potent competitive antagonist of the GIP receptor and effectively inhibits GIP-mediated insulin, glucagon, and somatostatin release. *Biochem. Pharmacol.* 131: 78–88. https://doi.org/10.1016/j.bcp.2017.02.012.

112 Gasbjerg, L.S., Helsted, M.M., Hartmann, B. et al. (2019). Separate and combined gluco-metabolic effects of endogenous glucose-dependent insulinotropic polypeptide and glucagon-like peptide-1 in healthy individuals. *Diabetes* 68 (5): 906–917. https://doi.org/10.2337/db18-1123.

113 Drucker, D.J. and Holst, J.J. (2023). The expanding incretin universe: from basic biology to clinical translation. *Diabetologia* 66 (10): 1765–1779. https://doi.org/10.1007/s00125-023-05906-7.

114 Deacon, C.F., Danielsen, P., Klarskov, L. et al. (2001). Dipeptidyl peptidase IV inhibition reduces the degradation and clearance of GIP and potentiates its insulinotropic and antihyperglycemic effects in anesthetized pigs. *Diabetes* 50 (7): 1588–1597. http://www.ncbi.nlm.nih.gov/pubmed/11423480.

115 Kieffer, T.J., McIntosh, C.H., and Pederson, R.A. (1995). Degradation of glucose-dependent insulinotropic polypeptide and truncated glucagon-like peptide 1 in vitro and in vivo by dipeptidyl peptidase IV. *Endocrinology* 136 (8): 3585–3596.

116 Vilsboll, T., Agerso, H., Lauritsen, T. et al. (2006). The elimination rates of intact GIP as well as its primary metabolite, GIP 3–42, are similar in type 2 diabetic patients and healthy subjects. *Regul. Pept.* 137 (3): 168–172. http://www.ncbi.nlm.nih.gov/pubmed/16934887.

117 Takeda, J., Seino, Y., Tanaka, K. et al. (1987). Sequence of an intestinal cDNA encoding human gastric inhibitory polypeptide precursor. *Proc. Natl. Acad. Sci. USA* 84 (20): 7005–7008. http://www.ncbi.nlm.nih.gov/pubmed/2890159.

118 Fehmann, H.C. and Goke, B. (1995). Characterization of GIP (1–30) and GIP (1–42) as stimulators of proinsulin gene transcription. *Peptides* 16 (6): 1149–1152.

119 Krogh, L.S.L., Henriksen, K., Stensen, S. et al. (2023). The naturally occurring GIP (1–30) NH2 is a GIP receptor agonist in humans. *Eur. J. Endocrinol.* 188 (1): https://doi.org/10.1093/ejendo/lvac015.

120 Deacon, C.F., Nauck, M.A., Meier, J. et al. (2000). Degradation of endogenous and exogenous gastric inhibitory polypeptide in healthy and in type 2 diabetic subjects as revealed using a new assay for the intact peptide. *J. Clin. Endocrinol. Metab.* 85 (10): 3575–3581. http://www.ncbi.nlm.nih.gov/pubmed/11061504.

121 Krarup, T., Holst, J.J., Lindorff Larsen, K., and Madsbad, S. (1987). Heterogeneity of IR-GIP in normal subjects and insulin-dependent diabetics. In: *Gut Regulatory Peptides: Their Role in Health and Disease*, vol. 16 (ed. E. Blázquez), 167–174. Karger.

122 Usdin, T.B., Mezey, E., Button, D.C. et al. (1993). Gastric inhibitory polypeptide receptor, a member of the secretin- vasoactive intestinal peptide receptor family, is widely distributed in peripheral organs and the brain. *Endocrinology* 133 (6): 2861–2870. http://www.ncbi.nlm.nih.gov/pubmed/8243312.

123 Campbell, J.E., Beaudry, J.L., Svendsen, B. et al. (2022). GIPR is predominantly localized to nonadipocyte cell types within white adipose tissue. *Diabetes* 71 (5): 1115–1127. https://doi.org/10.2337/db21-1166.

124 Killion, E.A., Chen, M., Falsey, J.R. et al. (2020). Chronic glucose-dependent insulinotropic polypeptide receptor (GIPR) agonism desensitizes adipocyte GIPR activity mimicking functional GIPR antagonism. *Nat. Commun.* 11 (1): 4981. https://doi.org/10.1038/s41467-020-18751-8.

125 Liskiewicz, A., Khalil, A., Liskiewicz, D. et al. (2023). Glucose-dependent insulinotropic polypeptide regulates body weight and food intake via GABAergic neurons in mice. *Nat. Metab.* 5 (12): 2075–2085. https://doi.org/10.1038/s42255-023-00931-7.

126 Adriaenssens, A., Broichhagen, J., de Bray, A. et al. (2023). Hypothalamic and brainstem glucose-dependent insulinotropic polypeptide receptor neurons employ distinct mechanisms to affect feeding. *JCI Insight* 8 (10): https://doi.org/10.1172/jci.insight.164921.

127 Krarup, T., Saurbrey, N., Moody, A.J. et al. (1987). Effect of porcine gastric inhibitory polypeptide on beta-cell function in type I and type II diabetes mellitus. *Metabolism* 36 (7): 677–682. https://doi.org/10.1016/0026-0495(87)90153-3.

128 Coskun, T., Sloop, K.W., Loghin, C. et al. (2018). LY3298176, a novel dual GIP and GLP-1 receptor agonist for the treatment of type 2 diabetes mellitus: from discovery to clinical proof of concept. *Mol. Metab* 18: 3–14. https://doi.org/10.1016/j.molmet.2018.09.009.

129 Aronne, L.J., Sattar, N., Horn, D.B. et al. (2024). Continued treatment with tirzepatide for maintenance of weight reduction in adults with obesity: the SURMOUNT-4 randomized clinical trial. *JAMA* 331 (1): 38–48. https://doi.org/10.1001/jama.2023.24945.

130 Frias, J.P., Davies, M.J., Rosenstock, J. et al. (2021). Tirzepatide versus semaglutide once weekly in patients with type 2 diabetes. *N. Engl. J. Med.* 385 (6): 503–515. https://doi.org/10.1056/NEJMoa2107519.

131 Marks, V. (1988). GIP – the obesity hormone. In: *Current Approaches: Obesity* (ed. W.P.T. James and S.W. Parker), 13–19. Duphar Medical Relations.

132 Yip, R.G. and Wolfe, M.M. (2000). GIP biology and fat metabolism. *Life Sci.* 66 (2): 91–103. http://www.ncbi.nlm.nih.gov/pubmed/0010666005.

133 Miyawaki, K., Yamada, Y., Ban, N. et al. (2002). Inhibition of gastric inhibitory polypeptide signaling prevents obesity. *Nat. Med.* 8 (7): 738–742. http://www.ncbi.nlm.nih.gov/pubmed/12068290.

134 Gasbjerg, L.S., Bergmann, N.C., Stensen, S. et al. (2019). Evaluation of the incretin effect in humans using GIP and GLP-1 receptor antagonists. *Peptides* 125: 170183. https://doi.org/10.1016/j.peptides.2019.170183.

135 Kizilkaya, H.S., Sorensen, K.V., Kibsgaard, C.J. et al. (2021). Loss of function glucose-dependent insulinotropic polypeptide receptor variants are associated with alterations in BMI, bone strength and cardiovascular outcomes. *Front. Cell Dev. Biol.* 9 (749): 607. https://doi.org/10.3389/fcell.2021.749607.

136 Finan, B., Ma, T., Ottaway, N. et al. (2013). Unimolecular dual incretins maximize metabolic benefits in rodents, monkeys, and humans. *Sci. Transl. Med.* 5 (209): 209ra151. https://doi.org/10.1126/scitranslmed.3007218.

137 Mroz, P.A., Finan, B., Gelfanov, V. et al. (2019). Optimized GIP analogs promote body weight lowering in mice through GIPR agonism not antagonism. *Mol. Metab* 20: 51–62. https://doi.org/10.1016/j.molmet.2018.12.001.

138 Veniant, M.M., Lu, S.C., Atangan, L. et al. (2024). A GIPR antagonist conjugated to GLP-1 analogues promotes weight loss with improved metabolic parameters in preclinical and phase 1 settings. *Nat. Metab.* 6 (2): 290–303. https://doi.org/10.1038/s42255-023-00966-w.

139 Bergmann, N.C., Lund, A., Gasbjerg, L.S. et al. (2019). Effects of combined GIP and GLP-1 infusion on energy intake, appetite and energy expenditure in overweight/obese individuals: a randomised, crossover study. *Diabetologia* 62 (4): 665–675. https://doi.org/10.1007/s00125-018-4810-0.

140 Bergmann, N.C., Gasbjerg, L.S., Heimburger, S.M. et al. (2020). No acute effects of exogenous glucose-dependent insulinotropic polypeptide on energy intake, appetite, or energy expenditure when added to treatment with a long-acting glucagon-like peptide 1 receptor agonist in men with type 2v diabetes. *Diabetes Care* 43 (3): 588–596. https://doi.org/10.2337/dc19-0578.

141 Willard, F.S., Douros, J.D., Gabe, M.B. et al. (2020). Tirzepatide is an imbalanced and biased dual GIP and GLP-1 receptor agonist. *JCI Insight* 5 (17): https://doi.org/10.1172/jci.insight.140532.

142 Kojima, M., Hosoda, H., Date, Y. et al. (1999). Ghrelin is a growth-hormone-releasing acylated peptide from stomach. *Nature* 402 (6762): 656–660. http://www.ncbi.nlm.nih.gov/pubmed/10604470.

143 Asakawa, A., Inui, A., Kaga, T. et al. (2001). Ghrelin is an appetite-stimulatory signal from stomach with structural resemblance to motilin. *Gastroenterology* 120 (2): 337–345. http://www.ncbi.nlm.nih.gov/pubmed/11159873.

144 Cummings, D.E., Weigle, D.S., Frayo, R.S. et al. (2002). Plasma ghrelin levels after diet-induced weight loss or gastric bypass surgery. *N. Engl. J. Med.* 346 (21): 1623–1630. https://doi.org/10.1056/NEJMoa012908.

145 Shiiya, T., Nakazato, M., Mizuta, M. et al. (2002). Plasma ghrelin levels in lean and obese humans and the effect of glucose on ghrelin secretion. *J. Clin. Endocrinol. Metab.* 87 (1): 240–244. https://doi.org/10.1210/jcem.87.1.8129.

146 Gross, J.D., Zhou, Y., Barak, L.S., and Caron, M.G. (2023). Ghrelin receptor signaling in health and disease: a biased view. *Trends Endocrinol. Metab.* 34 (2): 106–118. https://doi.org/10.1016/j.tem.2022.12.001.

147 Alex Thomas, M., Cui, X., Artinian, L.R. et al. (2023). Crosstalk between gut sensory ghrelin signaling and adipose tissue sympathetic outflow regulates metabolic homeostasis. *bioRxiv*. https://doi.org/10.1101/2023.11.25.568689.

148 Decarie-Spain, L. and Kanoski, S.E. (2021). Ghrelin and glucagon-like peptide-1 : a gut-brain axis battle for food reward. *Nutrients* 13 (3): 977. https://doi.org/10.3390/nu13030977.

149 Wren, A.M., Seal, L.J., Cohen, M.A. et al. (2001). Ghrelin enhances appetite and increases food intake in humans. *J. Clin. Endocrinol. Metab.* 86 (12): 5992. https://doi.org/10.1210/jcem.86.12.8111.

150 Wren, A.M., Small, C.J., Abbott, C.R. et al. (2001). Ghrelin causes hyperphagia and obesity in rats. *Diabetes* 50 (11): 2540–2547. https://doi.org/10.2337/diabetes.50.11.2540.

151 Tschop, M., Weyer, C., Tataranni, P.A. et al. (2001). Circulating ghrelin levels are decreased in human obesity. *Diabetes* 50 (4): 707–709. https://doi.org/10.2337/diabetes.50.4.707.

152 Adriaenssens, A.E., Svendsen, B., Lam, B.Y. et al. (2016). Transcriptomic profiling of pancreatic alpha, beta and delta cell populations identifies delta cells as a principal target for ghrelin in mouse islets. *Diabetologia* 59 (10): 2156–2165. https://doi.org/10.1007/s00125-016-4033-1.

153 Rahman, Q.F.A., Jufri, N.F., and Hamid, A. (2023). Hyperphagia in prader-willi syndrome with obesity: from development to pharmacological treatment. *Intractable Rare Dis Res* 12 (1): 5–12. https://doi.org/10.5582/irdr.2022.01127.

154 Muller, T.D., Nogueiras, R., Andermann, M.L. et al. (2015). Ghrelin. *Mol Metab* 4 (6): 437–460. https://doi.org/10.1016/j.molmet.2015.03.005.

155 Druce, M.R., Wren, A.M., Park, A.J. et al. (2005). Ghrelin increases food intake in obese as well as lean subjects. *Int. J. Obes.* 29 (9): 1130–1136. https://doi.org/10.1038/sj.ijo.0803001.
156 le Roux, C.W., Neary, N.M., Halsey, T.J. et al. (2005). Ghrelin does not stimulate food intake in patients with surgical procedures involving vagotomy. *J. Clin. Endocrinol. Metab.* 90 (8): 4521–4524. https://doi.org/10.1210/jc.2004-2537.
157 Huda, M.S., Dovey, T., Wong, S.P. et al. (2009). Ghrelin restores "lean-type" hunger and energy expenditure profiles in morbidly obese subjects but has no effect on postgastrectomy subjects. *Int. J. Obes.* 33 (3): 317–325. https://doi.org/10.1038/ijo.2008.270.
158 Lippl, F., Erdmann, J., Steiger, A. et al. (2012). Low-dose ghrelin infusion--evidence against a hormonal role in food intake. *Regul. Pept.* 174 (1–3): 26–31. https://doi.org/10.1016/j.regpep.2011.11.005.
159 De Smet, B., Depoortere, I., Moechars, D. et al. (2006). Energy homeostasis and gastric emptying in ghrelin knockout mice. *J. Pharmacol. Exp. Ther.* 316 (1): 431–439. https://doi.org/10.1124/jpet.105.091504.
160 Sun, Y., Ahmed, S., and Smith, R.G. (2003). Deletion of ghrelin impairs neither growth nor appetite. *Mol. Cell. Biol.* 23 (22): 7973–7981. https://doi.org/10.1128/MCB.23.22.7973-7981.2003.
161 Sun, Y., Wang, P., Zheng, H., and Smith, R.G. (2004). Ghrelin stimulation of growth hormone release and appetite is mediated through the growth hormone secretagogue receptor. *Proc. Natl. Acad. Sci. USA* 101 (13): 4679–4684. https://doi.org/10.1073/pnas.0305930101.
162 Zigman, J.M., Nakano, Y., Coppari, R. et al. (2005). Mice lacking ghrelin receptors resist the development of diet-induced obesity. *J. Clin. Invest.* 115 (12): 3564–3572. https://doi.org/10.1172/JCI26002.
163 Albarran-Zeckler, R.G., Sun, Y., and Smith, R.G. (2011). Physiological roles revealed by ghrelin and ghrelin receptor deficient mice. *Peptides* 32 (11): 2229–2235. https://doi.org/10.1016/j.peptides.2011.07.003.
164 Giorgioni, G., Del Bello, F., Quaglia, W. et al. (2022). Advances in the development of nonpeptide small molecules targeting ghrelin receptor. *J. Med. Chem.* 65 (4): 3098–3118. https://doi.org/10.1021/acs.jmedchem.1c02191.
165 Cummings, D.E. (2009). Endocrine mechanisms mediating remission of diabetes after gastric bypass surgery. *Int. J. Obes.* 33 Suppl 1: S33–S40. https://doi.org/10.1038/ijo.2009.15.
166 Fatima, F., Hjelmesaeth, J., Birkeland, K.I. et al. (2022). Gastrointestinal hormones and beta-cell function after gastric bypass and sleeve gastrectomy: a randomized controlled trial (oseberg). *J. Clin. Endocrinol. Metab.* 107 (2): e756–e766. 10.1210/clinem/dgab643.
167 Hedbäck, N., Dichman, M.L., Hindsø, M. et al. (2024). Effect of ghrelin on glucose tolerance, gut hormones, appetite, and food intake after sleeve gastrectomy. *Am J Physiol Endocrinol Metab* 327 (3): E396–E410. https://doi.org/10.1152/ajpendo.00177.2024.

168 Ge, X., Yang, H., Bednarek, M.A. et al. (2018). LEAP2 is an endogenous antagonist of the ghrelin receptor. *Cell Metab.* 27 (2): 461–469.e6. https://doi.org/10.1016/j.cmet.2017.10.016.

169 Hagemann, C.A., Jensen, M.S., Holm, S. et al. (2022). LEAP2 reduces postprandial glucose excursions and ad libitum food intake in healthy men. *Cell Rep Med* 3 (4): 100582. https://doi.org/10.1016/j.xcrm.2022.100582.

2

Agonists and Antagonists of the Human GIP Receptor

Hüsün S. Kizilkaya[1,2], Lærke S. Gasbjerg[1,2], Jens J. Holst[2,3], and Mette M. Rosenkilde[1]

[1] University of Copenhagen, Faculty of Health and Medical Sciences, Department of Biomedical Sciences, Molecular and Translational Pharmacology, Blegdamsvej 3B, 2200 Copenhagen, Denmark
[2] University of Copenhagen, Faculty of Health and Medical Sciences, Department of Biomedical Sciences, Endocrinology and Metabolism, Blegdamsvej 3B, 2200 Copenhagen, Denmark
[3] University of Copenhagen, Novo Nordisk Foundation Center for Basic Metabolic Research, Faculty of Health and Medical Sciences, Blegdamsvej 3B, 2200 Copenhagen, Denmark

Introduction

Metabolic diseases such as type 2 diabetes and obesity are probably best treated with a multimodal approach. Today, treatments usually includes recommendations regarding appropriate dieting and exercise habits combined with one or more pharmaceutical compounds [1]. In severe cases, patients with treatment-resistant obesity and related complications can also be treated with bariatric surgery [2]. One of the more recently introduced drug targets for the treatment of metabolic diseases is the glucose-dependent insulinotropic polypeptide (GIP) receptor (GIPR), and even though treatments with several different GIPR-targeting compounds may lead to reduced weight and improved glycemic control, it is still not fully understood what happens when the GIPR is stimulated (agonism) or blocked (antagonism). As we will present in this chapter, investigations of both modalities have led to similar clinical results, leaving the question why both GIPR agonism and antagonism are beneficial for these patient groups unanswered.

The physiological actions of endogenous GIP are mainly displayed in the postprandial state and include potentiation of glucose-induced insulin secretion from the pancreas [3, 4], stimulation of intestinal blood flow [5], and inhibition of postprandial bone resorption [6–8]. In addition, administration of exogenous GIP in humans causes an increase in heart rate [9, 10], increases the blood flow and triglyceride deposition in the subcutaneous adipose tissue [11, 12], and may enhance glucagon secretion [13, 14]. A therapeutic potential for either GIPR agonists or antagonists was revealed in animal models, and in rodents and nonhuman primates, both modalities result in resistance toward diet-induced weight gain and modest reduction in body weight [15–20].

This chapter was primarily written in 2024 and has been lightly updated prior to publication in 2026.

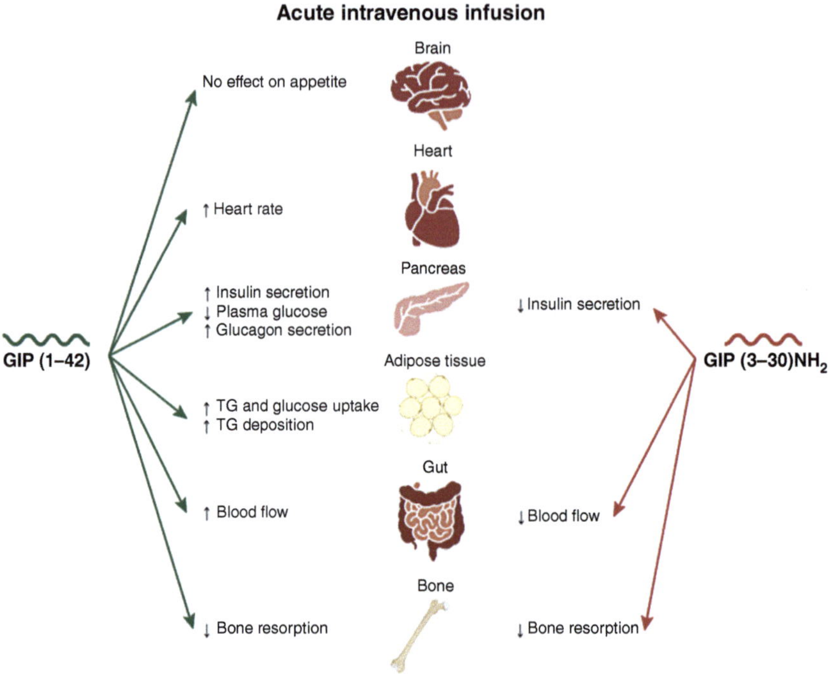

Figure 2.1 Physiological effects following acute intravenous infusion with GIPR agonist GIP(1–42) and GIPR antagonist GIP(3–30)NH_2 on organ systems in humans. GIP, glucose-dependent insulinotropic polypeptide; GIPR, glucose-dependent insulinotropic polypeptide receptor.

An increasing number of unimolecular compounds targeting GIPR, often combined with GLP-1R agonism, are emerging. The most established is tirzepatide, a coagonist of the GIPR and GLP-1R, which has demonstrated impressive improvement in glucose control in patients with type 2 diabetes and reduction in body weight in patients with obesity [21–26]. However, similar results are seen following treatment with a GIPR antagonist combined with a GLP-1R agonist [27, 28], an example of which is in late clinical development. Understanding the extent to which GIPR targeting contributes to the therapeutic benefits of these multi-targeting compounds has been difficult. Given there are no approved agonistic or antagonistic agents available, most of our knowledge about physiological and pathophysiological conditions of the human GIP system stems from clinical studies involving short-term infusions of native GIPR agonist, GIP(1–42), and/or the antagonist GIP(3–30)NH_2 (Figure 2.1) as well as studies of the phenotypic traits of persons carrying *GIPR* genetic variants.

Objective of the Chapter

Despite the increasing recognition of the GIPR as a promising therapeutic target, uncertainty remains regarding how both agonism and antagonism of the GIP system in some settings can produce similar clinical outcomes. This chapter will provide an overview of GIP and GIPR biology, from ligand binding and cellular signaling to physiological effects. It will draw insights from genetic studies and examine the current landscape of available GIPR agonists and antagonists.

Background

Glucose-Dependent Insulinotropic Polypeptide – Rationale for Initial Therapeutic Interest

GIP was discovered in 1970 from impurities of porcine cholecystokinin as a peptide involved in inhibiting stomach acid secretion in dogs, which is why it was first named "gastric inhibitory polypeptide" [29, 30]. Shortly after its isolation, it was revealed that GIP possessed the ability to stimulate insulin secretion in humans [31], whereas the inhibitory effect of gastric secretion turned out to be of uncertain physiological relevance in humans [32]. This prompted renaming the hormone to "glucose-dependent insulinotropic polypeptide" while retaining its acronym GIP. Over a decade later, in 1986, another insulinotropic hormone was discovered as a fragment of the glucagon precursor, proglucagon. Because of sequence similarity with glucagon, it was named glucagon-like peptide-1 (GLP-1) [33]. Based on infusions of the hormones and specific antagonists of the hormone receptors, GIP and GLP-1 were established as the most important incretin hormones accounting for two-thirds of postprandial insulin secretion in healthy individuals [3, 4].

Even though GIP was the first incretin hormone to be discovered, research into GLP-1 biology quickly surpassed that of GIP, and the interest in GIP as a therapeutic target in treating type 2 diabetes and obesity was limited for many years. This was mainly due to early studies demonstrating impaired insulinotropic action of GIP in individuals with type 2 diabetes, even at high (pharmacological) doses [34]. In contrast GLP-1 maintains its insulinotropic properties in patients with type 2 diabetes at higher hormone doses [35]. Compared to GLP-1, another disadvantage of GIP is its ability to stimulate glucagon secretion, feared to exacerbate hyperglycemia in type 2 diabetes in a therapeutic setting [36, 37]. Combined with the resistance toward diet-induced weight gain of mice with global knockout[1] of the GIPR [38] and clinical studies showing GIP-induced triglyceride deposition in adipose tissue [11] GIP was considered an obesogenic hormone [38]. Thus, the interest in GIPR agonism as a therapeutic option was dampened, and antagonism of the receptor was instead proposed as a potential treatment strategy for obesity [38]. Now more than 50 years after its discovery, both agonism and antagonism of the GIPR in combination with GLP-1R agonism have proven to be effective in the management of obesity and related metabolic diseases. In the following sections, we will explore how this development occurred.

---

1 This term refers to the genetic modification where the gene of interest is deleted from all cells of the body.

GIP – Posttranslational Processing, Secretion, and Degradation

Mature GIP is a 42-amino acid polypeptide (GIP(1–42)). It derives from the proteolytic processing of the precursor prohormone, proGIP, which consists of 153 amino acids encoding a signal peptide, an N-terminal peptide, GIP, and a C-terminal peptide (Figure 2.2) [39]. The cleavage of proGIP to GIP(1–42) is catalyzed by prohormone convertase (PC) 1/3 [40]. The functional roles, if any, of the N- or C-terminal regions encoded by proGIP are yet to be elucidated. The precursor prohormone, proGIP, can also be cleaved by another convertase, PC2, yielding GIP(1–30)NH_2 that has similar agonistic properties to full-length GIP(1–42) [41, 42]. In transiently transfected COS-7 cells, expressing the human GIPR, stimulation with GIP(1–30)NH_2 displays the same maximal response (efficacy) and a potency (EC_{50})[2] of 11.2 pmol/l compared to GIP(1–42), which has an EC_{50} of 6 pmol/l. Binding experiments with radioactively labeled GIP (^{125}I-GIP(1–42)) reveal a similar binding affinity[3] of GIP(1–30)NH_2 and GIP(1–42) to the GIPR with K_i[4] of 0.89 and 0.67 nmol/l, respectively [43]. When infused in healthy individuals, GIP(1–30)NH_2 displays similar effects on insulin secretion and bone metabolism as GIP(1–42) [44]. However, GIP(1–30)NH_2 circulates in very low concentrations both during fasting and following food ingestion and is therefore expected to have less physiological impact compared to GIP(1–42) that reaches 5–10-fold higher postprandial levels [45].

GIP is synthesized by enteroendocrine K-cells [46], mainly found in the duodenum and proximal part of the jejunum of the gastrointestinal tract [47, 48]. It is released in response to oral intake of carbohydrates and fats [49] and, to a lesser extent, proteins [50, 51] and possibly bile [52, 53]. GIP is secreted shortly after

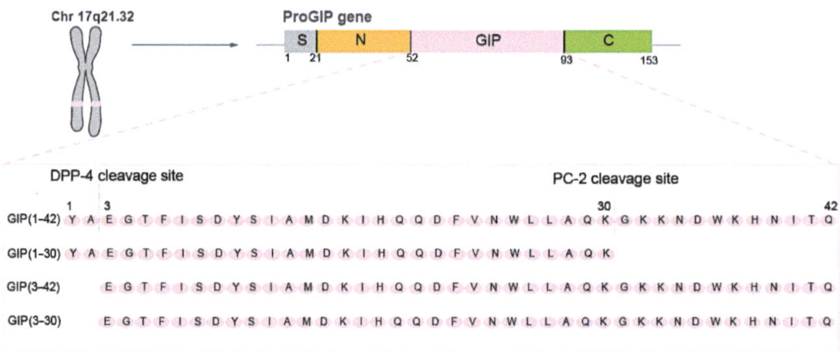
Chr 17q21.32
ProGIP gene
S
N
GIP
C
1
21
52
93
153
DPP-4 cleavage site
PC-2 cleavage site
1
3
30
42
GIP(1–42) Y A E G T F I S D Y S I A M D K I H Q Q D F V N W L L A Q K G K K N D W K H N I T Q
GIP(1–30) Y A E G T F I S D Y S I A M D K I H Q Q D F V N W L L A Q K
GIP(3–42) E G T F I S D Y S I A M D K I H Q Q D F V N W L L A Q K G K K N D W K H N I T Q
GIP(3–30) E G T F I S D Y S I A M D K I H Q Q D F V N W L L A Q K G K K N D W K H N I T Q

Figure 2.2 ProGIP and sequence of processed GIP. ProGIP is located on the human chromosome (Chr) 17 on the long arm (q) at position 21.32. ProGIP comprises 153 amino acids with a signal peptide (S) and an N- and C-terminal part. GIP, glucose-dependent insulinotropic polypeptide.

---

2 Potency refers to the half maximal effective concentration (EC_{50}) that is required to produce 50% of the maximum possible effect.

3 The molecular strength with which a ligand interacts with the receptor.

4 Inhibitory constant (K_i) is the concentration of nonlabeled GIP that is needed to displace 50% of the radioactively labeled GIP from its receptor.

nutrient intake and reaches peak levels after 30–45 minutes [54]. The half-life of GIP in humans ranges from five to seven minutes due to the cleavage of the first two amino acids by the ubiquitous enzyme, dipeptidylpeptidase-4 (DPP-4) [55]. The cleavage by DPP-4 terminates the agonistic activity of GIP(1–42), and the metabolite GIP(3–42) has been established as a very weak GIP receptor antagonist at pharmacological doses; antagonistic effect are not observed at physiological concentrations [56]. GIP(3–42) constitutes a significant part of the circulating GIP in plasma [57], alongside a much lower quantity of GIP(3–30)NH_2 (DPP-4 cleavage product of GIP(1–30)NH_2). GIP(3–30)NH_2, however, is a potent antagonist of the GIPR and shows a 26-fold higher potency for GIPR inhibition compared to GIP(3–42) [43, 56, 58, 59]. The two inactive metabolites of GIP have been reported to have a plasma half-life of 17–20 minutes [57] with a primary route of clearance through the kidneys [60].

Glucose-Dependent Insulinotropic Polypeptide Receptor (GIPR)

Receptor Activation and Signaling

The GIPR belongs to the largest class of membrane-expressed proteins, the G protein-coupled receptors (GPCRs), which have more than 800 members in the human genome [61] (Figure 2.3(a)). GPCRs can be divided into five major classes in vertebrates: Class A (rhodopsin) consists of 719 members, class B1 (secretin) of 15 members, class B2 (adhesion) of 33 members, class C (glutamate) of 22 members, and class F (frizzled) of 11 members [62] (Figure 2.3(b)). The GIPR belongs to class B1 [63]. Like all GPCRs, the GIPR has seven transmembrane domains (TM1–7) consisting of α-helices that span the cell membrane connected by three extracellular and three intracellular loops, an extracellular N-terminal and an intracellular C-terminal domain [64]. In class B1, the N-terminal part is larger, relative to most class A GPCR, and forms the well-structured extracellular N-terminal domain, which protrudes from the cell membrane and facilitates the initial receptor-ligand interaction [65].

In recent years, advancements in cryogenic electron microscopy (cryo-EM) have given further insight into specific residues that are involved in the activation mechanism of the GIPR [66, 67]. Like the other class B1 receptors, the activation of the GIPR follows the overall so-called *two-step binding and activation model* (Figure 2.3(c)). This model was originally proposed for the human parathyroid hormone 1 receptor [68] and is now refined with further atomic and molecular resolution provided by cryo-EM structures for all 15 class B1 receptors as of August 2024 [69].

In contrast to a high degree of promiscuity among the most closely related class B1 receptors, the GLP-1, GLP-2, and the glucagon receptor [70–72], GIP does not bind to other class B1 GPCRs besides the GIPR [67]. During initial receptor engagement, GIP adopts a single α-helical conformation in its middle part (from

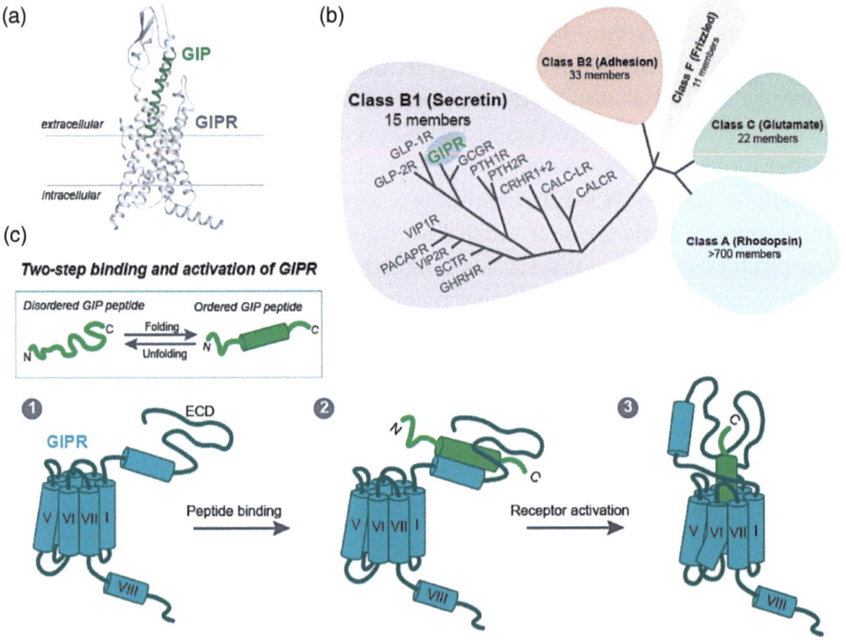

Figure 2.3 Overview of GIPR structure, family, and activation. (a) Structure of GIPR bound to GIP (Protein Data Bank accession number: 7DTY). (b) The five major classes of GPCRs, consisting of class A (rhodopsin) with over >700 members, class B1 (secretin) with 15 members including the GIPR, class B2 (adhesion) with 33 members, class C (glutamate) with 22 members, and class F (frizzled) with 11 members. (c) The binding and activation of the GIPR follows the general *two-step binding model* of class B1 GPCRs. GIP is in equilibrium between disordered and ordered state. Binding of GIP to the GIPR is initiated when ECD of the receptor tethers to the C-terminal part of GIP, in which the N-terminal part of GIP is then docked into the TMD. This results in activation of the receptor. CALCR, calcitonin receptor; CALCRL, calcitonin receptor-like receptor; CRHR1, corticotropin-releasing hormone receptor 1; CRHR2, corticotropin-releasing hormone receptor 2; ECD, extracellular domain; GCGR, glucagon receptor; GIPR, glucose-dependent insulinotropic polypeptide receptor; GLP1R, glucagon-like peptide 1; GLP2R, glucagon-like peptide 2; GPCR, G protein-coupled receptor; PACAPR, pituitary adenylate cyclase-activating polypeptide type I receptor; PTH1R, parathyroid hormone 1 receptor; PTH2R, parathyroid hormone 2 receptor; SCTR, secretin receptor; TMD, transmembrane domain; VIPR1, vasoactive intestinal peptide receptor 1; VIPR2, vasoactive intestinal peptide receptor 2.

amino acid 5 to 30) [66], which interacts with the extracellular domain (ECD) and extracellular loop 1 (ECL1) of the receptor. In the α-helix, the C-terminal part (residues 16–30) has the strongest engagement with the extracellular receptor regions, whereas the N-terminal half (residues 5–15) docks deeper into the TM domain core of the receptor, forming the main ligand-binding crevice. This results in the outward movement of TM6 at the intracellular side accompanied by a slight movement of the intracellular tip of TM5 toward TM6, which creates an intracellular cavity for G protein coupling [67].

The GIPR mainly couples to $G\alpha_s$ to exert its further downstream effects by activating adenylyl cyclase, which leads to a rise in intracellular levels of the second

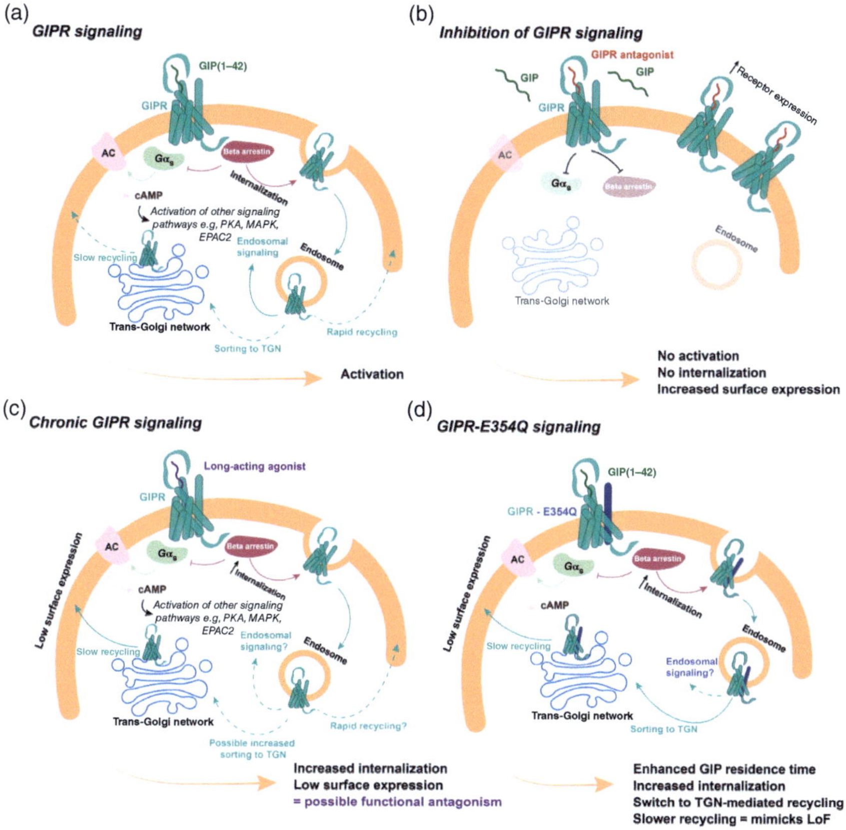

Figure 2.4 Overview of glucose-dependent insulinotropic polypeptide (GIP) receptor (GIPR) signaling and possible post-activation properties in response to (a) GIP agonist, (b) antagonist, (c) long-acting GIPR agonist, and (d) *GIPR* variant E354Q. AC, adenylyl cyclase; cAMP, cyclic adenosine monophosphate; EPAC2, exchange protein directly activated by cAMP 2; MAPK, mitogen-activated protein kinase; PKA, protein kinase A; TGN, trans-golgi network.

messenger cyclic adenosine monophosphate (cAMP) (Figure 2.4(a)). The increase in cAMP levels activates protein kinase A (PKA), which subsequently phosphorylates a series of proteins, thereby initiating multiple signaling cascades [73, 74]. cAMP can also activate *exchange protein directly activated by cAMP 2* (EPAC2), which is directly involved in insulin secretion in the pancreatic beta cell [73]. Another signaling pathway downstream of cAMP and PKA is the mitogen-activated protein kinase (MAPK), which can phosphorylate and activate extracellular-signal-regulated kinase 1 and 2 (ERK1/2). ERK1/2 is involved in regulating gene expression related to cellular responses like proliferation and apoptosis [75–77]. Minor coupling to $G\alpha_q$ by the GIPR has also been reported in few studies [78, 79]; however, the literature is ambiguous, and more studies are required to establish productive interaction with other G proteins by the GIPR.

An important aspect of GIPR signaling is the receptor expression levels at the cell surface. Investigations of naturally occurring genetic variants of the human *GIPR* gene as well as gene dose titration of wild-type GIPR in cell studies have revealed a linear correlation between receptor surface expression and cAMP production [80]. Intriguingly, compared to the GLP-1R, the increase in receptor activation for increasing receptor expression levels is higher for the GIPR [81].

Per definition, a receptor antagonist is a molecule that blocks the action of an agonist [64, 82], as illustrated in Figure 2.4(b). Since the N-terminus of GIP is necessary for GIPR activation, N-terminal truncations of GIP result in loss of agonistic properties. While GIP(3–42) is a low-affinity antagonist of the GIPR, the product of a similar N-terminal truncation of GIP(1–30)NH_2, GIP(3–30)NH_2, displays considerably higher affinity [43]. GIP(3–30)NH_2 was the first GIPR antagonist to be administered to humans [83, 84]. The results of the human studies will be described in detail later. Several truncated variants of GIP have been characterized over the years with respect to GIPR binding, activation, and biological effects. These studies revealed the importance of the N-terminus for receptor activation and the middle part for high-affinity binding, whereas the role of the C-terminus is less clear (Table 2.1).

Desensitization, Internalization, and Receptor Trafficking

An important aspect of GPCR activation is the desensitization of the receptor following agonist-mediated activation. The desensitization is thought to turn off the signaling. This ensures balanced cellular responses and protects against "overstimulation" of the system [100]. Desensitization may be followed by receptor resensitization through recycling back to the cell surface. Conventionally, β-arrestins are considered essential proteins for GPCR desensitization and internalization, *arresting the signaling*, hence the name of the protein family – arrestins [101, 102]. Once a receptor is internalized, it can - in some cases - continue signaling from endosomes by forming stable receptor-arrestin-G protein complexes, enabling sustained cAMP production, before being recycled to the cell surface (resensitization) or trafficked further intracellularly. This can involve being sorted to trans-Golgi network for slower recycling to the cell surface or getting degraded by lysosomes. Besides their role in GPCR desensitization and internalization, β-arrestins can also modulate receptor signaling as scaffolding proteins by interacting with a wide range of signaling pathways and facilitating intracellular signaling from different compartments, e.g., endosomes. For some GPCRs, receptor trafficking can occur independently of arrestins by direct interactions with other cellular players [103]. This is, for instance, the case for the GLP-1R and the GLP-2R, where arrestins are not needed for internalization after agonist binding (which is nevertheless pronounced) [71, 104, 105], whereas the GIPR, as evident from the next section, is dependent on arrestins for internalization [80, 105, 106].

Upon GIP-mediated activation of the GIPR, the conformational changes in the receptor promote phosphorylation of specific residues by G protein-coupled receptor kinases (GRKs), which results in recruitment of β-arrestins to the GIPR [107, 108]. The phosphorylation of specific residues by GRKs acts as a barcode for

Table 2.1 Overview of the various existing truncated and modified ligands of the GIPR.

Ligand	Origin of species			Binding	Activation (cAMP production)	Biological effect
	Ligand	Radioligand	Receptor			
GIP(1–3) [85]	Bovine	Porcine ^{125}I-GIP	Hamster	–		
GIP(1–6)NH_2 [86]	Unknown	Porcine ^{125}I-GIP	Rat	–	–	
GIP(1–7)NH_2 [86]	Unknown	Porcine ^{125}I-GIP	Rat	–	–	
GIP(1–13)NH_2 [86]	Porcine	Porcine ^{125}I-GIP	Rat	+	+	
GIP(1–14)NH_2 [86]	Porcine	Porcine ^{125}I-GIP	Rat	+	+++	Rat: induces 26% insulin release at 5 nM and reduces glucose levels
GIP(1–14) [86]	Hamster	Porcine ^{125}I-GIP	Rat	++	++++	
GIP(1–15)NH_2 [86]	Porcine	Porcine ^{125}I-GIP	Rat	+	+	
GIP(1–15) [86]	Porcine	Porcine ^{125}I-GIP	Rat	–	–	
GIP(1–16) [87]	Unknown		Rat			Obese mice: no effect on glucose regulation
GIP(1–30)NH_2 [43, 44]	Human	Human ^{125}I-GIP	Human	++++	++++	Humans: similar effects on glucose and bone metabolism in healthy humans as GIP(1–42)
GIP(1–30)OH [88]	Human	Porcine ^{125}I-GIP	Porcine	+		Rat pancreas perfusion: full insulin secretion
GIP(1–38) [89]						Rat pancreas perfusion: full insulin secretion
GIP(1–39) [90]						Rat pancreas perfusion: full insulin secretion
GIP(2–30) NH_2 [43]	Human	Human ^{125}I-GIP	Human	+	+	
GIP(3–30)NH_2 [5, 6, 12, 43, 91–94]	Human	Human ^{125}I-GIP	Human	++++	–	Humans: GIP(3–30)NH_2 reduces GIP-induced: (1) insulin secretion, (2) adipose tissue blood flow and triglyceride and glucose uptake in adipose tissue during hyperglycemia/insulinemia, (3) bone resorption, (4) glucagon secretion, (5) postprandial splanchnic blood flow, and (6) gallbladder relaxation
GIP(6–30)NH_2 [95]	Porcine	Porcine ^{125}I-GIP	Rat	++++	++	

(Continued)

Table 2.1 (Continued)

Ligand	Origin of species			Binding	Activation (cAMP production)	Biological effect
	Ligand	Radioligand	Receptor			
GIP(7–30)NH_2 [86, 96]	Porcine	Porcine ^{125}I-GIP	Rat	+	–	Anaesthetized rat: reduced insulin secretion
GIP(10–30) [95]	Porcine	Porcine ^{125}I-GIP	Rat	+	++	
GIP(15–30)NH_2 [86, 97]	Porcine	Porcine ^{125}I-GIP	Rat	+	–	Rat pancreas perfusion: no insulin release
GIP(16–30)NH_2 [86]	Porcine	Porcine ^{125}I-GIP	Rat	+	–	
GIP(17–30)NH_2 [86, 97, 98]	Porcine	Porcine ^{125}I-GIP	Rat	+	–	BRIN-BD11 cells: 1 μM inhibits insulin secretion Rat pancreas perfusion: 38% maintained insulin release at 1 ng/ml
GIP(18–28) [88]	Human	Porcine ^{125}I-GIP	Porcine	–		
GIP(19–30)NH_2 [86, 97]	Porcine	Porcine ^{125}I-GIP	Rat	++	++	Rat pancreas perfusion: 60% insulin secretion at 1 ng/ml and significant glucose decrease
GIP(21–30)NH_2 [96]	Porcine		Rat	–	–	
GIP(21–26) [88]	Human	Porcine ^{125}I-GIP	Porcine	–		
GIP(3–42) [56]	Porcine		Rat	+	–	Rat pancreas perfusion: inhibition of insulin release
GIP(4–42) [58]	Unknown		Rat		++	Obese mice: glucose increase at 25 nmol/kg
GIP(5–42) [58]	Unknown		Rat		++	Obese mice: increased plasma glucose levels at 25 nmol/kg
GIP(6–42) [58]	Unknown		Rat		+++	

GIP(7–42) [58]	Unknown		Rat		++	Obese mice: increased plasma glucose levels at 25 nmol/kg
GIP(8–42) [58]	Unknown		Rat		+	Obese mice: increase in plasma glucose levels and significantly decrease in insulin levels at 25 nmol/kg
GIP(9–42) [58]	Unknown		Rat		+++	BRIN-BD11 cells: 100% maintained insulin secretion
GIP(13–42) [99]	Human		Human	+		
GIP(15–42) [58, 86]				+	–	Rat pancreas perfusion: 40% maintained insulin response at 10 ng/ml
GIP(17–42) [85]	Bovine	Porcine ^{125}I-GIP	Hamster	+		Rat pancreas perfusion: 32% maintained insulin response at 5 ng/ml
GIP(19–42) [99]	Human		Human	+		
GIP(21–42) [99]	Human		Human	+		
GIP(23–42) [99]	Human		Human	–		
GIP(31–44) [96]	Porcine		Rat	–	–	

+: <30% binding or activation, ++: 30–60% binding or activation, +++: 60–90%, ++++: 90–100% binding or activation. –: no binding or activation.

β-arrestins and their distinct downstream actions [109, 110]. While – as mentioned - not all receptors depend on β-arrestin recruitment for internalization [103], the GIPR strongly depends on this [80, 105–107]. However, even in the absence of an agonist, the GIPR still exhibits high basal internalization, independent of β-arrestin recruitment, with rapid recycling back to the cell membrane [105, 107]. Compared to the GLP-1R and GLP-2R, the GIPR has a lower overall β-arrestin recruitment and degree of internalization [104, 108]. Yet its strong dependency on β-arrestin for ligand-mediated internalization is not shared by the other two receptors [71, 105]. This underscores the importance of β-arrestins for the regulation of GIPR signaling. Additionally, the GIPR has been reported to have faster recycling to the plasma membrane compared to the GLP-1R [81, 104]. Importantly, both receptors are able to continue their $G\alpha_s$-mediated signaling intracellularly from the endosomes [80, 111, 112].

Maintained activation is thought to result in interruption of GIPR trafficking, in turn desensitizing the GIP system (Figure 2.4(c)). An example of this is highlighted by the prevalent missense[5] variant of the *GIPR (rs1800437)* that leads to amino acid substitution of glutamic acid to glutamine at position 354 (E354Q) in TM6 (Figure 2.4(d)). Multiple in vitro studies have been carried out in different cell types through the last 30 years, all showing maintained, and some even slightly enhanced GIP-mediated receptor activation through $G\alpha_s$, β-arrestin recruitment and GIP binding to the mutated receptor relative to the wild-type background receptor [113–119]. However, when looking at the binding kinetics, the GIP ligand displays an enhanced residence time (defined as the reciprocal value of the off rate [K_{off}]), on the E354Q variant [117]. The variant is also associated with a faster receptor internalization [117], which may be related to altered ligand-receptor interaction dynamics and the prolonged residence time of GIP on the mutated receptor [120]. Furthermore, it recycles more slowly to the cell surface due to prolonged intracellular retention in the trans-golgi network compared to WT GIPR [107, 113, 121]. Combined, these effects are believed to result in impaired receptor function, mimicking a loss-of-function (LoF) genetic variant. An important lesson learned from the investigation of the molecular properties of 47 *GIPR* variants, identified in four Danish diabetes study cohorts, is the crucial role of β-arrestin recruitment for sustained intracellular GIPR signaling [80]. By investigating $G\alpha_s$ protein recruitment to endosomes in *GIPR* variants with varying degrees of cAMP production and β-arrestin recruitment, it was discovered that only variants with retained β-arrestin recruitment maintained internalization and intracellular signaling from the endosomes, even in variants with diminished overall cAMP production [80]; this establishes β-arrestin as a crucial regulator of GIPR signaling and its postactivation properties. Substantiating this, mice with genetic ablation of β-arrestin (both global knockout and specific knockout of β-arrestin in pancreatic beta cells), demonstrated higher blood glucose levels in response to GIP administration, while the blood-glucose-lowering effect of GLP-1 remained intact [80, 122].

5 Missense mutations result in an amino acid change in the protein sequence due to single nucleotide changes.

Expression in Humans and Animals

The GIPR has been found in several different tissues in both human and animal tissue with varying confidence [123]. According to the *Tissue Expression Database* [124, 125], GIPR is only reported to be present with high confidence in human pancreas tissue. GIPR messenger ribonucleic acid (RNA) expression has also been demonstrated on primary human osteoclasts and osteoblast-like cell-lines, implying the occurrence of GIPR on bone tissue [126]. Additionally, GIPR is expressed, with less confidence, in other tissues e.g., adipocytes, adrenal gland, brain, stomach, colon, liver, lung, heart, vasculature, and kidney.

In mice, GIPR is expressed with high confidence in several areas of the brain [127–129], while in tissues, e.g., pancreatic beta and alpha cells, adipocytes, intestine, and blood cells, GIPR expression is observed with moderate confidence.

Important Species Differences in the GIP System

Studies involving the use of GIPR antagonists have revealed that GIP and its receptor are less conserved across species compared to the more conserved GLP-1-system [130]. There is 81% sequence alignment between the human and rodent (rat and mouse) GIPR, whereas the alignment with the human GLP-1R is up to 91% for the rat GLP-1R and 93% for the mouse GLP-1R [130]. Although there are only two amino acid differences between the human GIP peptide sequence and the rat and mouse GIP sequences (Figure 2.5(a)), these are apparently sufficient to cause

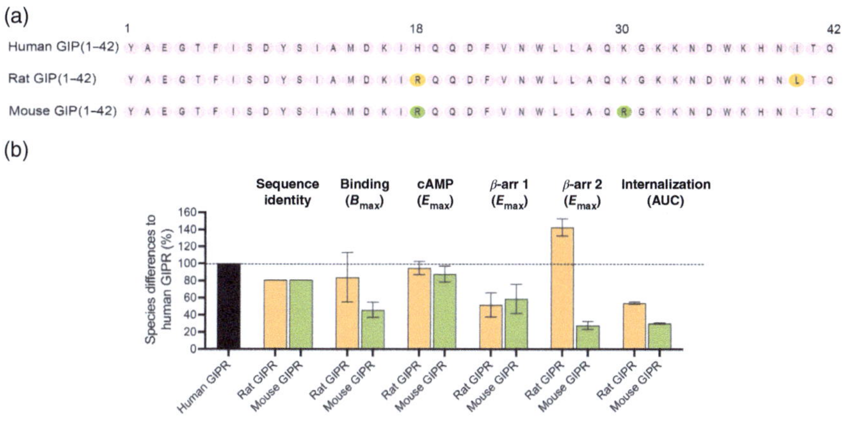

Figure 2.5 Differences between human, rat, and mouse GIP and GIPR. (a) Sequence difference between human, rat, and mouse GIP(1–42). (b) Percentage difference between human, rat, and mouse GIPR in (from the left) sequence identity, maximal binding capacity (B_{max}), maximal cAMP production (E_{max}), maximal β-arrestin 1 and 2 recruitment, and internalization (AUC). AUC, area under the curve; cAMP, cyclic adenosine monophosphate; GIP, glucose-dependent insulinotropic polypeptide; GIPR, glucose-dependent insulinotropic polypeptide receptor; SEM, standard error of the mean. Data represent mean ± SEM. Adapted from [130, 131].

species-specific functional alterations. A notable example is GIP(3–30)NH_2, which, based on the human GIP sequence, has threefold lower potency on the rat GIPR than GIP(3–30)NH_2 based on rat GIP [106, 132]. Thus, inhibition of the human GIPR is more effectively achieved with human GIP(3–30)NH_2 than with rat or mouse GIP(3–30)NH_2, and vice versa [132].

Another N-terminally modified version of GIP, with an amino acid substitution from glutamate to proline at position three, Pro3-GIP, used as a GIPR antagonist in rodent studies, also shows species-dependent pharmacological differences. Thus, human Pro3-GIP acts as a partial agonist on the human GIPR with maximal activation (E_{max}) reaching 90% of human GIP(1–42), while rat and mouse Pro3-GIP displayed E_{max} of 64 and 59%, respectively. A corresponding impaired potency was also observed across the species, with 4.7 nM for human, 13 nM for rat, and 29 nM for mouse Pro3-GIP, respectively [130].

Besides the ligand differences, molecular differences exist among the species in their GIPR postactivation properties regarding receptor desensitization and internalization (Figure 2.5(b)). Compared to the human GIPR, which strongly depends on β-arrestin 2 recruitment for receptor internalization upon GIP stimulation, the mouse GIPR barely recruits any β-arrestin 2 or undergoes internalization [131]. This has made it challenging to evaluate the pharmacodynamics of compounds targeting the GIPR across species.

Physiological Actions of GIP

The GIP hormone has several actions across different organs and tissues. Evaluating the current evidence, it is important to emphasize the distinction between the physiological and pharmacological effects of GIP. Pharmacological regimes usually involve the administration of supraphysiological concentrations of a compound with a long half-life, while the physiological role of a hormone can be explored through short-term administration of exogenous hormone at doses and timing that reflect natural levels or by using a selective antagonist to block the effects of the endogenous hormone. This section will focus on GIP's physiological role by examining studies involving short-term administration of exogenous GIP(1–42) and/or using GIPR antagonists.

GIP's Effect on the Pancreas of Healthy Individuals

One of the main physiological functions of GIP, if not the most important, is its potentiation of insulin secretion from the pancreatic beta cells in response to nutrient intake [3, 4]. In healthy individuals, the combined insulinotropic action of GIP and GLP-1 accounts for up to 70% of postprandial insulin release [133, 134], constituting the so-called *incretin effect*. This effect can be demonstrated by the two- to threefold increase in insulin secretion in response to oral glucose intake compared to intravenous isoglycemic glucose administration [135, 136]. The size of the incretin effect depends on the amount of glucose ingested, with clinical studies demonstrating the highest incretin-induced insulin secretion during the highest glucose consumption, illustrating the potentiating effect of GIP and GLP-1 on glucose-induced insulin secretion [3, 137–139]. There is no effect of the hormones without glucose co-stimulation. Glucose stimulation of beta cells increases the intracellular adenosine triphosphate/adenosine diphosphate ratio, resulting in the closure of K^+ channels, leading to depolarization[6] of the cell membrane and the opening of voltage-gated Ca^{2+} channels. The influx of Ca^{2+} triggers the fusion of insulin-containing vesicles with the plasma membrane for subsequent release of insulin [73, 140, 141]. This glucose dependency is a crucial aspect of the minimal risk of hypoglycemia during treatment with incretin-based therapies, and GIP administration during fasting plasma glucose levels only stimulates insulin secretion minimally, which results in a very small plasma glucose reduction [13, 142].

Investigation of the relative contribution of GIP versus GLP-1 revealed GIP to be the main incretin hormone in studies using the GIP-based GIPR antagonist, GIP(3–30)NH_2, and the GLP-1R antagonist, exendin(9–39)NH_2, where the GIPR antagonist reduced postprandial insulin secretion more than the GLP-1R antagonist in healthy participants [4, 94, 143].

During hypoglycemic conditions, GIP enhances glucagon secretion from pancreatic alpha cells [13, 14]. In some instances, supraphysiological doses of GIP have been shown to induce glucagon secretion during elevated glucose levels in patients with type 2 diabetes [144] in contrast to GLP-1 that suppresses glucagon secretion [145].

In animal models, a similar incretin effect to that in humans has been described in many species like mice [146, 147], rats [148], and pigs [149], while the evidence is less convincing in dogs [150]. Additionally, GIP is found to induce somatostatin release in rat pancreata and dogs [151, 152]. Somatostatin is a gut hormone that inhibits the release of pancreatic hormones, and this effect is independent of plasma glucose levels. The interplay between GIP and somatostatin is yet to be elucidated in humans but may be less pronounced than seen for GLP-1 [153].

GIP'S EFFECT ON THE PANCREAS OF HEALTHY INDIVIDUALS

AGONISM: Potent insulin secretion (eu-/hyperglycemia), minor glucagon secretion (eu-/hypoglycemia), overall glucose-lowering effect

ANTAGONISM: Reduced GIP-induced insulin and glucagon secretion

GIP's Effect on the Pancreas of Individuals with Type 2 Diabetes

Individuals with type 2 diabetes are characterized by partially or completely lost incretin effect, which includes a reduced insulinotropic activity toward GIP infusion [154]. Although acute infusion of GIP may initially cause a modest rise in insulin secretion during the early phase of glucose administration, this effect is lost in the late phase [137]. GLP-1, on the other hand, displays reduced beta cell sensitivity.

---

6 The process where the electrical charge inside cells becomes less negative compared to outside for initiation of action potentials.

However, supraphysiological concentrations of GLP-1 infusion can restore insulin secretion to levels observed in healthy individuals in response to glucose alone [155], making an agonist of the GLP-1R a possible therapeutic treatment option for individuals with type 2 diabetes. The differential insulinotropic response of GIP and GLP-1 in type 2 diabetes remains unexplained, but it has been suggested that low GIPR expression on pancreatic beta cells due to hyperglycemia may be a contributing factor [156]. The insulinotropic actions of GIP (and GLP-1) have also been demonstrated to improve in individuals with type 2 diabetes following insulin treatment, aiming at near-normalization of plasma glucose levels [157, 158], partly supporting the theory of glucotoxic effects on the beta cells being the mechanism behind the impaired actions of incretin hormones. However, the significant improvement in insulin secretion was far from full normalization, which challenges the notion that hyperglycemia and the consequent reduced GIP and GLP-1 receptor activity on pancreatic cells are the sole reason for the impaired insulinotropic activity observed in individuals with type 2 diabetes [159, 160]. A general reduction of the pancreatic beta cell activity due to insulin resistance, inflammation, and oxidative stress has also been proposed as an explanation for the impaired incretin effect in individuals with type 2 diabetes [161].

Interestingly, infusion of the GIPR antagonist in individuals with type 2 diabetes did reduce the postprandial insulin secretion to the same extent as in healthy individuals, but the changes in insulin did not result in blood glucose levels different from a saline infusion [162].

Whereas insulin secretion is impaired, GIP maintains its glucagonotropic action upon acute infusion in individuals with type 2 diabetes, even during simultaneous treatment with GLP-1. This has consequently resulted in elevated plasma glucose levels [36, 37, 163], and raised the question of whether long-acting GIPR agonists would have the same negative effect on glycemic control. However, this does not seem to be the case with the currently available dual GLP-1R and GIPR-targeting compound, tirzepatide [22], or long-acting GIPR agonist in preliminary clinical studies [164].

GIP'S EFFECT ON THE PANCREAS OF PATIENTS WITH TYPE 2 DIABETES

AGONISM: Weak insulin secretion (eu-/hyperglycemia), glucagon secretion (eu-/hypoglycemia), overall, very weak glucose-lowering effect

ANTAGONISM: Reduced GIP-induced insulin and glucagon secretion

GIP's Effect on the Pancreas of Individuals with Obesity

In obese individuals, GIP secretion has been shown to be increased both at fasting levels and after a meal intake [165]. Despite the higher plasma levels of GIP, a similar impairment in insulin sensitivity is also observed in obese individuals [166, 167], indicating a reduced, albeit not severely impaired, GIP sensitivity. Infusion of a GIPR antagonist in persons with obesity did, however, result in similar postprandial glucometabolic responses as persons with lower body mass index (BMI) included in the same study [54].

<u>**GIP'S EFFECT ON THE PANCREAS OF INDIVIDUALS WITH OBESITY**</u>
AGONISM: insulin secretion (eu-/hyperglycemia), glucagon secretion (eu-/hypoglycemia), overall, weak glucose-lowering effect
ANTAGONISM: reduced GIP-induced insulin and glucagon secretion

Extrapancreatic Physiological Effects of GIP

Adipose Tissue

Already in 1988, GIP was introduced as an "obesity hormone", acting as a lipogenic hormone to promote lipid deposition in adipose tissue [168]. This hypothesis received further support from studies of *Gipr* knockout mice which are resistant to diet-induced obesity [38]. Similarly, deletion of the *proGIP* gene (resulting in reduced GIP production) also resulted in resistance toward diet-induced obesity in mice [169], further reinforcing the hypothesis of GIP being an obesogenic hormone.

GIP's role in adipose tissue is still elusive. In healthy lean individuals, administration of GIP has been shown to increase blood flow to subcutaneous adipose tissue and enhance triglyceride clearance and glucose uptake during hyperinsulinemic and hyperglycemic clamps designed to mimic postprandial conditions [12]. The augmentation of blood flow and changes in triglyceride uptake induced by GIP were impaired in individuals with obesity [170], but could partly be restored by weight loss [171], implying a loss of sensitivity toward GIP in obese individuals.

The GIP-mediated augmentation of postprandial adipose tissue blood flow could explain a potential mechanism behind GIP's lipogenic action in humans because it is thought that the uptake of fat in the adipose tissue is dependent on the local blood flow. The lipogenic actions of GIP were supported in human ex vivo cultured adipocytes and 3T3-L1 cells (adipocytes of mouse origin) by the activation of lipoprotein lipase (LPL), which is an enzyme important for lipid metabolism by hydrolyzing triglycerides and facilitating the uptake of circulating free fatty acids [172, 173]. Thus, a common hypothesis for the obesity-protective role in *Gipr* knockout mice was attributed to the loss of GIPR activity in white adipose tissue, which led to limited lipogenesis. However, most of these studies on cultured cell lines utilized supraphysiological insulin levels in combination with high GIP doses, as GIP stimulation alone did not induce lipogenesis [38, 172, 173]. Noticeably, in adipocyte cell lines of both human and mouse origin, GIP has lipolytic activity in the absence of insulin through activation of hormone-sensitive lipase (HSL) [106, 174]. In contrast to LPL, HSL breaks down stored triglycerides into free fatty acids and glycerol. This suggests that GIP cooperates with insulin to regulate the adipose tissue by augmenting glucose and lipid clearance in the postprandial state while increasing lipolysis in the fasted state.

<u>**GIP'S EFFECTS IN ADIPOSE TISSUE**</u>
AGONISM: augment blood flow to adipose tissue and enhance triglyceride clearance and glucose uptake (hyperglycemia/insulinemia), GIP-induced postprandial lipogenesis and lipolysis in the fasting state
ANTAGONISM: resistance toward diet-induced obesity

Body Weight

Investigating genetic variants of the human *GIPR* has contributed to our understanding of the metabolic benefits and disadvantages of altered GIPR signaling and the impact on adiposity-related traits in humans. Early genome-wide association studies (GWAS) have identified the gene of *GIPR* as being associated with BMI [175]. The noncoding intron variant, rs2287019, a commonly occurring variant with an allele frequency of 18% worldwide (gnomAD v4.0 [176]), was found to be associated with increased BMI and fasting glucose levels [175]. Another prevalent coding variant of the *GIPR* (rs1800437) with an allele frequency of 19% among the world population (gnomAD, v4.0 [176]) and in linkage disequilibrium[7] with rs2287019 has been associated with lower BMI and C-peptide levels [115, 177–180]. Through GWAS, also more rare variants that are pharmacologically classified as *LoF* variants with low cAMP recruitment, low β-arrestin recruitment and low surface expression were associated with lower adiposity-related traits, including BMI [181–183]. Based on phenotypic data of 47 *GIPR* variant carriers, the β-arrestin recruitment to the GIPR was found to be crucial for the metabolic phenotype of *GIPR* variant carriers [80]. When both the cAMP accumulation ($G\alpha_s$ recruitment) and β-arrestin recruitment to GIPR are considered, only carriers of *GIPR* variants with loss of both $G\alpha_s$ signaling and β-arrestin recruitment (LoF_{cAMP}/LoF_{arr}) were associated with lower BMI and improvements of other adiposity-related traits (Figure 2.6(a)). In contrast, when the *GIPR* variants resulted in lost $G\alpha_s$ signaling but retained β-arrestin recruitment (LoF_{cAMP}/WT-like$_{arr}$), the individuals did not display any phenotypic changes compared to the wild-type GIPR (Figure 2.6(b)). Interestingly, a third group of *GIPR* variants displayed gain-of-function (GoF) in

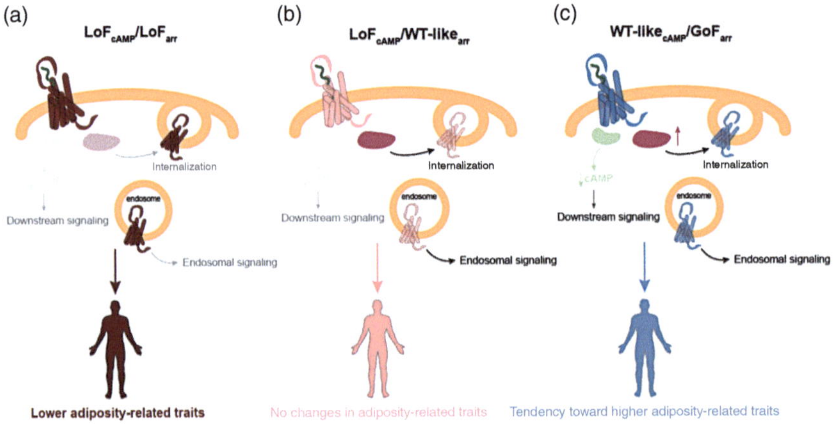

Figure 2.6 Human *GIPR* genetic variant groups with altered molecular activation and phenotypic consequences in adiposity-related traits. (a) Loss-of-function (LoF) *GIPR* variants in both cAMP and β-arrestin recruitment display diminished internalization and endosomal signaling, resulting in lower adiposity-related traits in the carriers. (b) Variants with wild-type-like (WT-like) cAMP but LoF in β-arrestin recruitment exhibited maintained internalization and endosomal signaling, while the carriers of these variants had no changes in their adiposity-related traits. (c) Carriers of WT-like cAMP and gain-of-function (GoF) *GIPR* variant had a tendency toward higher adiposity-related traits. GIPR, glucose-dependent insulinotropic polypeptide receptor; cAMP, cyclic adenosine monophosphate.

7 Nonrandom association of inheriting one single nucleotide variant with another.

β-arrestin recruitment with wild-type-like cAMP production (WT-like$_{cAMP}$/GoF$_{arr}$), and carriers of these variants tended to impact adiposity-related measures in the opposite direction of the LoF group with increased BMI, body fat percentage, and waist and hip circumference (Figure 2.6(c)). Supporting this hypothesis, meta-regression analyses of single-variant phenotype association estimates against variant-specific signaling parameters demonstrated that β-arrestin recruitment was associated with metabolic traits, including BMI and hip circumference, whereas cAMP signaling showed no such association. Conversely, cardiovascular traits, particularly systolic and diastolic blood pressure, were associated with cAMP signaling but not with β-arrestin recruitment.

Paradoxically, treatment with a long-acting GIPR agonist was also reported to cause modest weight reduction in individuals with obesity [184]. The ligand-receptor interaction properties and the molecular details are not yet disclosed, and the mechanism of action is also still unclarified.

GIP'S EFFECTS ON BODY WEIGHT REGULATION
AGONISM: reduced body weight
ANTAGONISM: overall reduced adiposity-related traits

Energy Expenditure

A repeated observation behind the weight loss in murine studies with genetic loss of *Gipr* is increased energy expenditure of the mice, potentially due to increased thermogenesis or locomotive activity rather than a direct effect of GIP on adipose tissue [20]. The GIPR is also found to be expressed in murine brown adipose tissue [185]. Mice with targeted knockout of *Gipr* in brown adipose tissue displayed increased body temperature during an acute cold challenge, implying a role for GIP in mouse thermogenesis via brown adipose tissue. However, in short-duration clinical infusion studies, neither GIPR agonists nor antagonists have affected resting energy expenditure [92, 167].

Taken together, based on clinical, animal, and in vitro studies, it is still challenging to create a cohesive explanation for GIP's role in body weight regulation and energy expenditure, and more studies are needed to understand it better.

GIP'S EFFECTS ON ENERGY EXPENDITURE
AGONISM: no effect on energy expenditure
ANTAGONISM: increased energy expenditure, potentially through regulation of thermogenesis in brown adipose tissue

Cardiovascular System

In humans, GIP is involved in regulating blood flow to the splanchnic region [186, 187] and adipose tissue [12]. Correspondingly, GIP infusion results in an increase in heart rate by 5–12 beats per minute while lowering the arterial blood pressure [9, 10]. However, it is uncertain whether these changes result from altered splanchnic blood flow or direct effects on the heart or blood vessels. Genetic variants of the *GIPR* have also been associated with cardiovascular traits. A genetic association study found a nominal association between heterozygous carriers of E354Q and the risk of cardiovascular disease [188]. The carriers of the LoF missense variants, R190Q and E288G, had significantly increased systolic blood pressure [183]. However, in the larger study, no alterations were found in systolic- and/or diastolic blood pressure in the carriers of LoF_{cAMP}/LoF_{arr} [80]. In the same study, additional 105 *GIPR* variants, detected in UK Biobank, were predicted to be LoF variants based on computational analysis, and the carriers of these variants were associated with significantly lower diastolic blood pressure [80]. As mentioned above, the large study, phenotyping 47 human *GIPR* variants, found a correlation between the ability to induce coupling to Gs and the blood pressure with increasing cAMP signaling correlating to increased diastolic and systolic blood pressure. Interestingly, a recent genetic study including individuals from UK Biobank and FinGen consortium assessed the cardiovascular effects of GIP signaling using variants in *GIP* and *GIPR* with reduced signaling as indicators of lower body weight and HbA1C (glycated hemoglobin) levels. Attenuated GIP signaling was linked to reduced risk of coronary artery disease and heart failure, suggesting that GIP may influence cardiovascular risk both indirectly via adiposity and potentially through direct effects on the cardiovascular system [189].

There are many animal studies with conflicting effects of GIP on the cardiovascular system. In one animal study, whole-body loss of *Gipr* and selective loss on cardiomyocytes have shown a cardioprotective effect [189]. However, another study in *Gipr* knockout mice demonstrated elevated aortic inflammation and atherosclerosis [190]. Overall, GIP's cardiovascular effects are complex with both increased and decreased GIPR signaling producing beneficial and adverse effects depending on the genetic and experimental model.

GIP'S EFFECTS IN THE CARDIOVASCULAR SYSTEM

AGONISM: augmentation of blood flow to the splanchnic region and subcutaneous adipose tissue, increased heart rate, and lower blood pressure

ANTAGONISM: alterations in blood pressure and heart rate, favorable cardiometabolic profile

Bones

Remodeling of the bone tissue is a continuous process that varies throughout the day, with a reduction in bone resorption during the daytime compared to nighttime due to the differential activity in the gut-bone axis [191].

While rodents are suitable for studying the skeletal system, the translation to humans should be done carefully due to species differences in bone remodeling [192]. In an earlier study, administration of GIP diminished the loss of bone density in ovariectomized rats as a model for postmenopausal osteoporosis [193]. Similarly, clinical studies indicate an anabolic role of GIP on bone tissue as indicated by a decrease in circulating levels of the bone resorption marker, carboxy-terminal type 1 collagen crosslinks (CTX) [6–8, 194] and short-lasting increases in bone formation marker procollagen type 1 amino-terminal propeptide (P1NP) in both healthy individuals and individuals with type 1 diabetes [8, 93]. Interestingly, the effects of endogenous GIP on the bones are maintained in individuals with type 2 diabetes that exhibit similar decrease, as healthy individuals, in CTX levels postprandially [162]. Supporting the direct role of GIP in human bone tissue, the presence of

GIPR has been demonstrated on primary human osteoclasts and osteoblast-like cell lines [126]. GIP was found to decrease osteoclast activity and differentiation while enhancing osteoblast survival [195], indicating a positive impact of GIP on the skeletal system. The long-term effect of GIPR-targeting compounds' role on bone tissue is not known. Investigating LoF *GIPR* variants as models for the prolonged impact of GIP on bone metabolism, the missense variants R190Q, E288G, and E354Q have all been associated with slightly lower bone mineral density [183, 196]. Additionally, in a clinical study of 1686 perimenopausal women followed over the course of 10 years, carriers of the "LoF mimicking" E354Q variant were associated with lower bone mineral density, and those who were homozygous for the variant had a higher risk of nonvertebral fractures [196]. However, a large meta-analysis of 1.2 million participants found no significant association with lower bone mineral or increased fracture risk in carriers of the *GIPR* variants R190Q, E288G, and E354Q [179].

GIP'S EFFECTS IN BONES
AGONISM: reduced bone resorption and increased bone formation
ANTAGONISM: lower bone mineral density and possible higher fracture risk

Central Nervous System

Although many experiments have been conducted to address the potential effects of GIP in the central nervous system, the effect of GIP in the human brain is yet to be determined. Involvement in appetite regulation and memory functions has been suggested, but no clear therapeutic mechanisms or physiological roles have been confirmed. In humans, no reduction in food intake and appetite has been observed during exogenous GIP infusions [197], and the antagonism of the GIPR has not led to any changes in food intake or appetite sensations [83, 84]. Intriguingly, when GIP was administered with GLP-1 on one occasion, it counteracted the appetite suppression induced by GLP-1 [163], implying an appetite-stimulating effect of GIP in humans. Otherwise, only pharmacological targeting of the GIPR (as presented in the following sections) has implied involvement in appetite regulation. The other incretin hormone, GLP-1, has well-described anorexigenic actions [198] both in animal models and humans, and since the coadministration of GLP-1 and GIP in animal models improved the anorexigenic actions of GLP-1, the *Gipr* location and implications have been investigated [199]. Recent years' technical advancements have confirmed the expression of the *Gipr* in the hypothalamus and hindbrain of mice [200, 201], which are regions involved in energy regulation. Studies using single-cell RNA sequencing have shown that most *Gipr*-expressing cells in the brain are mural cells, specifically pericytes, which are specialized vascular support cells implied in regulating blood flow to the brain [128, 200, 202]. Additionally, *Gipr* expression is high in the area postrema [127, 203], which, along with the nucleus tractus solitarius (NTS) and the vagus nerve's dorsal motor nucleus, forms the hindbrain's dorsal vagal complex. Although *Gipr* is reported to be expressed in the NTS, primarily in non-neuronal cells, its presence is much less abundant than in the area postrema [200]. Area postrema is important in detecting toxins and triggering the vomiting reflex. It has been shown that *Gipr* in the area postrema is present in the inhibitory gamma-aminobutyric acid (GABA) neurons [129, 200, 204], implying that GIP has a suppressive activity in this mouse brain region. Furthermore, a neuroprotective role has been proposed for GIP, as subcutaneous administration was associated with improvements in cognitive function and hippocampal synaptic plasticity in animal models [205].

GIP'S EFFECTS IN THE CENTRAL NERVOUS SYSTEM
AGONISM: reduced food intake, reduced GLP-1-induced emesis, and possible neuroprotective role
ANTAGONISM: no changes in food intake and appetite sensation

Pharmacological GIPR Agonism

Animal Studies

While earlier animal studies using GIPR agonism in the treatment of preexisting obesity seemed to be ineffective, studies starting from 2010 have shown greater efficacy with respect to lowering body weight and reducing food intake in mice [15, 17, 206]. This shift is believed to be due to the development and use of high-affinity GIPR agonists with a slower elimination rate providing better exposure than compounds used in the older studies.

In a study from 2010, a long-acting GIP analog, D-Ala2-GIP, which is resistant toward DPP-4 degradation, was administered subchronically/daily into lean and obese mice. This resulted in a decrease in body weight and LPL activity in both the lean and obese mice [207]. Similarly, another potent long-acting fatty acid acylated GIP (acyl-GIP) analog resulted in moderate weight reduction combined with decreased food intake in obese mice receiving daily administration of the GIP agonist [15, 208]. Noticeably, this decrease in body weight induced by acyl-GIP was not observed in *Gipr* knockout mice [15], supporting the weight-lowering properties of GIPR agonists with molecular pharmacological properties similar to native GIP(1–42) in terms of binding and cAMP production. Other studies using long-acting GIPR agonists, which had further molecular modifications, have been reported to either produce no changes or lead to moderate weight loss in obese mice [17, 209]. Hence, chronic administration of different GIPR agonists either appear to be weight neutral or slightly weight decreasing in preclinical models, depending on the level of GIPR agonism, which is influenced by the compound's potency, efficacy, and prolonged half-life. One of the hypotheses for the weight-reducing properties is believed to be due to the involvement of GIPR activation in appetite regulation in the brain of mice (see section titled "Central Nervous System"). GIP has been shown to increase neuronal activity in the area postrema of the hindbrain [127, 203, 210], in which *Gipr* is predominantly expressed in inhibitory GABAergic neurons [129, 200, 204]. The weight-reducing effects of chronic treatment with acyl-GIP were not observed in mice deficient in *Gipr* expression in GABAergic neurons [211], supporting a role for GIPR in the regulation of body weight and food intake. Similarly, the enhanced weight-lowering effect of MAR709, a potent dual GIPR and GLP-1R agonist developed by Novo Nordisk, could not be recapitulated in mice with *Gipr* deletion in GABAergic neurons [211]. Direct administration of acyl-GIP into the brain of mice has resulted in decreased weight and food intake [95]. The mechanism by which GIP regulates appetite through the inhibitory GABA system and area postrema is not yet fully understood, but it has been suggested that GIP may, via these pathways, transmit satiety signals from the area postrema to brain regions such as the amygdala and hypothalamus, which regulate food intake [202]. Recent reports show that GIPR agonism engages neural circuits that are molecularly and functionally distinct from those recruited by GIPR antagonism, helping to explain why both approaches can reduce food intake and body weight in vivo (particularly with GLP-1R coactivation) [212, 213]. These data reinforce that the anorectic actions of GIPR agonists reflect active engagement of specific hindbrain inhibitory pathways rather than peripheral metabolic effects.

The same neuronal axis was suggested to be implicated in alleviating nausea and emesis caused by GLP-1R-targeting compounds through the activation of GIPR in the area postrema's inhibitory circuit; this was studied in preclinical models e.g., shrews that unlike mice and rats are capable of vomiting [210, 212, 213].

PHARMACOLOGICAL EFFECTS OF GIPR AGONISTS IN ANIMALS
Weight neutral or slightly weight-decreasing
CNS involvement
Beneficial in combination with GLP-1

Human Studies

No long-acting GIPR agonist is available for therapeutic use in humans. However, similar therapeutic effects to those observed during acute activation of the GIPR with native GIP in clinical studies could be expected with long-term activation of the GIP system. As mentioned earlier, these effects include potentiation of insulin secretion in a glucose-dependent manner, increased blood flow to adipose tissue and the splanchnic region, enhanced lipid deposition and postprandial decrease in bone resorption [3–8, 11, 12].

While Novo Nordisk and Eli Lilly have developed long-acting GIPR agonists and evaluated them in early preclinical and clinical trials, publicly available information on their current developmental status is limited (Table 2.2). NNC0480-0389, a long-acting once-weekly GIPR agonist developed by Novo Nordisk, was according to their financial report terminated in May 2023 due to insufficient additional effect on glycemia and weight loss in participants with type 2 diabetes when administered together with the GLP-1R agonist, semaglutide [236, 237]. LY3537021, a long-acting GIPR agonist developed by Eli Lilly, demonstrated modest weight reduction in both healthy participants and individuals with type 2 diabetes compared to those receiving placebo [184, 216]. Additionally, the compound has also been shown to improve insulin sensitivity alone, and more than an additive augmentation of insulin

Table 2.2 Overview of GIPR-targeting compounds and their developmental stages.

Compound name	Target	Company	Administration	Indication	Stage of development
NNC0480-0389 [214, 215]	GIP-RA	Novo Nordisk	Once-weekly SC injection with semaglutide	T2D (dose-finding with semaglutide); exploratory weight endpoints	Phase 2 completed (dose-finding combo with semaglutide)
LY3537021 [184, 216–218]	GIP-RA	Eli Lilly	Once-weekly SC injection	Obesity, T2D, antiemetic	Phase 2
ZP6590 [219]	GIP-RA	Zealand Pharma	NA	Obesity, antiemetic	Preclinical (FIH planned)
AT-7687 [18]	GIPR antagonist	Antag Therapeutics	Once-weekly SC injection	Obesity ± combination with GLP-1-RA	Phase 1
Tirzepatide [21, 220, 221]	GIP-RA/GLP-1RA	Eli Lilly	Once-weekly SC injection	T2D, obesity, HFpEF, OSA, CV outcome in T2D, MASH, CKD	Approved (FDA/EMA) for T2D and obesity Approved (FDA) for OSA Ongoing: HFpEF, CKD, CV outcome in T2D
MariTide [28, 222, 223]	Antagonistic monoclonal antibody of GIPR conjugated to two peptide-based GLP1-RA	Amgen	Once-monthly SC injection	Obesity ± T2D, ASCVD, heart failure, OSA, CKD	Phase 3
CT-388 [224]	GIP-RA/GLP1-RA	Carmot Therapeutics	Once-daily SC injection	Obesity, T2D	Phase 2 Phase 3 (planned 2026)

CT-868 [225]	GIP-RA/GLP1-RA	Carmot Therapeutics	Once-weekly SC injection	Obesity, T1D	Phase 2 completed
VK2735 [226, 227]	GIP-RA/GLP1-RA	Viking Therapeutics	Both oral and once-weekly SC injections are under development	Obesity (±T2D), MASH	Phase 3 (SC) Phase 2 (oral)
SCO-094 [228, 229]	GIP-RA/GLP1-RA	Scohia Pharma	SC, oral formulation under investigation	Obesity (±T2D), MASH	Phase 1
Retatrutide [230–233]	GIP-RA/GLP1-RA/GCG-RA	Eli Lilly	Once-weekly SC injection	Obesity, T2D, osteoarthritis, CVD, CKD	Phase 3 (obesity/T2D) Phase 2 (select comorbidities)
HM15211 [234, 235]	GIP-RA/GLP1-RA/GCG-RA	Hanmi Pharmaceuticals	NA	MASH	Phase 2

ASCVD, atherosclerotic cardiovascular disease; CKD, chronic kidney disease; CV, cardiovascular; CVD, cardiovascular diseases; FDA, Food and Drug Administration; GIP-RA, glucose-dependent insulinotropic polypeptide receptor agonist; GLP-1RA, glucagon-like peptide 1 receptor agonist; GCG-RA, glucagon receptor agonist; HFpEF, heart failure with preserved ejection fraction; FIH, first in human; OSA, obstructive sleep apnea; T1D, type 1 diabetes; T2D, type 2 diabetes; MASH, metabolic dysfunction-associated steatohepatitis; NA, not available; SC, subcutaneous.

sensitivity is observed in combination with the GLP-1-based dulaglutide [164]. Interestingly, LY3537021 was also suggested to have greater tolerability without causing nausea and vomiting, than seen with treatment with GLP-1R agonists alone [216, 217, 238]. This might suggest similar antiemetic properties in humans as in preclinical models, but more studies are needed to understand GIP's effects in the human brain, if any. Consistent with this hypothesis, Eli Lilly is currently conducting a phase 2 trial to assess the antiemetic effects of LY3537021 in adults with cancer receiving chemotherapy, with an expected completion date in September 2026 [218].

Currently, the most efficacious therapeutic effect of GIPR agonism is achieved when combined with GLP-1R agonism, demonstrated by tirzepatides' apparently superior effects on glycemic control and weight loss [239, 240], although the importance of the difference in dosing should be noted, for instance 1–2 mg for semaglutide versus 10–15 mg for tirzepatide. Tirzepatide, which has now received approval from the US Food and Drug Administration and the European Medicines Agency in the treatment of type 2 diabetes and obesity, has demonstrated >20% weight reduction in obese individuals in the latest clinical study [241]. Functional studies have revealed that tirzepatide is an imbalanced agonist, meaning it does not activate the two receptors equally, although the importance of this is unclear. It has similar pharmacological properties to native GIP on the GIPR in terms of binding, cAMP production, β-arrestin recruitment, and internalization [81]. However, it has lower affinity and potency on the GLP-1R and a preference for $G\alpha_s$ protein signaling over β-arrestin recruitment, which makes it a biased agonist of the GLP-1R. As a result of this bias, the GLP-1R displays reduced internalization and increased receptor cell surface expression, while the GIPR has maintained internalization [81]. While the clinical results of tirzepatide speak for themselves, the extent to which the GIPR-activating component of the dual agonist contributes to these effects remains unclear. In clinical studies with type 2 diabetes patients, combinations of exogenous GIP and GLP-1 infusion have shown a similar insulinotropic effect as GLP-1 infusion alone [198–200]. Hence, the superiority of tirzepatide cannot immediately be attributed to the dual activation of both incretin systems. Although, a possible explanation could be that GIP enhances insulin sensitivity, as demonstrated by the long-acting GIPR agonist [164]; however, further studies are needed to confirm this effect. It should also be noted that most recent clinical data (Phase 3b STEP UP obesity trial) on ~7.2 mg once-weekly semaglutide demonstrated up to ~20.7% body weight loss matching the effects of tirzepatide [242].

Nonetheless, the clinical success of tirzepatide and its biased nature has spurred the development of more multi-targeting compounds, including G protein-biased agonists of both receptors (Figure 2.7). One such compound, CT-388 developed by Carmot Therapeutics, which displays minimal β-arrestin recruitment to both the GIPR and GLP-1R, was recently tested in a phase 1 clinical study and demonstrated up to 8.5% weight-lowering effect and enhanced glycemic control after four weeks in obese individuals [243]. The same company also has another G protein-biased compound, CT-868, in a phase 2 clinical trial for the treatment of obesity in participants with type 1 diabetes (clinical trial gov: NCT06062069).

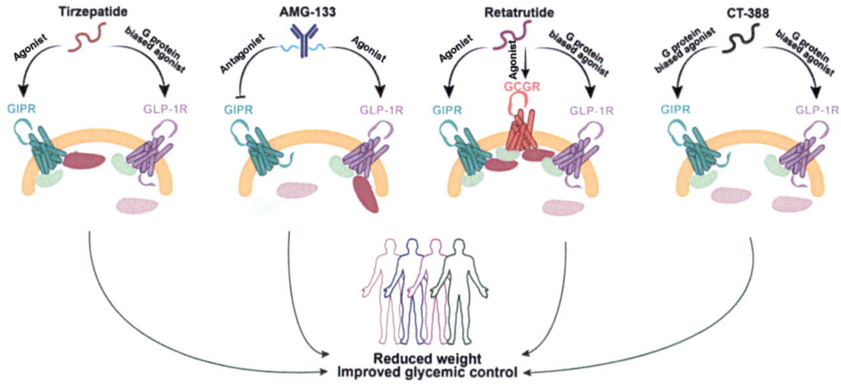

Figure 2.7 The distinct modes of action of dual and triple agonists of GIPR-targeting compounds and the clinical outcome. Tirzepatide is an imbalanced unimolecular peptide-based coagonist of the GIPR and the GLP-1R with a G protein-bias on the latter receptor with little arrestin recruitment. AMG-133 is an antagonistic GIPR antibody conjugated to two GLP-1 analogs. Retatrutide is a peptide-based unimolecular triple agonist of the GIPR, GLP-1R, and GCGR with similar pharmacology as tirzepatide on the GIPR and the GLP-1R, while also being an unbiased agonist on the GCGR. CT-388 is a peptide-based unimolecular $G\alpha_s$ biased agonist of both the GIPR and the GLP-1R with very little arrestin recruitment. All four compounds demonstrate varied degrees of weight reduction and improved glycemic control in clinical studies with type 2 diabetes patients and obese individuals. GIPR, glucose-dependent insulinotropic polypeptide receptor; GLP-1R, glucagon-like peptide-1; GCGR, glucagon receptor.

In addition to the combined targeting of the incretin receptors, triple agonism, including the glucagon receptor, has metabolic benefits perhaps surpassing those of dual agonism [230, 234, 244, 245]. A prominent example of this is retatrutide, a clinically promising unimolecular triple agonist developed by Eli Lilly. Retatrutide shares similarly unbalanced pharmacology with tirzepatide on the GIPR and GLP-1R while being less potent and unbiased agonist of the glucagon receptor [244]. In patients with type 2 diabetes, retatrutide improves HbA1c levels after 36 weeks of treatment and reduces body weight by close to 17% [230]. In a phase 2 study including individuals with obesity, up to 24% weight loss was achieved at the end of a 48-week treatment with retatrutide [245], exceeding the weight loss observed with any incretin-based therapy to date.

Currently, there are also unimolecular compounds targeting up to four and five receptors under development, exemplified by the tetra-agonist of the GLP-1R, GIPR, amylin, and calcitonin receptors, PTT-A, which has shown promising effects in preclinical studies in reducing body weight and glycemic control [246].

PHARMACOLOGICAL EFFECTS OF GIPR AGONISTS IN HUMANS
Slight weight reduction
Possible antiemetic effect
Reduced GLP-1-induced gastrointestinal side effects
Improved insulin sensitivity

Pharmacological GIPR Antagonism

Currently, GIPR antagonism refers to the inhibition of GIP-induced signaling. Since GIPR mainly couples to $G\alpha_s$, antagonism of the GIPR most often refers to blocking the cAMP response. However, for the GIPR, the balance between receptor signaling, desensitization, and intracellular signaling and recycling is central for interpreting the physiological consequences of GIP. Hence, the basic pharmacological term for an antagonist might be insufficient for compound characterization.

Animal Studies

Early efforts to antagonize the GIPR involved modifying the N-terminus of GIP at position three, resulting in the creation of Pro3-GIP by substituting glutamate with proline. This modification was developed to protect GIP from DPP-4 degradation and thereby prolong its plasma half-life, but the amino acid substitution was also reported to result in antagonistic properties at the GIPR [247, 248]. Intraperitoneal administration of Pro3-GIP into obese diabetic mice resulted in decreased insulin levels [248]. Likewise, chronic intraperitoneal administration of Pro3-GIP produced weight loss in obese mice on a high-fat diet [249] and protected against the development of age-related diabetes [250]. However, as mentioned previously, subsequent molecular pharmacological characterization of Pro3-GIP revealed that it is a partial agonist of the human GIPR with maximal activation reaching 90%, although it is 180-fold less potent compared to GIP(1–42) [130]. Thus, the physiological consequences of Pro3-GIP should not be attributed solely to GIPR antagonism.

As mentioned earlier, another peptide-based GIPR antagonist that is naturally occurring is GIP(3–30), which has been shown to retain its antagonistic properties in a species-specific manner in rodents and humans [106, 251]. Extensive functional characterization of this peptide in vitro has revealed that it suppresses cAMP accumulation and arrestin recruitment to the GIPR in a competitive manner. GIP(3–30)NH_2 also reduces receptor internalization, thereby increasing GIPR cell surface expression [106]. In pancreas perfusion studies with rats, GIP(3–30)NH_2 successfully blocked GIP-mediated insulin, glucagon, and somastostatin secretion [132]. A modified version of GIP(3–30)NH_2, AT364, that was designed for the mouse GIPR with higher binding affinity and has a half-life of seven hours, inhibited GIP-induced glucagon and insulin secretion with a reduction in body weight and fat mass during subchronic treatment in female ovariectomized mice on high-fat diet [252].

The antagonistic properties of GIP(3–30)NH_2 resulted in the development of an optimized long-acting peptide analog, AT-7687. Administration into nonhuman primates has shown prevention against diet-induced weight gain, and the combination of the antagonist with liraglutide (long-acting GLP-1R agonist) led to improved weight reduction compared to mono-treatment with liraglutide [18]. The nonhuman primates also displayed lower lipid profiles [18].

Around the same time as the first studies of GIP(3–30)NH_2, two other modified GIP(3–30) analogs were evaluated as long-acting GIPR antagonists,

GIP(3–30)Cex-K^{40}[Pal] and Pro^3GIP(3–30)Cex-K^{40}[Pal]. Both peptides were shown to reduce body weight, circulating glucose and insulin concentration in obese mice following once-daily injection for 21 days [19].

In addition to peptide-based antagonists of the GIPR, antagonistic antibodies have been developed to evaluate the metabolic benefits of GIPR inhibition. Antibodies designed to antagonize the mouse GIPR resulted in a modest reduction in body weight with slightly reduced food intake in obese mice models [16, 253]. A monoclonal GIPR antibody generated for the human GIPR was similarly effective in antagonizing GIPR in nonhuman obese primates, and did – combined with GLP-1 agonism – result in profound weight loss and substantial reduction in food intake in obese primates [16]. Like the peptide-based antagonist, the antagonistic antibody combined with GLP-1R agonism produced a synergistic effect, resulting in a greater weight loss observed with GLP-1R agonism alone in studies with both mice and nonhuman primates [16]. Consistent with these observations, recent reports demonstrate that GIPR antagonism potentiates GLP-1R-mediated weight loss via complementary neural networks (distinct from those activated by GIPR agonism) [212, 213], providing a mechanistic rationale for the synergy seen with peptide and antibody antagonists in animal studies.

PHARMACOLOGICAL EFFECTS OF GIPR ANTAGONISTS IN ANIMALS
Inhibition of insulin, glucagon, and somatostatin secretion
Reduced body weight and food intake
Lower blood lipid levels
Synergistic effect on body weight reduction when combined with GLP-1R agonism

Human Studies

GIP(3–30)NH_2 is the only peptide-based antagonist of the GIPR administered intravenously in clinical studies. Infusion of GIP(3–30)NH_2 in clinical studies has demonstrated reduced GIP-induced insulin secretion and higher postprandial plasma glucose levels, reduced adipose tissue blood flow and triglyceride and glucose uptake in adipose tissue, reduced attenuation of bone resorption marker, CTX, reduced glucagon secretion, and reduced splanchnic blood flow [6, 12, 54, 94, 142, 187].

However, to date, no long-term studies exceeding five hours have been performed with GIP(3–30)NH_2; hence, it has mostly been used as a tool compound to gain a better understanding of the endogenous GIP in human physiology (see Table 2.1). Our knowledge of chronic mono-treatment with GIPR antagonist in humans is limited and the most effective outcome of GIPR antagonism seems to be achieved when combined with GLP-1R agonism as with GIPR agonism. Recently, an antagonistic GIPR antibody conjugated to two GLP-1 peptide analogs, AMG-133 (maridebart cafraglutide [MariTide]), developed by Amgen [27, 254], completed phase 2 clinical study. This randomized trial showed that once-monthly injection of this compound led to weight loss of up to 16% at 52 weeks in adults with obesity, with or without type 2 diabetes, compared with placebo. Weight loss efficacy was similar whether or not dose escalation was used. However, escalation improved gastrointestinal tolerability and reduced discontinuations [28]. A phase 3 study is already initiated and currently enrolling, with additional planned and ongoing studies designed to evaluate the effects of AMG-133 in related conditions [222].

PHARMACOLOGICAL EFFECTS OF GIPR ANTAGONISTS IN HUMANS
Reduced body weight and improved glycemic control together with GLP-1R agonism

Theories Bridging GIPR Agonism and Antagonism

How is it biologically possible that both agonism and antagonism of the GIPR result in weight loss as described earlier? While a unifying answer to this question is still under debate, several theories have been proposed to explain the paradoxical effect of GIP agonism and antagonism.

One explanation could be that the pharmacological characterizations in vitro, evaluating $G\alpha_s$ signaling and cAMP accumulation, are insufficient to predict the mode of action for GIPR-targeting treatments. An increasing number of studies emphasize the importance of β-arrestin recruitment and possibly GRK phosphorylation in regulating GIPR signaling, particularly in receptor internalization, recycling, and sustained signaling from intracellular compartments such as the endosomes [105–107, 111, 121]. Hence, balanced β-arrestin recruitment to the GIPR may also be an important factor to consider under drug development, as highlighted by the genetic association study that points to the level of β-arrestin recruitment as the main driver of the adiposity-related traits in *GIPR* variant carriers [80]. Additionally, under hyperglycemic conditions, it has been demonstrated that pancreatic beta cells remain chronically depolarized, causing the GLP-1R to switch from $G\alpha_s$ to $G\alpha_q$-mediated signaling pathway to stimulate insulin secretion [255]. While this has not been observed for GIPR, it suggests a potential for the GIPR to engage with alternative effector molecules under pathophysiological conditions that could be part of explaining the effects of GIP agonism and antagonism.

Another hypothesis is that long-lasting activation of the GIPR will result in chronic desensitization and hence mimic GIPR antagonism, similar to the phenotype observed in the *GIPR* variant, E354Q. As mentioned, this genetic variant has a faster internalization [117] and slower recycling rate (longer residence time in the trans-golgi network) to the plasma membrane following GIP-induced activation compared to the wild-type GIPR [107, 113, 121], which ultimately leads to lower GIPR presence on the cell surface for further activation. In line, carriers of E354Q are also associated with lower adiposity-related traits, reinforcing the proposition that enhanced activation of the GIP-system results in inactivation of GIPR signaling. To further support this hypothesis, in vitro studies have demonstrated that prolonged activation of the GIPR results in receptor desensitization [17, 131]. Treatment with a long-acting GIPR agonist resulted in receptor desensitization in differentiated preadipocytes of human or mouse origin, measured as lower levels of cAMP production following subsequent exposure to the agonist [17]. Similar to the E354Q variant, chronic activation of the GIPR also resulted in increased internalization followed by reduced receptor availability on the cell surface in the adipocytes [17]. Given the distinct trafficking properties of the GIPR post-activation, prolonged agonism of the system appears to result in functional outcomes that highlight the complexity of GIPR pharmacology, where enhanced activation does not equate to straightforward agonism.

A third area requiring more investigation is the interplay between the GIPR and GLP-1R, for instance, in pancreatic beta cells, the only known tissue where the receptors are coexpressed. In vitro studies with coexpression of both receptors have shown that GIPR expression suppresses GLP-1R signaling and surface expression, while the GIPR remains unaffected by the presence of GLP-1R [256, 257]. A new mouse study using global and targeted knockouts and transcriptomics showed that intact neuronal coexpression of GIPR and GLP-1R is required for full weight-lowering effects of combined incretin-based therapies, suggesting mechanistic interplay between the receptors within the same neuronal population [212, 213]. However, whether this also applies to humans remains unknown, further underscoring that understanding the implications of this crosstalk between the incretin receptors could enhance our comprehension of cotargeting compounds.

Lastly, an aspect to consider when therapeutically targeting the GIP system is its effect on other tissues besides the pancreas. An explanation for the paradox observed for the weight-reducing effects of GIPR agonism and antagonism might result from GIP's action to augment intestinal blood flow, potentially affecting nutrient uptake and its involvement in adipose tissue metabolism [5, 11, 12]. Additionally, the central role of GIP agonism in the regulation of appetite as seen in animal models remains to be further explored in humans.

Conclusion

The GIP system has gained attention as a valuable complement to GLP-1-based treatments following the development of the GLP-1R/GIPR coagonist tirzepatide and its subsequent therapeutic success. However, several possible treatment candidate drugs (e.g., MariTide) block the GIPR and result in the same clinical outcomes as tirzepatide (weight loss and improved glycemic control). We are, therefore, in a pharmacological conundrum where better understanding of each molecule will be necessary to fully appreciate the results of all GIPR-targeting treatments. Furthermore, it is also important to acknowledge the impact of species differences in the GIP system, exemplified by the involvement of GIP in appetite regulation in mice, whereas this does not seem to be the case in human studies. Nevertheless, exciting times lie ahead as the development of GIPR-targeting compounds continues to advance, and a deeper understanding of their mechanisms of action will pave the way for optimizing GIP pharmacology, unlocking its full therapeutic potential.

References

1 Davies, M.J., Aroda, V.R., Collins, B.S. et al. (2022). Management of hyperglycaemia in type 2 diabetes, 2022. A consensus report by the American Diabetes Association (ADA) and the European Association for the Study of Diabetes (EASD). *Diabetologia* 65 (65): 1925–1966. https://doi.org/10.1007/s00125-022-05787-2.

2 Holst, J.J., Madsbad, S., Bojsen-Møller, K.N. et al. (2018). Mechanisms in bariatric surgery: gut hormones, diabetes resolution, and weight loss. *Surg. Obes. Relat. Dis.* 14: 708–714. https://doi.org/10.1016/J.SOARD.2018.03.003.

3 Nauck, M.A., Bartels, E., Orskov, C. et al. (1993). Additive insulinotropic effects of exogenous synthetic human gastric inhibitory polypeptide and glucagon-like peptide-1-(7–36) amide infused at near-physiological insulinotropic hormone and glucose concentrations. *J. Clin. Endocrinol. Metab.* 76: 912–917. https://doi.org/10.1210/jcem.76.4.8473405.

4 Gasbjerg, L.S., Bergmann, N.C., Stensen, S. et al. (2020). Evaluation of the incretin effect in humans using GIP and GLP-1 receptor antagonists. *Peptides* 125: 170183. https://doi.org/10.1016/j.peptides.2019.170183.

5 Rasmussen, R.S., Langberg, L.S., Østergaard, F. et al. (2025). Glucose-dependent insulinotropic polypeptide is involved in postprandial regulation of splanchnic blood supply. *Diabetes* 74 (8): 1355–1366.

6 Helsted, M.M., Gasbjerg, L.S., Lanng, A.R. et al. (2020). The role of endogenous GIP and GLP-1 in postprandial bone homeostasis. *Bone* 140: 115553. https://doi.org/10.1016/j.bone.2020.115553.

7 Nissen, A., Christensen, M., Knop, F.K. et al. (2014). Glucose-dependent insulinotropic polypeptide inhibits bone resorption in humans. *J. Clin. Endocrinol. Metab.* 99: E2325–E2329. https://doi.org/10.1210/jc.2014-2547.

8 Christensen, M.B., Lund, A., Calanna, S. et al. (2018). Glucose-dependent insulinotropic polypeptide (GIP) inhibits bone resorption independently of insulin and glycemia. *J. Clin. Endocrinol. Metab.* 103: 288–294. https://doi.org/10.1210/jc.2017-01949.

9 Karstoft, K., Mortensen, S.P., Knudsen, S.H. et al. (2015). Direct effect of incretin hormones on glucose and glycerol metabolism and hemodynamics. *Am. J. Physiol.-Endocrinol. Metab.* 308: E426–E433. https://doi.org/10.1152/ajpendo.00520.2014.

10 Wang, S., Oestricker, L.Z., Wallendorf, M.J. et al. (2018). Cholinergic signaling mediates the effects of xenin-25 on secretion of pancreatic polypeptide but not insulin or glucagon in humans with impaired glucose tolerance. *PLoS One* 13: e0192441. https://doi.org/10.1371/journal.pone.0192441.

11 Asmar, M., Simonsen, L., Madsbad, S. et al. (2010). Glucose-dependent insulinotropic polypeptide may enhance fatty acid re-esterification in subcutaneous abdominal adipose tissue in lean humans. *Diabetes* 59: 2160–2163. https://doi.org/10.2337/db10-0098.

12 Asmar, M., Asmar, A., Simonsen, L. et al. (2017). The gluco- and liporegulatory and vasodilatory effects of glucose-dependent insulinotropic polypeptide

(GIP) are abolished by an antagonist of the human GIP receptor. *Diabetes* 66: 2363–2371. https://doi.org/10.2337/db17-0480.

13 Christensen, M., Vedtofte, L., Holst, J.J. et al. (2011). Glucose-dependent insulinotropic polypeptide a bifunctional glucose-dependent regulator of glucagon and insulin secretion in humans. *Diabetes* 60: 3103–3109. https://doi.org/10.2337/dB11-0979.

14 Christensen, M., Calanna, S., Sparre-Ulrich, A.H. et al. (2015). Glucose-dependent insulinotropic polypeptide augments glucagon responses to hypoglycemia in type 1 diabetes. *Diabetes* 64: 72–78. https://doi.org/10.2337/db14-0440.

15 Mroz, P.A., Finan, B., Gelfanov, V. et al. (2019). Optimized GIP analogs promote body weight lowering in mice through GIPR agonism not antagonism. *Mol. Metab.* 20: 51–62. https://doi.org/10.1016/j.molmet.2018.12.001.

16 Killion, E.A., Wang, J., Yie, J. et al. (2018). Anti-obesity effects of GIPR antagonists alone and in combination with GLP-1R agonists in preclinical models [internet]. *Sci. Transl. Med.* 10: 3392; https://www.science.org.

17 Killion, E.A., Chen, M., Falsey, J.R. et al. (2020). Chronic glucose-dependent insulinotropic polypeptide receptor (GIPR) agonism desensitizes adipocyte GIPR activity mimicking functional GIPR antagonism. *Nat. Commun.* 11: 4981. https://doi.org/10.1038/s41467-020-18751-8.

18 Jensen, M.H., Sanni, S.J., Riber, D. et al. (2024). AT-7687, a novel GIPR peptide antagonist, combined with a GLP-1 agonist, leads to enhanced weight loss and metabolic improvements in cynomolgus monkeys. *Mol. Metab.* 88: 102006. https://doi.org/10.1016/j.molmet.2024.102006.

19 Pathak, V., Gault, V.A., Flatt, P.R., and Irwin, N. (2015). Antagonism of gastric inhibitory polypeptide (GIP) by palmitoylation of GIP analogues with N- and C-terminal modifications improves obesity and metabolic control in high fat fed mice. *Mol. Cell. Endocrinol.* 401: 120–129. https://doi.org/10.1016/j.mce.2014.10.025.

20 Campbell, J.E. (2021). Targeting the GIPR for obesity: to agonize or antagonize? Potential mechanisms. *Mol. Metab.* 46: 101139. https://doi.org/10.1016/j.molmet.2020.101139.

21 Jastreboff, A.M., Aronne, L.J., Ahmad, N.N. et al. (2022). Tirzepatide once weekly for the treatment of obesity. *N. Engl. J. Med.* 387: 205–216. https://doi.org/10.1056/NEJMoa2206038.

22 Rosenstock, J., Wysham, C., Frías, J.P. et al. (2021). Efficacy and safety of a novel dual GIP and GLP-1 receptor agonist tirzepatide in patients with type 2 diabetes (SURPASS-1): a double-blind, randomised, phase 3 trial. *Lancet Lond. Engl.* 398: 143–155. https://doi.org/10.1016/S0140-6736(21)01324-6.

23 Frías, J.P., Davies, M.J., Rosenstock, J. et al. (2021). Tirzepatide versus semaglutide once weekly in patients with type 2 diabetes. *N. Engl. J. Med.* 385: 503–515. https://doi.org/10.1056/NEJMoa2107519.

24 Ludvik, B., Giorgino, F., Jódar, E. et al. (2021). Once-weekly tirzepatide versus once-daily insulin degludec as add-on to metformin with or without SGLT2 inhibitors in patients with type 2 diabetes (SURPASS-3): a randomised, open-label, parallel-group, phase 3 trial. *Lancet Lond. Engl.* 398: 583–598. https://doi.org/10.1016/S0140-6736(21)01443-4.

25 Del Prato, S., Kahn, S.E., Pavo, I. et al. (2021). Tirzepatide versus insulin glargine in type 2 diabetes and increased cardiovascular risk (SURPASS-4): a randomised, open-label, parallel-group, multicentre, phase 3 trial. *Lancet Lond. Engl.* 398: 1811–1824. https://doi.org/10.1016/S0140-6736(21)02188-7.

26 Dahl, D., Onishi, Y., Norwood, P. et al. (2022). Effect of subcutaneous tirzepatide vs placebo added to titrated insulin glargine on glycemic control in patients with type 2 diabetes. *JAMA* 327: 534–545. https://doi.org/10.1001/jama.2022.0078.

27 Véniant, M.M., Lu, S.-C., Atangan, L. et al. (2024). A GIPR antagonist conjugated to GLP-1 analogues promotes weight loss with improved metabolic parameters in preclinical and phase 1 settings. *Nat. Metab. Nature. Publishing Group* 1–14. https://doi.org/10.1038/s42255-023-00966-w.

28 Jastreboff, A.M., Ryan, D.H., Bays, H.E. et al. (2025). Once-monthly maridebart cafraglutide for the treatment of obesity – a phase 2 trial. *N. Engl. J. Med.* 393: 843–857. https://doi.org/10.1056/NEJMoa2504214.

29 Brown, J.C. and Pederson, R.A. (1970). A multiparameter study on the action of preparations containing cholecystokinin-pancreozymin. *Scand. J. Gastroenterol.* 5: 537–541. https://doi.org/10.1080/00365521.1970.12096632.

30 Brown, J.C. and Dryburgh, J.R. (1971). A gastric inhibitory polypeptide. II. The complete amino acid sequence. *Can. J. Biochem.* 49: 867–872. https://doi.org/10.1139/o71-122.

31 Dupre, J., Ross, S.A., Watson, D., and Brown, J.C. (1973). Stimulation of insulin secretion by gastric inhibitory polypeptide in man. *J. Clin. Endocrinol. Metab.* 37: 826–828. https://doi.org/10.1210/jcem-37-5-826.

32 Nauck, M.A., Bartels, E., Orskov, C. et al. (2004). Lack of effect of synthetic human gastric inhibitory polypeptide and glucagon-like peptide 1 [7–36 amide] infused at near-physiological concentrations on pentagastrin-stimulated gastric acid secretion in normal human subjects. *Digestion* 52: 214–221. https://doi.org/10.1159/000200956.

33 Holst, J.J., Ørskov, C., Vagn Nielsen, O., and W, S.T. (1987). Truncated glucagon-like peptide I, an insulin-releasing hormone from the distal gut. *FEBS Lett.* 211: 169–174. https://doi.org/10.1016/0014-5793(87)81430-8.

34 Vilsbøll, T., Knop, F.K., Krarup, T. et al. (2003). The pathophysiology of diabetes involves a defective amplification of the late-phase insulin response to glucose by glucose-dependent insulinotropic polypeptide-regardless of etiology and phenotype. *J. Clin. Endocrinol. Metab.* 88: 4897–4903. https://doi.org/10.1210/jc.2003-030738.

35 Nauck, M.A., Heimesaat, M.M., Orskov, C. et al. (1993). Preserved incretin activity of glucagon-like peptide 1 [7–36 amide] but not of synthetic human gastric inhibitory polypeptide in patients with type-2 diabetes mellitus. *J. Clin. Invest.* 91: 301–307. https://doi.org/10.1172/JCI116186.

36 Lund, A., Vilsbøll, T., Bagger, J.I. et al. (2011). The separate and combined impact of the intestinal hormones, GIP, GLP-1, and GLP-2, on glucagon secretion in type 2 diabetes. *Am. J. Physiol. Endocrinol. Metab.* 300: E1038–E1046. https://doi.org/10.1152/ajpendo.00665.2010.

37 Chia, C.W., Carlson, O.D., Kim, W. et al. (2009). Exogenous glucose-dependent insulinotropic polypeptide worsens post prandial hyperglycemia in T ype 2 diabetes. *Diabetes* 58: 1342–1349. https://doi.org/10.2337/db08-0958.

38 Miyawaki, K., Yamada, Y., Ban, N. et al. (2002). Inhibition of gastric inhibitory polypeptide signaling prevents obesity. *Nat. Med.* 8: 738–742. https://doi.org/10.1038/nm727.

39 Takeda, J., Seino, Y., Tanaka, K. et al. (1987). Sequence of an intestinal cDNA encoding human gastric inhibitory polypeptide precursor. *Proc. Natl. Acad. Sci. USA* 84: 7005–7008. https://doi.org/10.1073/pnas.84.20.7005.

40 Ugleholdt, R., Poulsen, M.-L.H., Holst, P.J. et al. (2006). Prohormone convertase 1/3 is essential for processing of the glucose-dependent insulinotropic polypeptide precursor. *J. Biol. Chem.* 281: 11050–11057. https://doi.org/10.1074/jbc.M601203200.

41 Fujita, Y., Wideman, R.D., Asadi, A. et al. (2010). Glucose-dependent insulinotropic polypeptide is expressed in pancreatic islet α-cells and promotes insulin secretion. *Gastroenterology* 138: 1966–1975.e1. https://doi.org/10.1053/j.gastro.2010.01.049.

42 Fujita, Y., Asadi, A., Yang, G.K. et al. (2010). Differential processing of pro-glucose-dependent insulinotropic polypeptide in gut. *Am. J. Physiol.-Gastrointest. Liver Physiol.* 298: G608–G614. https://doi.org/10.1152/ajpgi.00024.2010.

43 Hansen, L.S., Sparre-Ulrich, A.H., Christensen, M. et al. (2016). N-terminally and C-terminally truncated forms of glucose-dependent insulinotropic polypeptide are high-affinity competitive antagonists of the human GIP receptor. *Br. J. Pharmacol.* 173: 826–838. https://doi.org/10.1111/BPH.13384.

44 Krogh, L.S.L., Henriksen, K., Stensen, S. et al. (2023). The naturally occurring GIP(1–30)NH2 is a GIP receptor agonist in humans. *Eur. J. Endocrinol.* 188: 48–58. https://doi.org/10.1093/ejendo/lvac015.

45 Lund, A., Bagger, J.I., Wewer Albrechtsen, N.J. et al. (2016). Evidence of extrapancreatic glucagon secretion in man. *Diabetes* 65: 585–597. https://doi.org/10.2337/db15-1541.

46 Buchan, A.M.J., Polak, J.M., Capella, C. et al. (1978). Electronimmunocytochemical evidence for the *K* cell localization of gastric inhibitory polypeptide (GIP) im man. *Histochemistry* 56: 37–44. https://doi.org/10.1007/BF00492251.

47 Buffa, R., Polak, J.M., Pearse, A.G.E. et al. (1975). Identification of the intestinal cell storing gastric inhibitory peptide. *Histochemistry* 43: 249–255. https://doi.org/10.1007/BF00499706.

48 Polak, J.M., Bloom, S.R., Kuzio, M. et al. (1973). Cellular localization of gastric inhibitory polypeptide in the duodenum and jejunum. *Gut* 14: 284–288. https://doi.org/10.1136/gut.14.4.284.

49 Morgan, L.M., Flatt, P.R., and Marks, V. (1988). Nutrient regulation of the entero-insular axis and insulin secretion. *Nutr. Res. Rev.* 1: 79–97. https://doi.org/10.1079/NRR19880008.

50 Carr, R.D., Larsen, M.O., Winzell, M.S. et al. (2008). Incretin and islet hormonal responses to fat and protein ingestion in healthy men. *Am. J. Physiol.-Endocrinol. Metab.* 295: E779–E784. https://doi.org/10.1152/ajpendo.90233.2008.

51 Lindgren, O., Pacini, G., Tura, A. et al. (2015). Incretin effect after oral amino acid ingestion in humans. *J. Clin. Endocrinol. Metab.* 100: 1172–1176. https://doi.org/10.1210/jc.2014-3865.

52 Kuhre, R.E., Wewer Albrechtsen, N.J., Larsen, O. et al. (2018). Bile acids are important direct and indirect regulators of the secretion of appetite- and metabolism-regulating hormones from the gut and pancreas. *Mol. Metab.* 11: 84–95. https://doi.org/10.1016/j.molmet.2018.03.007.

53 Rohde, U., Sonne, D.P., Christensen, M. et al. (2016). Cholecystokinin-induced gallbladder emptying and metformin elicit additive glucagon-like peptide-1 responses. *J. Clin. Endocrinol. Metab.* 101: 2076–2083. https://doi.org/10.1210/jc.2016-1133.

54 Gasbjerg, L.S., Helsted, M.M., Hartmann, B. et al. (2019). Separate and combined glucometabolic effects of endogenous glucose-dependent insulinotropic polypeptide and glucagon-like peptide 1 in healthy individuals. *Diabetes* 68: 906–917. https://doi.org/10.2337/db18-1123.

55 Deacon, C.F., Nauck, M.A., Meier, J. et al. (2000). Degradation of endogenous and exogenous gastric inhibitory polypeptide in healthy and in type 2 diabetic subjects as revealed using a new assay for the intact peptide. *J. Clin. Endocrinol. Metab.* 85: 3575–3581. https://doi.org/10.1210/jcem.85.10.6855.

56 Deacon, C.F., Plamboeck, A., Rosenkilde, M.M. et al. (2006). GIP-(3–42) does not antagonize insulinotropic effects of GIP at physiological concentrations. *Am. J. Physiol.-Endocrinol. Metab.* 291: E468–E475. https://doi.org/10.1152/ajpendo.00577.2005.

57 Vilsbøll, T., Agersø, H., Lauritsen, T. et al. (2006). The elimination rates of intact GIP as well as its primary metabolite, GIP 3–42, are similar in type 2 diabetic patients and healthy subjects. *Regul. Pept.* 137: 168–172. https://doi.org/10.1016/j.regpep.2006.07.007.

58 Kerr, B.D., Flatt, A.J.S., Flatt, P.R., and Gault, V.A. (2011). Characterization and biological actions of N-terminal truncated forms of glucose-dependent insulinotropic polypeptide. *Biochem. Biophys. Res. Commun.* 404: 870–876. https://doi.org/10.1016/j.bbrc.2010.12.077.

59 Gault, V., Parker, J., Harriott, P. et al. (2002). Evidence that the major degradation product of glucose-dependent insulinotropic polypeptide, GIP(3–42), is a GIP receptor antagonist in vivo. *J. Endocrinol.* 175: 525–533. https://doi.org/10.1677/joe.0.1750525.

60 Meier, J.J., Nauck, M.A., Kranz, D. et al. (2004). Secretion, degradation, and elimination of glucagon-like peptide 1 and gastric inhibitory polypeptide in patients with chronic renal insufficiency and healthy control subjects. *Diabetes* 53: 654–662. https://doi.org/10.2337/diabetes.53.3.654.

61 Takeda, S., Kadowaki, S., Haga, T. et al. (2002). Identification of G protein-coupled receptor genes from the human genome sequence. *FEBS Lett.* 520: 97–101. https://doi.org/10.1016/S0014-5793(02)02775-8.

62 Yang, D., Zhou, Q., Labroska, V. et al. (2021). G protein-coupled receptors: structure- and function-based drug discovery. *Signal Transduct. Target. Ther.* 6: 1–27. https://doi.org/10.1038/s41392-020-00435-w.

63 Fredriksson, R., Lagerström, M.C., Lundin, L.-G., and Schiöth, H.B. (2003). The G-protein-coupled receptors in the human genome form five main families. Phylogenetic analysis, paralogon groups, and fingerprints. *Mol. Pharmacol.* 63: 1256–1272. https://doi.org/10.1124/mol.63.6.1256.

64 Alexander, S.P.H., Christopoulos, A., Davenport, A.P. et al. (2019). The concise guide to pharmacology 2019/20: G protein-coupled receptors [internet]. *Br. J. Pharmacol.* 176: S21–S141. https://doi.org/10.1111/bph.14748.

65 Cary, B.P., Zhang, X., Cao, J. et al. (2023). New insights into the structure and function of class B1 GPCRs. *Endocr. Rev.* 44: 492–517. https://doi.org/10.1210/endrev/bnac033.

66 Smit, F.X., van der Velden, W.J.C., Kizilkaya, H.S. et al. (2021). Investigating GIPR (ant)agonism: a structural analysis of GIP and its receptor. *Structure* 29: 679. https://doi.org/10.1016/j.str.2021.04.001–693.e6.

67 Zhao, F., Zhang, C., Zhou, Q. et al. (2021). Structural insights into hormone recognition by the human glucosedependent insulinotropic polypeptide receptor. *elife* 10: e68719. https://doi.org/10.7554/ELIFE.68719.

68 Hoare, S.R.J. (2005). Mechanisms of peptide and nonpeptide ligand binding to class B G-protein-coupled receptors. *Drug Discov. Today* 10: 417–427. https://doi.org/10.1016/S1359-6446(05)03370-2.

69 Pándy-Szekeres, G., Munk, C., Tsonkov, T.M. et al. (2018). GPCRdb in 2018: adding GPCR structure models and ligands. *Nucleic Acids Res.* 46: D440–D446. https://doi.org/10.1093/nar/gkx1109.

70 Svendsen, B., Larsen, O., Gabe, M.B.N. et al. (2018). Insulin secretion depends on intra-islet glucagon signaling. *Cell Rep.* 25: 1127–1134.e2. https://doi.org/10.1016/j.celrep.2018.10.018.

71 Gabe, M.B.N., von Voss, L., Hunt, J.E. et al. (2023; https://doi.org/10.1111/bph.16040). Biased GLP-2 agonist with strong G protein-coupling but impaired arrestin recruitment and receptor desensitization enhances intestinal growth in mice. *Br. J. Pharmacol.* 180: 1674–1689.

72 Gadgaard, S., van der Velden, W.J.C., Schiellerup, S.P. et al. (2022). Novel agonist and antagonist radioligands for the GLP-2 receptor. Useful tools for studies of basic GLP-2 receptor pharmacology. *Br. J. Pharmacol.* 179: 1998–2015. https://doi.org/10.1111/bph.15766.

73 McIntosh, C.H., Widenmaier, S., and Kim, S. (2012). Glucose-dependent insulinotropic polypeptide signaling in pancreatic β-cells and adipocytes. *J. Diabetes Investig.* 3: 96–106. https://doi.org/10.1111/j.2040-1124.2012.00196.x.

74 Kashima, Y., Miki, T., Shibasaki, T. et al. (2001). Critical role of cAMP-GEFII – Rim2 complex in incretin-potentiated insulin secretion. *J. Biol. Chem.* 276: 46046–46053. https://doi.org/10.1074/jbc.M108378200.

75 Ehses, J.A., Pelech, S.L., Pederson, R.A., and McIntosh, C.H.S. (2002). Glucose-dependent insulinotropic polypeptide activates the Raf-Mek1/2-ERK1/2 module via a cyclic AMP/cAMP-dependent protein kinase/Rap1-mediated pathway. *J. Biol. Chem.* 277: 37088–37097. https://doi.org/10.1074/jbc.M205055200.

76 Yuliantie, E., Darbalaei, S., Dai, A. et al. (2020). Pharmacological characterization of mono-, dual- and tri-peptidic agonists at GIP and GLP-1 receptors. *Biochem. Pharmacol.* 177: 114001. https://doi.org/10.1016/j.bcp.2020.114001.

77 Jones, B., McGlone, E.R., Fang, Z. et al. (2021). Genetic and biased agonist-mediated reductions in β-arrestin recruitment prolong cAMP signaling at glucagon family receptors [internet]. *J. Biol. Chem.* 296: 100133. https://doi.org/10.1074/JBC.RA120.016334.

78 Novikoff, A., O'Brien, S.L., Bernecker, M. et al. (2021). Spatiotemporal GLP-1 and GIP receptor signaling and trafficking/recycling dynamics induced by selected receptor mono- and dual-agonists. *Mol. Metab.* 49: 101181. https://doi.org/10.1016/j.molmet.2021.101181.

79 Avet, C., Mancini, A., Breton, B. et al. (2022). Effector membrane translocation biosensors reveal G protein and parrestin coupling profiles of 100 therapeutically relevant GPCRs. *elife* 11: e74101. https://doi.org/10.7554/ELIFE.74101.

80 Kizilkaya, H.S., Sørensen, K.V., Madsen, J.S. et al. (2024). Characterization of genetic variants of GIPR reveals a contribution of β-arrestin to metabolic phenotypes. *Nat. Metab.* 6: 1268–1281. https://doi.org/10.1038/s42255-024-01061-4.

81 Willard, F.S., Douros, J.D., Gabe, M.B.N. et al. (2020). Tirzepatide is an imbalanced and biased dual GIP and GLP-1 receptor agonist [internet]. *JCI Insight* 5: https://doi.org/10.1172/JCI.INSIGHT.140532.

82 Harding, S.D., Armstrong, J.F., Faccenda, E. et al. (2024). The IUPHAR/BPS guide to PHARMACOLOGY in 2024. *Nucleic Acids Res.* 52: D1438–D1449. https://doi.org/10.1093/nar/gkad944.

83 Lynggaard, M.B., Gasbjerg, L.S., Christensen, M.B., and Knop, F.K. (2020). GIP(3–30)NH2 – a tool for the study of GIP physiology. *Curr. Opin. Pharmacol.* 55: 31–40. https://doi.org/10.1016/J.COPH.2020.08.011.

84 Rosenkilde, M.M., Lindquist, P., Kizilkaya, H.S., and Gasbjerg, L.S. (2024). GIP-derived GIP receptor antagonists – a review of their role in GIP receptor pharmacology. *Peptides* 177: 171212. https://doi.org/10.1016/j.peptides.2024.171212.

85 Maletti, M., Carlquist, M., Portha, B. et al. (1986). Structural requirements for gastric inhibitory polypeptide (GIP) receptor binding and stimulation of insulin release. *Peptides* 7: 75–78. https://doi.org/10.1016/0196-9781(86)90167-1.

86 Hinke, S.A., Manhart, S., Pamir, N. et al. (2001). Identification of a bioactive domain in the amino-terminus of glucose-dependent insulinotropic polypeptide (GIP). *Biochim. Biophys. Acta* 1547: 143–155. https://doi.org/10.1016/S0167-4838(01)00181-9.

87 Irwin, N., Green, B.D., Parker, J.C. et al. (2006). Biological activity and antidiabetic potential of synthetic fragment peptides of glucose-dependent insulinotropic polypeptide, GIP(1–16) and (Pro3)GIP(1–16). *Regul. Pept.* 135: 45–53. https://doi.org/10.1016/j.regpep.2006.03.006.

88 Wheeler, M.B., Gelling, R.W., McIntosh, C.H. et al. (1995). Functional expression of the rat pancreatic islet glucose-dependent insulinotropic polypeptide receptor: ligand binding and intracellular signaling properties. *Endocrinology* 136: 4629–4639. https://doi.org/10.1210/endo.136.10.7664683.

89 Moroder, L., Thamm, P., Wilschowitz, L. et al. (1978). Studies on gastric inhibitory polypeptide: synthesis of the octatricontapeptide GIP(1–38) with full insulinotropic activity. *Scand. J. Gastroenterol.* 49: 129.

90 Sandberg, E., Ahrén, B., Tendler, D. et al. (1986). Potentiation of glucose-induced insulin secretion in the perfused rat pancreas by porcine GIP (gastric inhibitory polypeptide), bovine GIP, and bovine GIP(1–39). *Acta Physiol. Scand.* 127: 323–326. https://doi.org/10.1111/j.1748-1716.1986.tb07911.x.

91 Gasbjerg, L.S., Christensen, M.B., Hartmann, B. et al. (2018). GIP(3–30)NH2 is an efficacious GIP receptor antagonist in humans: a randomised, double-blinded, placebo-controlled, crossover study. *Diabetologia* 61: 413–423. https://doi.org/10.1007/s00125-017-4447-4.

92 Stensen, S., Krogh, L.L., Sparre-Ulrich, A.H. et al. (2022). Acute concomitant glucose-dependent insulinotropic polypeptide receptor antagonism during glucagon-like peptide 1 receptor agonism does not affect appetite, resting energy expenditure or food intake in patients with type 2 diabetes and overweight/obesity. *Diabetes. Obes. Metab.* 24: 1882–1887. https://doi.org/10.1111/dom.14736.

93 Gasbjerg, L.S., Hartmann, B., Christensen, M.B. et al. (2020). GIP's effect on bone metabolism is reduced by the selective GIP receptor antagonist GIP(3–30)NH2. *Bone* 130: 115079. https://doi.org/10.1016/j.bone.2019.115079.

94 Gasbjerg, L.S., Helsted, M.M., Hartmann, B. et al. (2020). GIP and GLP-1 receptor antagonism during a meal in healthy individuals. *J. Clin. Endocrinol. Metab.* 105: e725–e738. https://doi.org/10.1210/clinem/dgz175.

95 Gelling, R.W., Coy, D.H., Pederson, R.A. et al. (1997). GIP(6–30amide) contains the high affinity binding region of GIP and is a potent inhibitor of GIP1–42 action in vitro. *Regul. Pept.* 69: 151–154. https://doi.org/10.1016/s0167-0115(97)00009-8.

96 Tseng, C.C., Kieffer, T.J., Jarboe, L.A. et al. (1996). Postprandial stimulation of insulin release by glucose-dependent insulinotropic polypeptide (GIP). Effect of a specific glucose-dependent insulinotropic polypeptide receptor antagonist in the rat. *J. Clin. Invest.* 98: 2440–2445. https://doi.org/10.1172/JCI119060.

97 Morrow, G.W., Kieffer, T.J., McIntosh, C.H. et al. (1996). The insulinotropic region of gastric inhibitory polypeptide; fragment analysis suggests the bioactive site lies between residues 19 and 30. *Can. J. Physiol. Pharmacol.* 74: 65–72.

98 Gault, V.A., Harriott, P., Flatt, P.R., and O'Harte, F.P.M. (2002). Cyclic AMP production and insulin releasing activity of synthetic fragment peptides of glucose-dependent insulinotropic polypeptide. *Biosci. Rep.* 22: 523–528. https://doi.org/10.1023/a:1022073819618.

99 Parthier, C., Kleinschmidt, M., Neumann, P. et al. (2007). Crystal structure of the incretin-bound extracellular domain of a G protein-coupled receptor. *Proc. Natl. Acad. Sci. USA* 104: 13942–13947. https://doi.org/10.1073/pnas.0706404104.

100 Hausdorff, W.P., Caron, M.G., and Lefkowitz, R.J. (1990). Turning off the signal: desensitization of β-adrenergic receptor function. *FASEB J.* 4: 2881–2889. https://doi.org/10.1096/fasebj.4.11.2165947.

101 Ferguson, S.S.G., Downey, W.E., Colapietro, A.-M. et al. (1996). Role of β-arrestin in mediating agonist-promoted G protein-coupled receptor internalization. *Science* 271: 363–366. https://doi.org/10.1126/science.271.5247.363.

102 Gurevich, V.V. and Gurevich, E.V. (2019). GPCR signaling regulation: the role of GRKs and arrestins [internet]. *Front. Pharmacol.* 10: 125. https://doi.org/10.3389/fphar.2019.00125.

103 Moo, E.V., van Senten, J.R., Bräuner-Osborne, H. et al. (2021). Arrestin-dependent and -independent internalization of G protein–coupled receptors: methods, mechanisms, and implications on cell signaling. *Mol. Pharmacol.* 99: 242–255. https://doi.org/10.1124/MOLPHARM.120.000192.

104 Manchanda, Y., Bitsi, S., Chen, S. et al. (2023). Enhanced endosomal signaling and desensitization of GLP-1R vs GIPR in pancreatic beta cells [internet]. *Endocrinology* 164: 164. https://doi.org/10.1210/endocr/bqad028.

105 Møller, T.C., Moo, E.V., Inoue, A. et al. (2024). Characterization of the real-time internalization of nine GPCRs reveals distinct dependence on arrestins and G proteins. *Biochim. Biophys. Acta* 1871: 119584. https://doi.org/10.1016/j.bbamcr.2023.119584.

106 Gabe, M.B.N., Sparre-Ulrich, A.H., Pedersen, M.F. et al. (2018). Human GIP(3–30)NH2 inhibits G protein-dependent as well as G protein-independent signaling and is selective for the GIP receptor with high-affinity binding to primate but not rodent GIP receptors. *Biochem. Pharmacol.* 150: 97–107. https://doi.org/10.1016/j.bcp.2018.01.040.

107 Abdullah, N., Beg, M., Soares, D. et al. (2016). Downregulation of a GPCR by β-arrestin2-mediated switch from an endosomal to a TGN recycling pathway. *Cell Rep.* 17: 2966–2978. https://doi.org/10.1016/j.celrep.2016.11.050.

108 Al-Sabah, S., Al-Fulaij, M., Shaaban, G. et al. (2014). The GIP receptor displays higher basal activity than the GLP-1 receptor but does not recruit GRK2 or arrestin3 effectively. *PLoS One* 9: e106890. https://doi.org/10.1371/journal.pone.0106890.

109 Mayer, D., Damberger, F.F., Samarasimhareddy, M. et al. (2019). Distinct G protein-coupled receptor phosphorylation motifs modulate arrestin affinity and activation and global conformation. *Nat. Commun.* 10: 1261. https://doi.org/10.1038/s41467-019-09204-y.

110 Maharana, J., Sano, F.K., Sarma, P. et al. (2024). Molecular insights into atypical modes of b-arrestin interaction with seven transmembrane receptors. *Science* 383 (6678): 101–108.

111 Ismail, S., Gherardi, M.J., Froese, A. et al. (2016). Internalized receptor for glucose-dependent insulinotropic peptide stimulates adenylyl cyclase on early endosomes. *Biochem. Pharmacol.* 120: 33–45. https://doi.org/10.1016/J.BCP.2016.09.009.

112 Wright, S.C., Motso, A., Koutsilieri, S. et al. (2023). GLP-1R signaling neighborhoods associate with the susceptibility to adverse drug reactions of incretin mimetics. *Nat. Commun.* 14: 6243. https://doi.org/10.1038/s41467-023-41 893-4.

113 Mohammad, S., Patel, R.T., Bruno, J. et al. (2014). A naturally occurring GIP receptor variant undergoes enhanced agonist-induced desensitization, which impairs GIP control of adipose insulin sensitivity. *Mol. Cell. Biol.* 34: 3618–3629. https://doi.org/10.1128/MCB.00256-14.

114 Kubota, A., Yamada, Y., Hayami, T. et al. (1996). Identification of two missense mutations in the GIP receptor gene: a functional study and association analysis with NIDDM: no evidence of association with Japanese NIDDM subjects. *Diabetes* 45: 1701–1705.

115 Almind, K., Ambye, L., Urhammer, S.A. et al. (1998). Discovery of amino acid variants in the human glucose-dependent insulinotropic polypeptide (GIP) receptor: the impact on the pancreatic beta cell responses and functional expression studies in Chinese hamster fibroblast cells. *Diabetologia* 41: 1194–1198. https://doi.org/10.1007/s001250051051.

116 Fortin, J.-P., Schroeder, J.C., Zhu, Y. et al. (2010). Pharmacological characterization of human incretin receptor missense variants. *J. Pharmacol. Exp. Ther.* 332: 274–280. https://doi.org/10.1124/jpet.109.160531.

117 Gabe, M.B.N., van der Velden, W.J.C., Gadgaard, S. et al. (2020). Enhanced agonist residence time, internalization rate and signalling of the GIP receptor variant [E354Q] facilitate receptor desensitization and long-term impairment of the GIP system. *Basic Clin. Pharmacol. Toxicol.* 126: 122–132. https://doi.org/10.1111/bcpt.13289.

118 Saxena, R., Hivert, M.-F., Langenberg, C. et al. (2010). Genetic variation in GIPR influences the glucose and insulin responses to an oral glucose challenge. *Nat. Genet.* 42: 142–148. https://doi.org/10.1038/ng.521.

119 Ahlqvist, E., Osmark, P., Kuulasmaa, T. et al. (2013). Link between GIP and osteopontin in adipose tissue and insulin resistance. *Diabetes* 62: 2088–2094. https://doi.org/10.2337/db12-0976.

120 van der Velden, W.J.C., Heitman, L.H., and Rosenkilde, M.M. (2020). Perspective: implications of ligand-receptor binding kinetics for therapeutic targeting of G protein-coupled receptors. *ACS Pharmacol. Transl. Sci.* 3: 179–189. https://doi.org/10.1021/acsptsci.0c00012.

121 Yammine, L., Picatoste, B., Abdullah, N. et al. (2023). Spatiotemporal regulation of GIPR signaling impacts glucose homeostasis as revealed in studies of a common GIPR variant. *Mol. Metab.* 78: 101831. https://doi.org/10.1016/j.molmet.2023.101831.

122 Zaïmia, N., Obeid, J., Varrault, A. et al. (2023). GLP-1 and GIP receptors signal through distinct β-arrestin 2-dependent pathways to regulate pancreatic β cell function. *Cell Rep.* 42: 113326. https://doi.org/10.1016/j.celrep.2023.113326.

123 Nauck, M.A., Quast, D.R., Wefers, J., and AFH, P. (2021). The evolving story of incretins (GIP and GLP -1) in metabolic and cardiovascular disease: a pathophysiological update. *Diabetes. Obes. Metab.* 23: 5–29. https://doi.org/10.1111/dom.14496.

124 Santos, A., Tsafou, K., Stolte, C. et al. (2015). Comprehensive comparison of large-scale tissue expression datasets. *PeerJ.* 3: e1054. https://doi.org/10.7717/peerj.1054.

125 Palasca, O., Santos, A., Stolte, C. et al. (2018). TISSUES 2.0: an integrative web resource on mammalian tissue expression. *Database* 2018: bay003. https://doi.org/10.1093/database/bay003.

126 Skov-Jeppesen, K., Hepp, N., Oeke, J. et al. (2021). The antiresorptive effect of GIP, but not GLP-2, is preserved in patients with hypoparathyroidism-A randomized crossover study. *J. Bone Miner. Res. Off. J. Am. Soc. Bone Miner. Res.* 36: 1448–1458. https://doi.org/10.1002/jbmr.4308.

127 Costa, A., Ai, M., Nunn, N. et al. (2022). Anorectic and aversive effects of GLP-1 receptor agonism are mediated by brainstem cholecystokinin neurons, and modulated by GIP receptor activation. *Mol. Metab.* 55: 101407. https://doi.org/10.1016/j.molmet.2021.101407.

128 Adriaenssens, A.E., Biggs, E.K., Darwish, T. et al. (2019). Glucose-dependent insulinotropic polypeptide receptor-expressing cells in the hypothalamus regulate food intake. *Cell. Metab.* 30: 987–996.e6. https://doi.org/10.1016/j.cmet.2019.07.013.

129 Zhang, C., Kaye, J.A., Cai, Z. et al. (2021). Area postrema cell types that mediate nausea-associated behaviors. *Neuron* 109: 461–472.e5. https://doi.org/10.1016/j.neuron.2020.11.010.

130 Sparre-Ulrich, A.H., Hansen, L.S., Svendsen, B. et al. (2016). Species-specific action of (Pro3)GIP – a full agonist at human GIP receptors, but a partial agonist and competitive antagonist at rat and mouse GIP receptors. *Br. J. Pharmacol.* 173: 27–38. https://doi.org/10.1111/bph.13323.

131 Gasbjerg, L.S., Rasmussen, R.S., Dragan, A. et al. (2025). Altered desensitization and internalization patterns of rodent versus human glucose-dependent insulinotropic polypeptide (GIP) receptors. An important drug discovery challenge. *Br. J. Pharmacol.* 182: 3353. https://doi.org/10.1111/bph.16478–3370.

132 Sparre-Ulrich, A.H., Gabe, M.N., Gasbjerg, L.S. et al. (2017). GIP(3–30)NH2 is a potent competitive antagonist of the GIP receptor and effectively inhibits GIP-mediated insulin, glucagon, and somatostatin release. *Biochem Pharmacol. Biochem Pharmacol.* 131: 78–88. https://doi.org/10.1016/J.BCP.2017.02.012.

133 Perley, M.J. and Kipnis, D.M. (1967). Plasma insulin responses to oral and intravenous glucose: studies in normal and diabetic subjects. *J. Clin. Invest.* 46: 1954–1962.

134 Nauck, M., Stöckmann, F., Ebert, R., and Creutzfeldt, W. (1986). Reduced incretin effect in type 2 (non-insulin-dependent) diabetes. *Diabetologia* 29: 46–52. https://doi.org/10.1007/BF02427280.

135 McIntyre, N., Holdsworth, C.D., and Turner, D.S. (1965). Intestinal factors in the control of insulin secretion. *J. Clin. Endocrinol. Metab.* 25: 1317–1324. https://doi.org/10.1210/jcem-25-10-1317.

136 Nauck, M.A., Homberger, E., Siegel, E.G. et al. (1986). Incretin effects of increasing glucose loads in man calculated from venous insulin and C-peptide responses. *J. Clin. Endocrinol. Metab.* 63: 492–498. https://doi.org/10.1210/jcem-63-2-492.

137 Vilsbøll, T., Krarup, T., Madsbad, S., and Holst, J.J. (2002). Defective amplification of the late phase insulin response to glucose by GIP in obese Type II diabetic patients. *Diabetologia* 45: 1111–1119. https://doi.org/10.1007/s00125-002-0878-6.

138 Christensen, M.B., Calanna, S., Holst, J.J. et al. (2014). Glucose-dependent insulinotropic polypeptide: blood glucose stabilizing effects in patients with type 2 diabetes. *J. Clin. Endocrinol. Metab.* 99: E418–E426. https://doi.org/10.1210/jc.2013-3644.

139 Rudovich, N.N., Rochlitz, H.J., and Pfeiffer, A.F.H. (2004). Reduced hepatic insulin extraction in response to gastric inhibitory polypeptide compensates for reduced insulin secretion in normal-weight and normal glucose tolerant first-degree relatives of type 2 diabetic patients. *Diabetes* 53: 2359–2365. https://doi.org/10.2337/diabetes.53.9.2359.

140 Holst, J.J. and Gromada, J. (2004). Role of incretin hormones in the regulation of insulin secretion in diabetic and nondiabetic humans. *Am. J. Physiol.-Endocrinol. Metab.* 287: E199–E206. https://doi.org/10.1152/ajpendo.00545.2003.

141 Mayendraraj, A., Rosenkilde, M.M., and Gasbjerg, L.S. (2022). GLP-1 and GIP receptor signaling in beta cells – a review of receptor interactions and co-stimulation. *Peptides* 151: 170749. https://doi.org/10.1016/j.peptides.2022.170749.

142 Skov-Jeppesen, K., Svane, M.S., Martinussen, C. et al. (2019). GLP-2 and GIP exert separate effects on bone turnover: a randomized, placebo-controlled, crossover study in healthy young men. *Bone* 125: 178–185. https://doi.org/10.1016/j.bone.2019.05.014.

143 Holst, J.J., Gasbjerg, L.S., and Rosenkilde, M.M. (2021). The role of incretins on insulin function and glucose homeostasis. *Endocrinology* 162: 1–10. https://doi.org/10.1210/ENDOCR/BQAB065.

144 Christensen, M.B., Gasbjerg, L.S., Heimbürger, S.M. et al. (2020). GIP's involvement in the pathophysiology of type 2 diabetes. *Peptides* 125: 170178. https://doi.org/10.1016/j.peptides.2019.170178.

145 Ørskov, C., Holst, J.J., and Nielsen, O.V. (1988). Effect of truncated glucagon-like peptide-1 [proglucagon-(78–107) amide] on endocrine secretion from pig pancreas, antrum, and nonantral stomach. *Endocrinology* 123: 2009–2013. https://doi.org/10.1210/ENDO-123-4-2009.

146 Preitner, F., Ibberson, M., Franklin, I. et al. (2004). Gluco-incretins control insulin secretion at multiple levels as revealed in mice lacking GLP-1 and GIP receptors. *J. Clin. Invest.* 113: 635–645. https://doi.org/10.1172/JCI200420518.

147 Pacini, G. and Ahrén, B. (2017). Glucagon-like peptide-1 and glucose-dependent insulinotropic peptide: effects alone and in combination on insulin secretion and glucose disappearance in mice. *Physiol. Rep.* 5: e13280. https://doi.org/10.14814/phy2.13280.

148 Wang, Z., Wang, R.M., Owji, A.A. et al. (1995). Glucagon-like peptide-1 is a physiological incretin in rat. *J. Clin. Invest.* 95: 417–421.

149 Nauck, M., van Hoorn, W., Gubernatis, G. et al. (1985). Preserved incretin effect after complete surgical denervation of the pancreas in young pigs. *Res. Exp. Med. (Berl)* 185: 291–298. https://doi.org/10.1007/BF01851954.

150 Edgerton, D.S., Kraft, G., Smith, M.S. et al. (2019). Effect of portal glucose sensing on incretin hormone secretion in a canine model. *Am. J. Physiol. Endocrinol. Metab.* 317: E244–E249. https://doi.org/10.1152/ajpendo.00100.2019.

151 de Heer, J., Rasmussen, C., Coy, D.H., and Holst, J.J. (2008. https://doi.org/10.1007/s00125-008-1149-y). Glucagon-like peptide-1, but not glucose-dependent insulinotropic peptide, inhibits glucagon secretion via somatostatin (receptor subtype 2) in the perfused rat pancreas [internet]. *Diabetologia* 51: 2263–2270.

152 Ipp, E., Dobbs, R.E., Harris, V. et al. (1977). The effects of gastrin, gastric inhibitory polypeptide, secretin, and the octapeptide of cholecystokinin upon immunoreactive somatostatin release by the perfused canine pancreas [internet]. *J. Clin. Invest.* 60: 1216–1219. https://doi.org/10.1172/JCI108875.

153 Gasbjerg, L.S., Bari, E.J., Christensen, M., and Knop, F.K. (2021). Exendin(9–39)NH2: recommendations for clinical use based on a systematic literature review. *Diabetes. Obes. Metab.* 23: 2419–2436. https://doi.org/10.1111/dom.14507.

154 Nauck, M.A. and Meier, J.J. (2016). The incretin effect in healthy individuals and those with type 2 diabetes: physiology, pathophysiology, and response to therapeutic interventions. *Lancet Diabetes Endocrinol.* 4: 525–536. https://doi.org/10.1016/S2213-8587(15)00482-9.

155 Nauck, M.A., Kleine, N., Orskov, C. et al. (1993). Normalization of fasting hyperglycaemia by exogenous glucagon-like peptide 1 (7–36 amide) in type 2 (non-insulin-dependent) diabetic patients. *Diabetologia* 36: 741–744. https://doi.org/10.1007/BF00401145.

156 Xu, G., Kaneto, H., Laybutt, D.R. et al. (2007). Downregulation of GLP-1 and GIP receptor expression by hyperglycemia: possible contribution to impaired incretin effects in diabetes. *Diabetes* 56: 1551–1558. https://doi.org/10.2337/db06-1033.

157 Højberg, P.V., Zander, M., Vilsbøll, T. et al. (2008). Near normalisation of blood glucose improves the potentiating effect of GLP-1 on glucose-induced insulin secretion in patients with type 2 diabetes. *Diabetologia* 51: 632–640. https://doi.org/10.1007/s00125-008-0943-x.

158 Højberg, P.V., Vilsbøll, T., Rabøl, R. et al. (2009). Four weeks of near-normalisation of blood glucose improves the insulin response to glucagon-like peptide-1 and glucose-dependent insulinotropic polypeptide in

patients with type 2 diabetes. *Diabetologia* 52: 199–207. https://doi.org/10.1007/s00125-008-1195-5.
159 Holst, J.J. and Rosenkilde, M.M. (2020). GIP as a therapeutic target in diabetes and obesity: insight from incretin co.-agonists. *J. Clin. Endocrinol. Metab.* 105: e2710–e2716. https://doi.org/10.1210/clinem/dgaa327.
160 Nauck, M.A. and Müller, T.D. (2023). Incretin hormones and type 2 diabetes. *Diabetologia* 66: 1780–1795. https://doi.org/10.1007/s00125-023-05956-x.
161 Christensen, A.A. and Gannon, M. (2019). The beta cell in type 2 diabetes [internet]. *Curr. Diab. Rep.* 19: 81. https://doi.org/10.1007/s11892-019-1196-4.
162 Stensen, S., Gasbjerg, L.S., Krogh, L.L. et al. (2021). Effects of endogenous GIP in patients with type 2 diabetes. *Eur. J. Endocrinol.* 185: 33–45. https://doi.org/10.1530/EJE-21-0135.
163 Bergmann, N.C., Gasbjerg, L.S., Heimbürger, S.M. et al. (2020). No acute effects of exogenous glucose-dependent insulinotropic polypeptide on energy intake, appetite, or energy expenditure when added to treatment with a long-acting glucagon-like peptide 1 receptor agonist in men with type 2 diabetes. *Diabetes Care* 43: 588–596. https://doi.org/10.2337/dc19-0578.
164 Heise, T., Zijlstra, E., Mari, A. et al. A long-acting glucose dependent insulinotropic polypeptide receptor agonist improves insulin sensitivity and beta cell function in subjects with type 2 diabetes [internet]. *EASD 2024*, Madrid, Spain. https://cattendee.abstractsonline.com/meeting/20620/presentation/2938.
165 Creutzfeldt, W., Ebert, R., Willms, B. et al. (1978). Gastric inhibitory polypeptide (GIP) and insulin in obesity: increased response to stimulation and defective feedback control of serum levels. *Diabetologia* 14: 15–24. https://doi.org/10.1007/BF00429703.
166 Salera, M., Giacomoni, P., Pironi, L. et al. (1982). Gastric inhibitory polypeptide release after oral glucose: relationship to glucose intolerance, diabetes mellitus, and obesity. *J. Clin. Endocrinol. Metab.* 55: 329–336. https://doi.org/10.1210/jcem-55-2-329.
167 Bergmann, N.C., Lund, A., Gasbjerg, L.S. et al. (2019). Effects of combined GIP and GLP-1 infusion on energy intake, appetite and energy expenditure in overweight/obese individuals: a randomised, crossover study. *Diabetologia* 62: 665–675. https://doi.org/10.1007/s00125-018-4810-0.
168 Marks, V. (1988). GIP-the obesity hormone. *Obes. Curr. Approaches* 13–20.
169 Nasteska, D., Harada, N., Suzuki, K. et al. (2014). Chronic reduction of GIP secretion alleviates obesity and insulin resistance under high-fat diet conditions. *Diabetes* 63: 2332–2343. https://doi.org/10.2337/dB13-1563.
170 Asmar, M., Simonsen, L., Arngrim, N. et al. (2005). Glucose-dependent insulinotropic polypeptide has impaired effect on abdominal, subcutaneous adipose tissue metabolism in obese subjects. *Int. J. Obes.* 2014 (38): 259–265. https://doi.org/10.1038/ijo.2013.73.
171 Asmar, M., Arngrim, N., Simonsen, L. et al. (2016). The blunted effect of glucose-dependent insulinotropic polypeptide in subcutaneous abdominal adipose tissue in obese subjects is partly reversed by weight loss. *Nutr. Diabetes* 6: e208. https://doi.org/10.1038/nutd.2016.15.

172 Kim, S.-J., Nian, C., and McIntosh, C.H.S. (2007). Activation of lipoprotein lipase by glucose-dependent insulinotropic polypeptide in adipocytes. A role for a protein kinase B, LKB1, and AMP-activated protein kinase cascade. *J. Biol. Chem.* 282: 8557–8567. https://doi.org/10.1074/jbc.M609088200.

173 Kim, S.-J., Nian, C., and McIntosh, C.H.S. (2010). GIP increases human adipocyte LPL expression through CREB and TORC2-mediated trans-activation of the LPL gene. *J. Lipid Res.* 51: 3145–3157. https://doi.org/10.1194/jlr.M006841.

174 McIntosh, C.H.S., Bremsak, I., Lynn, F.C. et al. (1999). Glucose-dependent insulinotropic polypeptide stimulation of lipolysis in differentiated 3 T3-L1 cells: wortmannin-sensitive inhibition by insulin. *Endocrinology* 140: 398–404. https://doi.org/10.1210/endo.140.1.6464.

175 Speliotes, E.K., Willer, C.J., Berndt, S.I. et al. (2010). Association analyses of 249 796 individuals reveal eighteen new loci associated with body mass index. *Nat. Genet.* 42: 937–948. https://doi.org/10.1038/ng.686.

176 Chen, S., Francioli, L.C., Goodrich, J.K. et al. (2024). A genomic mutational constraint map using variation in 76 156 human genomes. *Nature* 625: 92–100. https://doi.org/10.1038/s41586-023-06045-0.

177 Almgren, P., Lindqvist, A., Krus, U. et al. (2017). Genetic determinants of circulating GIP and GLP-1 concentrations. *JCI Insight* 2: e93306. https://doi.org/10.1172/jci.insight.93306.

178 Trifonova, E.A., Popovich, A.A., Makeeva, O.A. et al. (2021). Replicative association analysis of genetic markers of obesity in the Russian population. *Russ. J. Genet.* 57: 620–625. https://doi.org/10.1134/S1022795421050136.

179 Styrkarsdottir, U., Tragante, V., Stefansdottir, L. et al. (2024). Obesity variants in the GIPR gene do not associate with risk of fracture or bone mineral density. *J. Clin. Endocrinol. Metab.* 109: e1608. https://doi.org/10.1210/clinem/dgad734–e1615.

180 Lyssenko, V., Eliasson, L., Kotova, O. et al. (2011). Pleiotropic effects of GIP on islet function involve osteopontin. *Diabetes* 60: 2424–2433. https://doi.org/10.2337/db10-1532.

181 Turcot, V., Lu, Y., Highland, H.M. et al. (2018). Protein-altering variants associated with body mass index implicate pathways that control energy intake and expenditure in obesity. *Nat. Genet.* 50: 26–41. https://doi.org/10.1038/s41588-017-0011-x.

182 Akbari, P., Gilani, A., Sosina, O. et al. (2021). Sequencing of 640 000 exomes identifies *GPR75* variants associated with protection from obesity. *Science* 373: 373. https://doi.org/10.1126/science.abf8683.

183 Kizilkaya, H.S., Sørensen, K.V., Kibsgaard, C.J. et al. (2021). Loss of function glucose-dependent insulinotropic polypeptide receptor variants are associated with alterations in BMI, bone strength and cardiovascular outcomes [internet]. *Front. Cell Dev. Biol.* 9: 749607. https://doi.org/10.3389/fcell.2021.749607.

184 Knop, F.K., Urva, S., Rettiganti, M. et al. (2023). A long-acting glucose-dependent insulinotropic polypeptide receptor agonist improves gastrointestinal tolerability of glucagon-like peptide 1 receptor agonist therapy – Media Centre | EASD [internet]. EASD 2023 Hambg Ger. https://www.easd.org/media-centre/home.html%20#!resources/a-long-acting-glucose-dependent-insulinotropic-polypeptide-receptor-agonist-improves-gastrointestinal-tolerability-of-glucagon-like-peptide-1-receptor-agonist-therapy-665f341f-3438-4504-8e74-73bff825d3e9 (cited 8 September 2024; accessed 8 September 2024).

185 Beaudry, J.L., Kaur, K.D., Varin, E.M. et al. (2019). Physiological roles of the GIP receptor in murine brown adipose tissue. *Mol. Metab.* 28: 14–25. https://doi.org/10.1016/j.molmet.2019.08.006.

186 Koffert, J., Honka, H., Teuho, J. et al. (2017). Effects of meal and incretins in the regulation of splanchnic blood flow. *Endocr. Connect.* 6: 179–187. https://doi.org/10.1530/EC-17-0015.

187 Rasmussen, R.S., Langberg, L.S., Østergaard, F. et al. (2025). Glucose-dependent insulinotropic polypeptide is involved in postprandial regulation of splanchnic blood supply. *Diabetes* 74: 1355–1366. https://doi.org/10.2337/db25-0149.

188 Nitz, I., Fisher, E., Weikert, C. et al. (2007). Association analyses of GIP and GIPR polymorphisms with traits of the metabolic syndrome. *Mol. Nutr. Food Res.* 51: 1046–1052. https://doi.org/10.1002/mnfr.200700048.

189 Ussher, J.R., Campbell, J.E., Mulvihill, E.E. et al. (2018). Inactivation of the glucose-dependent insulinotropic polypeptide receptor improves outcomes following experimental myocardial infarction. *Cell Metab.* 27: 450–460.e6. https://doi.org/10.1016/j.cmet.2017.11.003.

190 Pujadas, G., Baggio, L.L., Kaur, K.D. et al. (2022). Genetic disruption of the Gipr in Apoe−/− mice promotes atherosclerosis. *Mol. Metab.* 65: 101586. https://doi.org/10.1016/j.molmet.2022.101586.

191 Diemar, S.S., Dahl, S.S., West, A.S. et al. (2023). A Systematic review of the circadian rhythm of bone markers in blood. *Calcif. Tissue Int.* 112: 126–147. https://doi.org/10.1007/s00223-022-00965-1.

192 Allen, M.R. (2017). Preclinical models for skeletal research: how commonly used species mimic (or don't) aspects of human bone. *Toxicol. Pathol.* 45: 851–854. https://doi.org/10.1177/0192623317733925.

193 Bollag, R.J., Zhong, Q., Ding, K.H. et al. (2001). Glucose-dependent insulinotropic peptide is an integrative hormone with osteotropic effects. *Mol. Cell. Endocrinol.* 177: 35–41. https://doi.org/10.1016/s0303-7207(01)00405-1.

194 Bergmann, N.C., Lund, A., Gasbjerg, L.S. et al. (2019). Separate and combined effects of GIP and GLP-1 infusions on bone metabolism in overweight men without diabetes. *J. Clin. Endocrinol. Metab.* 104: 2953–2960. https://doi.org/10.1210/jc.2019-00008.

195 Hansen, M.S., Søe, K., Christensen, L.L. et al. (2023). GIP reduces osteoclast activity and improves osteoblast survival in primary human bone cells. *Eur. J. Endocrinol.* 188: 144–157. https://doi.org/10.1093/ejendo/lvac004.

196 Torekov, S.S., Harsløf, T., Rejnmark, L. et al. (2014). A functional amino acid substitution in the glucose-dependent insulinotropic polypeptide receptor

(GIPR) gene is associated with lower bone mineral density and increased fracture risk. *J. Clin. Endocrinol. Metab.* 99: E729–E733. https://doi.org/10.1210/jc.2013-3766.

197 Gasbjerg, L.S., Rosenkilde, M.M., Meier, J.J. et al. (2023). The importance of glucose-dependent insulinotropic polypeptide receptor activation for the effects of tirzepatide. *Diabetes. Obes. Metab.* 25: 3079–3092. https://doi.org/10.1111/dom.15216.

198 Trapp, S. and Brierley, D.I. (2022). Brain GLP-1 and the regulation of food intake: GLP-1 action in the brain and its implications for GLP-1 receptor agonists in obesity treatment. *Br. J. Pharmacol.* 179: 557–570. https://doi.org/10.1111/bph.15638.

199 Usdin, T.B., Mezey, E., Button, D.C. et al. (1993). Gastric inhibitory polypeptide receptor, a member of the secretin-vasoactive intestinal peptide receptor family, is widely distributed in peripheral organs and the brain. *Endocrinology* 133: 2861–2870. https://doi.org/10.1210/endo.133.6.8243312.

200 Ludwig, M.Q., Todorov, P.V., Egerod, K.L. et al. (2021). Single-cell mapping of GLP-1 and GIP receptor expression in the dorsal vagal complex. *Diabetes* 70: 1945–1955. https://doi.org/10.2337/dbi21-0003.

201 Smith, C., Patterson-Cross, R., Woodward, O. et al. (2022). A comparative transcriptomic analysis of glucagon-like peptide-1 receptor- and glucose-dependent insulinotropic polypeptide receptor-expressing cells in the hypothalamus. *Appetite* 174: 106022. https://doi.org/10.1016/j.appet.2022.106022.

202 Liskiewicz, A. and Müller, T.D. (2024). Regulation of energy metabolism through central GIPR signaling. *Peptides* 176: 171198. https://doi.org/10.1016/j.peptides.2024.171198.

203 Samms, R.J., Cosgrove, R., Snider, B.M. et al. (2022). GIPR agonism inhibits PYY-induced Nausea-Like Behavior. *Diabetes* 71: 1410–1423. https://doi.org/10.2337/db21-0848.

204 Ludwig, M.Q., Cheng, W., Gordian, D. et al. (2021). A genetic map of the mouse dorsal vagal complex and its role in obesity. *Nat. Metab.* 3: 530–545. https://doi.org/10.1038/s42255-021-00363-1.

205 Porter, D.W., Irwin, N., Flatt, P.R. et al. (2011). Prolonged GIP receptor activation improves cognitive function, hippocampal synaptic plasticity and glucose homeostasis in high-fat fed mice. *Eur. J. Pharmacol.* 650: 688–693. https://doi.org/10.1016/j.ejphar.2010.10.059.

206 Zhang, Q., Delessa, C.T., Augustin, R. et al. (2021). The glucose-dependent insulinotropic polypeptide (GIP) regulates body weight and food intake via CNS-GIPR signaling. *Cell. Metab.* 33: 833–844.e5. https://doi.org/10.1016/j.cmet.2021.01.015.

207 Szalowska, E., Meijer, K., Kloosterhuis, N. et al. (2011). Sub-chronic administration of stable GIP analog in mice decreases serum LPL activity and body weight. *Peptides* 32: 938–945. https://doi.org/10.1016/j.peptides.2011.02.011.

208 Finan, B., Yang, B., Ottaway, N. et al. (2015). A rationally designed monomeric peptide triagonist corrects obesity and diabetes in rodents. *Nat. Med.* 21: 27–36. https://doi.org/10.1038/nm.3761.

209 Nørregaard, P.K., Deryabina, M.A., Tofteng Shelton, P. et al. (2018). A novel GIP analogue, ZP4165, enhances glucagon-like peptide-1-induced body weight loss and improves glycaemic control in rodents. *Diabetes. Obes. Metab.* 20: 60–68. https://doi.org/10.1111/dom.13034.

210 Borner, T., Reiner, B.C., Crist, R.C. et al. (2023). GIP receptor agonism blocks chemotherapy-induced nausea and vomiting. *Mol. Metab.* 73: 101743. https://doi.org/10.1016/j.molmet.2023.101743.

211 Liskiewicz, A., Khalil, A., Liskiewicz, D. et al. (2023). Glucose-dependent insulinotropic polypeptide regulates body weight and food intake via GABAergic neurons in mice. *Nat. Metab.* 5: 2075–2085. https://doi.org/10.1038/s42255-023-00931-7.

212 Gutgesell, R.M., Khalil, A., Liskiewicz, A. et al. (2025). GIPR agonism and antagonism decrease body weight and food intake via different mechanisms in male mice. *Nat. Metab.* 7: 1282–1298. https://doi.org/10.1038/s42255-025-01294-x.

213 Liu, C.M., Killion, E.A., Hammoud, R. et al. (2025). GIPR-Ab/GLP-1 peptide–antibody conjugate requires brain GIPR and GLP-1R for additive weight loss in obese mice. *Nat. Metab.* 7: 1266–1281. https://doi.org/10.1038/s42255-025-01295-w.

214 Novo Nordisk A/S (2025). Investigation of the safety and efficacy of semaglutide s.c. in combination with NNC0480–0389 in participants with type 2 diabetes – a dose finding study [internet]. clinicaltrials.gov. https://clinicaltrials.gov/study/NCT05144984 (cited 23 January 2026; accessed 23 January 2026).

215 Novo Nordisk A/S NNC0480–0389 and semaglutide in diabetes mellitus, type 2 – clinical trials registry – ICH GCP [internet]. https://ichgcp.net/clinical-trials-registry/NCT05144984 (cited 23 January 2026; accessed 23 January 2026).

216 Roell, W., Alsina-Fernandez, J., Qu, H. et al. (2026). Long-acting GIPR agonist LY3537021 reduces body weight and fasting blood glucose in patients with T2D: preclinical development and phase 1 randomized ascending dose studies. *Mol. Metab.* 103: 102298. https://doi.org/10.1016/j.molmet.2025.102298.

217 Knop, F.K., Urva, S., Rettiganti, M. et al. (2023). 56-OR: a long-acting glucose-dependent insulinotropic polypeptide receptor agonist shows weight loss without nausea or vomiting. *Diabetes* 72: 56 OR. https://doi.org/10.2337/db23-56-OR.

218 Eli Lilly and Company (2026). A study to evaluate LY3537021 for the treatment of nausea and vomiting caused by chemotherapy in adults with cancer [internet]. https://ichgcp.net/clinical-trials-registry/NCT07169851 (cited 6 January 2026; accessed 6 January 2026).

219 Zealand Pharma ZP6590 2026 [internet]. https://www.zealandpharma.com/pipeline/zp6590/ (cited 23 January 2026; accessed 23 January 2026).

220 Chuang, M.-H., Chen, J.-Y., Wang, H.-Y. et al. (2024). Clinical outcomes of tirzepatide or GLP-1 receptor agonists in individuals with type 2 diabetes. *JAMA Netw. Open* 7: e2427258. https://doi.org/10.1001/jamanetworkopen.2024.27258.

221 Lillys-Tirzepatide Lilly's tirzepatide reduced the risk of worsening heart failure events by 38% in adults with heart failure with preserved ejection fraction (HFpEF) and obesity | Eli Lilly and Company [internet]. https://investor.lilly.com/news-releases/news-release-details/lillys-tirzepatide-reduced-risk-worsening-heart-failure-events (cited 23 January 2026; accessed 23 January 2026).

222 AMGEN (2026). Results from Amgen's phase 2 obesity study of monthly maritide presented at the American Diabetes Association 85th Scientific Sessions [internet]. https://www.amgen.com/newsroom/press-releases/2025/06/results-from-amgens-phase-2-obesity-study-of-monthly-maritide-presented-at-the-american-diabetes-association-85th-scientific-sessions.

223 AMGEN Inside Amgen's phase 3 MARITIME program: advancing the future of obesity care [internet]. https://www.amgen.com/stories/2025/06/inside-amgens-phase-3-maritime-program---advancing-the-future-of-obesity-care (cited 23 January 2026; accessed 23 January 2026).

224 Carmot Therapeutics, Inc A randomized, double-blind, placebo-controlled, parallel-group, multi-center phase 2 study to evaluate the efficacy, safety, and tolerability of once-weekly CT-388 administered subcutaneously for 48 weeks to participants who are overweight or obese with type 2 diabetes mellitus [internet]. clinicaltrials.gov. January 2026. Report No.: NCT06628362. https://clinicaltrials.gov/study/NCT06628362 (accessed 23 January 2026).

225 Carmot Therapeutics, Inc A phase 2, double-blind, randomized, placebo-controlled study to evaluate the efficacy, safety, tolerability, and pharmacokinetics of CT-868 administered for 16 weeks to overweight and obese adult participants with type 1 diabetes mellitus [internet]. clinicaltrials.gov. July 2025. Report No.: NCT06062069. https://clinicaltrials.gov/study/NCT06062069 (accessed 23 January 2026).

226 Viking Therapeutics VK2735 [internet]. https://vikingtherapeutics.com/pipeline/metabolic-disease-program/vk2735/ (cited 16 August 2024; accessed 16 August 2024).

227 Viking Therapeutics InvestorRoom Viking therapeutics announces publication of results from phase 2 VENTURE trial of dual GLP-1/GIP receptor agonist VK2735 in the journal obesity [internet]. https://ir.vikingtherapeutics.com/2026-2101-2112-Viking-Therapeutics-Announces-Publication-of-Results-from-Phase-2-VENTURE-Trial-of-Dual-GLP-1-GIP-Receptor-Agonist-VK2735-in-the-Journal-Obesity (cited 23 January 2026; accessed 23 January 2026).

228 SCOHIA PHARMA Inc SCO-094 [internet]. https://www.scohia.com/sco-094/ (cited 23 January 2026; accessed 23 January 2026).

229 Health Research Authority Safety, tolerability, PK and PD of SCO-094 in type 2 diabetic patients [internet]. https://www.hra.nhs.uk/planning-and-improving-research/application-summaries/research-summaries/safety-tolerability-pk-and-pd-of-sco-094-in-type-2-diabetic-patients/ (cited 23 January 2026; accessed 23 January 2026).

230 Rosenstock, J., Frias, J., Jastreboff, A.M. et al. (2023). Retatrutide, a GIP, GLP-1 and glucagon receptor agonist, for people with type 2 diabetes: a randomised, double-blind, placebo and active-controlled, parallel-group, phase 2 trial conducted in the USA. *Lancet* 402: 529–544. https://doi.org/10.1016/S0140-6736(23)01053-X.

231 Lilly, E. A study of retatrutide (LY3437943) once weekly in participants who have obesity or overweight and osteoarthritis of the knee (TRIUMPH-4) [internet]. Lilly Trials. https://trials.lilly.com/en-US/trial/408355 (cited 24 September 2024; accessed 24 September 2024).

232 Lilly, E. A study of retatrutide (LY3437943) in participants with obesity and cardiovascular disease (TRIUMPH-3) [internet]. Lilly Trials. https://trials.lilly.com/en-US/trial/405675 (cited 24 September 2024; accessed 24 September 2024).

233 Lilly, E. A study of retatrutide (LY3437943) on renal function in participants with overweight or obesity and chronic kidney disease with or without type 2 diabetes [internet]. Lilly Trials. https://trials.lilly.com/en-US/trial/410437 (cited 24 September 2024; accessed 24 September 2024).

234 Abdelmalek, M.F., Suzuki, A., Sanchez, W. et al. (2023). A phase 2, adaptive randomized, double-blind, placebo-controlled, multicenter, 52-week study of HM15211 in patients with biopsy-confirmed non-alcoholic steatohepatitis – study design and rationale of HM-TRIA-201 study. *Contemp. Clin. Trials* 130: 107176. https://doi.org/10.1016/j.cct.2023.107176.

235 Hanmi Hanmi | Hanmi Pharmaceutical's official site [internet]. https://www.hanmipharm.com/main.hm (cited 23 January 2026; accessed 23 January 2026).

236 Novo Nordisk (2023). Financial report for 1 January 2023 to 31 March 2023. pp. 1–29.

237 Novo Nordisk A/S En forskningsundersøgelse, der ser på, hvor godt en kombination af lægemidlerne semaglutid og NNC0480–0389 virker hos mennesker med type 2-diabetes [internet]. https://ichgcp.net/da/clinical-trials-registry/NCT05144984 (cited 6 January 2026; accessed 6 January 2026).

238 Douros, J.D., Flak, J.N., and Knerr, P.J. (2025). The agony and the efficacy: central mechanisms of GLP-1 induced adverse events and their mitigation by GIP. *Front. Endocrinol.* 16: 1530985. https://doi.org/10.3389/fendo.2025.1530985.

239 Melson, E., Ashraf, U., Papamargaritis, D., and Davies, M.J. (2024). What is the pipeline for future medications for obesity? *Int. J. Obes.* 1–19. https://doi.org/10.1038/s41366-024-01473-y.

240 Ala, M., Mohammad Jafari, R., Dehpour, A.R., and Poursalehian, M. (2024). Tirzepatide outcompetes long-acting insulin in managing type 2 diabetes: a meta-analysis of three phase 3 randomized controlled trials. *Int. J. Obes.* 1–12. https://doi.org/10.1038/s41366-024-01621-4.

241 Aronne, L.J., Horn, D.B., Le Roux, C.W. et al. (2025). Tirzepatide as compared with semaglutide for the treatment of obesity. *N. Engl. J. Med.* 393: 26–36. https://doi.org/10.1056/NEJMoa2416394.

242 Wharton, S., Freitas, P., Hjelmesæth, J. et al. (2025). Once-weekly semaglutide 7·2 mg in adults with obesity (STEP UP): a randomised, controlled, phase 3b trial. *Lancet Diabetes Endocrinol.* 13: 949–963. https://doi.org/10.1016/S2213-8587(25)00226-8.

243 Chakravarthy, M., Argüelles-Tello, F.A., Sun, A.L.A. et al. (2023). 75-LB: CT-388, a novel once-weekly dual GLP-1 and GIP receptor modulator, is safe, well-tolerated, and produces more than 8% weight loss in four weeks in overweight and obese adults. *Diabetes* 72: 75 LB. https://doi.org/10.2337/db23-75-LB.

244 Coskun, T., Urva, S., Roell, W.C. et al. (2022). LY3437943, a novel triple glucagon, GIP, and GLP-1 receptor agonist for glycemic control and weight loss: from discovery to clinical proof of concept. *Cell Metab.* 34: 1234–1247.e9. https://doi.org/10.1016/j.cmet.2022.07.013.

245 Jastreboff, A.M., Kaplan, L.M., Frías, J.P. et al. (2023). Triple–hormone-receptor agonist retatrutide for obesity – a phase 2 trial. *N. Engl. J. Med. Massachusetts Medical Society* 389: 514–526. https://doi.org/10.1056/NEJMoa2301972.

246 Rondinone, C.M., Valdecantos, M.P., Rada, P., et al. Novel unimolecular tetra-agonist peptides targeting GLP-1, GIP, amylin, and calcitonin receptors with enhanced metabolic benefits in animal models of obesity [internet]. *EASD 2024*, Madrid Spain. https://cattendee.abstractsonline.com/meeting/20620/presentation/1841.

247 Gault, V.A., O'Harte, F.P.M., Harriott, P., and Flatt, P.R. (2002). Characterization of the cellular and metabolic effects of a novel enzyme-resistant antagonist of glucose-dependent insulinotropic polypeptide. *Biochem. Biophys. Res. Commun.* 290: 1420–1426. https://doi.org/10.1006/bbrc.2002.6364.

248 Gault, V.A., O'Harte, F.P.M., Harriott, P. et al. (2003). Effects of the novel (Pro3)GIP antagonist and exendin(9–39)amide on GIP- and GLP-1-induced cyclic AMP generation, insulin secretion and postprandial insulin release in obese diabetic (ob/ob) mice: evidence that GIP is the major physiological incretin. *Diabetologia* 46: 222–230. https://doi.org/10.1007/s00125-002-1028-x.

249 McClean, P.L., Irwin, N., Cassidy, R.S. et al. (2007). GIP receptor antagonism reverses obesity, insulin resistance, and associated metabolic disturbances induced in mice by prolonged consumption of high-fat diet. *Am. J. Physiol. Endocrinol. Metab.* 293: E1746–E1755. https://doi.org/10.1152/ajpendo.00460.2007.

250 Irwin, N., McClean, P.L., O'Harte, F.P.M. et al. (2007). Early administration of the glucose-dependent insulinotropic polypeptide receptor antagonist (Pro3)GIP prevents the development of diabetes and related metabolic abnormalities associated with genetically inherited obesity in ob/ob mice. *Diabetologia* 50: 1532–1540. https://doi.org/10.1007/s00125-007-0692-2.

251 Gasbjerg, L.S., Gabe, M.B.N., Hartmann, B. et al. (2018). Glucose-dependent insulinotropic polypeptide (GIP) receptor antagonists as anti-diabetic agents. *Peptides* 100: 173–181. https://doi.org/10.1016/J.PEPTIDES.2017.11.021.

252 Boer, G.A., Hunt, J.E., Gabe, M.B.N. et al. (2022). Glucose-dependent insulinotropic polypeptide receptor antagonist treatment causes a reduction in weight gain in ovariectomised high fat diet-fed mice. *Br. J. Pharmacol.* 179: 4486–4499. https://doi.org/10.1111/bph.15894.

253 Svendsen, B., Capozzi, M.E., Nui, J. et al. (2020). Pharmacological antagonism of the incretin system protects against diet-induced obesity. *Mol. Metab.* 32: 44–55. https://doi.org/10.1016/j.molmet.2019.11.018.

254 Lu, S.-C., Chen, M., Atangan, L. et al. (2021). GIPR antagonist antibodies conjugated to GLP-1 peptide are bispecific molecules that decrease weight in obese mice and monkeys. *Cell Rep. Med.* 2: 100263. https://doi.org/10.1016/j.xcrm.2021.100263.

255 Oduori, O.S., Murao, N., Shimomura, K. et al. (2020). Gs/Gq signaling switch in β cells defines incretin effectiveness in diabetes. *J. Clin. Invest.* 130: 6639–6655. https://doi.org/10.1172/JCI140046.

256 Wang, Y., Yang, D., and Wang, M. (2022). Signaling profiles in HEK 293T cells co-expressing GLP-1 and GIP receptors. *Acta Pharmacol. Sin.* 43: 1453–1460. https://doi.org/10.1038/S41401-021-00758-6.

257 Roed, S.N., Nøhr, A.C., Wismann, P. et al. (2014). Functional consequences of glucagon-like peptide-1 receptor cross-talk and trafficking. *J. Biol. Chem.* 290 (2): 1233–1243. https://doi.org/10.1074/jbc.M114.592436.

3

Amylin – Biological Aspects

Thomas A. Lutz

University of Zurich, Institute of Veterinary Physiology, Winterthurerstrasse 260, Zurich, CH 8057, Switzerland

Introduction

Amylin is a member of the calcitonin family of peptides which also includes calcitonin, calcitonin gene-related peptide (CGRP), and adrenomedullin [1]. Amylin (also called islet amyloid polypeptide, IAPP) was originally discovered as the main constituent of pancreatic islet amyloid deposits in type 2 diabetics in primates including humans and in diabetic cats [2–7]. Different from this pathophysiologically important aspect [8], amylin is a physiologically relevant circulating peptide hormone. The main source of circulating amylin is the pancreatic beta-cell where it is cosynthesized with insulin and from where it is cosecreted with insulin [1]. Amylin has been known to reduce food intake for many years [9–13], but amylin also exerts additional functions in the control of energy homeostasis, e.g., by affecting food reward [14–18] and by sensitizing the brain to the catabolic actions of leptin [19–24]. All established metabolic effects of amylin seem to be mediated directly by the central nervous system, in particular via the area postrema (AP) in the caudal hindbrain [25]. However, in particular the sensitizing effect of amylin on leptin action may also depend on a direct interaction in the hypothalamus [21, 23], and a direct effect of amylin on reward mediating pathways has been proposed [17, 26, 27].

Amylin Synthesis and Secretion

Amylin had originally been discovered as the main constituent of pancreatic islet amyloid deposits isolated from patients with type 2 diabetes (T2D) and in diabetic cats [2, 3, 5]. In these species, amylin (because part of the amino acid sequence differs from nonaggregating amylin forms) has the propensity to aggregate into oligomers and eventually mature amyloid fibrils under certain pathophysiological conditions, and this aggregation probably plays an important pathophysiological role in T2D [28].

Monomeric and metabolically active amylin is mainly released by pancreatic beta-cells from where it is coreleased with insulin in response to food intake [29]. Postprandial concentrations (15–25 pmol/l) are approx. three to five times higher than fasting levels in rats (3–5 pmol/l) [30, 31]. Other neuroendocrine cells along the gastrointestinal tract are known to produce amylin but their contribution to meal-induced changes in circulating amylin is probably minimal [32–34].

Different Molecular Forms of Amylin

Similar to other bioactive peptides, the mature 37-amino acid amylin peptide is derived from a larger precursor peptide that results in various cellular products. Starting with a pre-pro form of amylin, initial cleavage of human amylin leads to a 67-residue pro-amylin that is further processed to pro-amylin(1-51) and pro-amylin(1-48), and finally to the mature 37-amino acid peptide amylin(1-37) [35]. Processing of human amylin is of particular interest because of its propensity to form oligomers and amyloid fibrils resulting in beta-cell damage [6, 8, 28, 36–40]. We currently know very little about the circulating concentrations of amylin forms other than the mature 37-amino acid peptide, but a recent study indicated that longer molecular forms of amylin, such as pro-amylin(1-48), may also have biological activity [41]. These two latter aspects will be discussed later in this review.

Amylin Signaling at the Amylin Receptor

Amylin receptors are heterodimers of the core receptor, the calcitonin receptor (CTR), and one (or several) receptor activity modifying proteins (RAMP) coexpressed in the same cell [33, 42, 43]. The CTR has various splice variants; the variant $CT_{(a)}$ is the best characterized and most likely mediates the known amylin actions, but knowledge on the physiological relevance of other variants is scarce [44]. RAMP expression changes receptor specificity and enhances the binding and potency of amylin so that physiological amylin concentrations in the picomolar range are able to activate the receptor [43, 45–49]. With the three RAMPs defined so far, the current understanding is that the amylin receptors 1–3 (AMY1–3) mediate amylin's biological actions. However, neurons in brain areas relevant to mediate the metabolic effects of amylin often seem to express more than one RAMP together with CTR [50, 51], potentially resulting in the generation of even more amylin receptor subtypes [33, 43, 44]. More research is necessary to define whether hetero "multi" mers of the CTR and more than one RAMP are physiologically relevant.

Amylin Receptor Activation and Intracellular Signaling

Activation of amylin receptors triggers several intracellular signaling systems. In transfected cells, this allowed the characterization of AMY-specific agonists (e.g., amylin, pramlintide, NN1213 [52, 53]) compared to less specific dual AMY and CTR-activating agonists (e.g., salmon calcitonin [sCT], cagrilintide, KBP-042 or -89, etc.), the so-called DACRAs (dual amylin calcitonin receptor agonists) [54–56]. Our understanding of the role of the different intracellular signals in mediating the physiological effects of amylin is still rudimentary but there is some evidence that intracellular cGMP and the activation of the extracellular-signal regulated kinase 1 and 2 pathways are linked to amylin's satiating effect [57, 58].

A recently developed technique to directly assess receptor activation confirmed that sCT has a higher potency than amylin at the CTR [59]. Interestingly, at the AMY1, sCT appeared to be a weaker agonist and had a lower maximal effect than amylin, but CGRP, which is a widespread neurotransmitter across the brain, was similarly potent to amylin, and the potency was much higher than at the CTR. This confirms that the AMY1 also acts as the "second" CGRP receptor [44]. Amylin and CGRP had a similar potency to sCT at the AMY2 receptor, but the maximal effect was higher for sCT. The same was true for sCT at the AMY3 [59]. Such results may help for the future development of receptor subtype-specific agonists (or antagonists), and they may also help us to better understand the specific roles and actions mediated by the different receptor subtypes [60].

Amylin's Effect on Energy Homeostasis

Amylin Effects on Eating; Induction of Satiation

The effect of amylin to inhibit eating was one of the first amylin actions identified after its discovery [9, 11], and it remains the effect that is best identified for its physiological relevance. Amylin's eating-inhibitory effect seems to rely mainly on a reduction in meal size, i.e., enhanced satiation [34, 61, 62]. Amylin dose-dependently reduces meal size and duration, and administration of an amylin antagonist increases meal size [58].

Data on the induction of satiety and hence an effect on the intermetal interval are less clear [63, 64]. It seems plausible that the long-acting amylin analogs like cagrilintide and others [55, 65–67] may also decrease eating via a satiety effect, but the findings that sCT that seems to activate the AMY receptor even longer than cagrilintide [55], also mainly affects meal size [68, 69], do not support this idea. Hence, increased satiation, i.e., a reduced average meal size which is not compensated by increased meal frequency, seems to be the major factor for amylin's overall effect to reduce eating. This effect combines with slowed gastric emptying and reduced pancreatic glucagon secretion to control nutrient fluxes [70].

An important feature of physiological satiation signals is that they specifically reduce eating without inducing visceral illness [62]. Amylin seems to fulfill this criterion [13, 71–75], which is different from glucagon-like peptide 1 (GLP-1) and its analogs [76] or cholecystokinin which may also cause aversion at high CCK doses [77]. A full understanding of the exact modes of action is important because the brain pathways that are affected by eating controls typically overlap significantly [78, 79], and these pathways are also involved in mediating aversive effects [80, 81].

Indeed, recent experiments confirmed that amylin reduces eating without signs of avoidance or aversion, but that sCT also activates aversive pathways [82]. The reason for this behavioral difference between amylin and sCT remains unclear. It may be due to the lower specificity of sCT versus amylin for signaling at AMY versus CTR [44, 54, 55, 83]; in other words, specific activation of the AMY may have a low propensity for the induction of avoidance and aversion. However, given the widespread distribution of the CTR and RAMPs across the brain, another potential explanation is that sCT may reach different receptor populations in the brain compared to amylin, and that some of these additional action sites may also engage aversive pathways [84]. Such a site-specific mechanism was recently shown for GLP-1 action [85]; this paper convincingly showed that activation of GLP-1 receptor neurons in the AP may induce aversion while activation of GLP-1 receptor neurons in the nucleus of the solitary tract (NTS) reduced eating without signs of aversion. This said, I do not want to postulate that amylin action in the AP has an aversive component; there is no indication for this, and I just want to point out the general importance to study site-specific effects for each of these signals. Please see the section titled "Caudal Hindbrain with the AP and the NTS" for further discussion. A third potential explanation for the different propensity to induce aversion by sCT but not amylin could lie in a specific characteristic of sCT when binding to AMY and CTR; sCT has a very slow off-rate at the respective receptors. In other words, once bound, sCT seems to bind to the receptor for extended periods of time, leading to a long-lasting activation [55, 69]; such neuronal "overstimulation" may potentially lead to side-effects that are not seen with receptor ligands showing more physiological on- and off-rates, like amylin.

It will be important in the future to distinguish among these possibilities, and to investigate whether the difference between nonaversive and aversive amylin receptor agonists lies in the activation of different pathways or in the way how receptors or specific pathways are influenced.

Amylin Effects on Energy Expenditure

Various studies investigated the effect of amylin receptor activation on energy expenditure. Based on experiments indicating that chronic amylin administration reduced body adiposity more than in rats pair-fed to amylin-treated rats, it was later shown that amylin indeed increases energy expenditure [74, 86–88], most likely by a central effect in the AP [89, 90]. At least in mice, the effect on energy expenditure involved an activation of brown adipose tissue activity and an upregulation of the major thermogenic protein uncoupling protein-1 via the sympathetic nervous system ([91, 92]; but see: [64, 86] for rats). Interestingly, transgenic mice overexpressing the RAMP1 component of the AMY1 receptor in the brain had an exaggerated effect of amylin on energy expenditure. This was associated with a leaner phenotype, increased energy expenditure, and higher body temperature. Despite the clear evidence that exogenous amylin affects energy expenditure, the physiological relevance of the effect and the contribution of the effect to total energy balance over extended treatment periods with amylin has so far not been substantiated.

Sex Differences in Amylin Action

Preclinical experiments revealed no striking sex-dependent differences in amylin's acute or chronic effects on eating and body weight [22, 86, 93, 94]. But interestingly, the interaction of amylin and other controls of eating appeared to be at least in part sex-dependent. In male but not female amylin-deficient mice, the response to exogenous leptin vanished after weeks of treatment [21] while melanocortin-4 receptor agonists reduced eating more in male than in female amylin-deficient mice [95].

Only few studies looked into the specific question whether the action of amylin may differ across the sexual cycle or in relation to the presence or absence of female sex hormones [96, 97]. Chronic amylin administration reduced eating and body weight more in ovariectomized rats, also resulting in a stronger decrease in body adiposity. The effects were reversed in estradiol-replaced females. Surprisingly, an acute single injection of amylin was less effective in ovariectomized female rats, and this effect was restored by estradiol replacement; hence, just the opposite compared to chronic amylin administration. Further, the effect of the amylin antagonist AC187 to increase eating was also stronger in estradiol-replaced rats [97]. The reasons for the apparent opposing role of estradiol in acute versus chronic amylin action have not yet been investigated; importantly, the eating-inhibitory effects of acute versus chronic amylin administration seem to be mediated by the same brain structures [68, 98]. Estradiol is known to increase the expression of the amylin receptor component RAMP3 [99]; whether this effect explains the increased effectiveness of acute amylin on eating in E2-replaced ovariectomized rats, and whether the effect might be different during chronic amylin stimulation, is currently unknown.

Brain Sites of Amylin Action

Caudal Hindbrain with the AP and the NTS

Amylin has been shown to be able to cross the blood-brain barrier [100, 101], but most available data indicate that the most relevant direct brain targets for amylin seem to lie in circumventricular organs which are not protected by the blood-brain barrier. This also seems to be true for amylin analogs like sCT or cagrilintide that mainly reach circumventricular organs when injected peripherally in rats [102, 103].

Of the circumventricular organs, the caudal hindbrain AP in particular plays a critical and necessary role for the direct mediation of peripheral amylin's effects; as a structural requisite, the AP has a high density of amylin receptors, and all critical amylin receptor components are expressed in single AP neurons [12, 50, 75, 98, 104–110]. A peripheral action of amylin seems unlikely, because a blockade of nerve transmission (vagal and nonvagal) from the periphery to the brain leaves peripheral amylin's effects unaltered [109–112]. Further, the local AP administration of amylin decreased eating while the administration of the amylin antagonist AC187 into the AP increased meal size [58]; lesions of the AP [98], specific deletion of the CTR core receptor in the AP [113], or a specific deletion of noradrenergic AP neurons which mediate amylin's action [114] was shown to block the effect of peripheral amylin on eating. In addition, electrophysiological and imaging experiments confirmed that AP neurons are directly responsive to amylin and probably constitute the direct target of circulating amylin [25, 115].

The AP neurons directly affected by amylin seem to show only some overlap with neurons activated by other stimuli, e.g., by GLP-1, by aversive stimuli (like LiCl) or by stimuli unrelated to ingestive control [116, 117]. A recent study suggested that amylin receptors may also be located on presynaptic terminals, and that glutamate released from these neurons may then act on AP neurons [107]. Further, we also observed a close proximity of amylin-activated neurons with VGLUT2-positive boutons [118]. However, the relevance and necessity for this presynaptic amylin signaling are currently unknown, given the direct effect of peripheral amylin action on AP neurons by a postsynaptic action [119], and because amylin action does not seem to require afferent nerve input from the periphery to the brain [109].

As mentioned, noradrenergic AP neurons seem to mediate at least part of amylin's effects. These neurons project to the NTS and also directly to the lateral parabrachial nucleus (LPBN) [114, 120]; even a partial lesion of these neurons was sufficient to block entirely the anorectic effect induced by a peripheral amylin injection [114, 118].

The CTR is also expressed in NTS neurons albeit at a lower density than in AP neurons [113]. A recent study showed that the selective activation of CTR-positive neurons in the NTS led to a decrease in eating and body weight, while their silencing led to the opposite effects in mice, pointing to the potential physiological relevance of the CTR in NTS neurons for weight control. Further, the deletion of the CTR from these neurons prevented the eating-inhibitory effect of sCT but, surprisingly, did not attenuate conditioned taste avoidance induced by peripheral sCT. Hence, it was postulated that these neurons may participate in mediating the physiological effects of amylin on energy balance but that they may be distinct from aversive pathways [84]. It is unclear at present whether these neurons indeed represent a population of target neurons that are activated separately from the AP and that may mediate the effects of endogenous amylin or potentially also of amylin receptor agonists.

Projections from the AP – Role of the Lateral Parabrachial Nucleus

Activation of AP neurons leads to the subsequent activation of a neural circuitry that projects rostrally to the forebrain and includes the NTS, LPBN, and possibly the central nucleus of the amygdala (CeA). The AP, NTS, and the LPBN all seem to be necessary for peripheral amylin to reduce eating because lesions in the respective brain areas abolished the effect of peripheral amylin on eating [25, 121, 122], and tract-tracing studies confirmed the structural presence of these projections [123].

When amylin is administered to animals with a chemotoxic lesion of the LPBN, an activation of AP neurons (gauged by cos expression) is still present, but this lesion blocked peripheral amylin's ability to reduce eating [121]. Hence, the projection from primarily activated AP neurons to the LPBN seems necessary for peripheral amylin to reduce eating. Part of the amylin-activated LPBN neurons express the neurotransmitter CGRP [124], which project to the CeA [125] and other brain areas [81, 124]. Despite the established role of CGRP neurons for the control of meal-ending satiation [81] and in meal-size control under normal conditions [81] but also in certain disease states [80, 126], it was not clear until recently whether CGRP is actually the critical neurotransmitter released from these neurons.

This is of particular interest in the context of amylin because the AMY1 receptor also acts as the second CGRP receptor [44]. Hence, it seemed plausible that CGRP-eric projections from LPBN neurons may mediate the effects of peripheral amylin in other brain areas. This could potentially be the structural correlate to the findings that local administration of amylin receptor antagonists (which are unable to distinguish between the different amylin receptor subtypes [33, 43, 44]) into various brain regions was able to block peripheral amylin's or sCT's effects (e.g., [15–17, 27, 127]). This could also mean that peripheral amylin does not necessarily have to reach some receptor sites after crossing the blood-brain barrier [100, 101] because the endogenous ligand of these AMY1-carrying neurons may actually be neuron-derived CGRP (potentially from LPBN neurons).

In an attempt to investigate the role of CGRP-eric LPBN neurons, we recently reported that noradrenergic depletion specifically reduced CGRP neural activation mediated by peripheral amylin, and that NA depletion did not reduce the activation of other non-CGRP expressing neurons activated by amylin [120]. Surprisingly, a later study showed that the acute or permanent inhibition of LPBN CGRP neurons had no effect on amylin's eating-inhibitory effect, but it did reduce sCT's effects in mice [82]. Further, knocking down CGRP expression in these neurons had no influence on the eating effect of neither amylin nor sCT in rats. More importantly, only sCT, but not amylin, reduced eating at least in part via triggering an aversive response, coupled with nausea and emesis, and these effects of sCT appeared to be mediated by CGRP-eric LPBN neurons in mice [82]. However, because knocking down CGRP expression in these LPBN neurons did not ablate sCT's effect on taste avoidance in rats, other neurotransmitters released from these neurons may be more relevant.

The potential specific role of CTR-expressing neurons in the NTS has been discussed earlier [84]. Interestingly, the latter study indicated that these neurons, which can be activated by sCT, project to non-CGRP neurons in the LPBN and may not be involved in mediating aversive pathways in mice. Future work will therefore have to define in detail the exact role of amylin-activated AP versus NTS neurons that project to the LPBN; potential species differences between mice and rats may also have to be considered.

Single Cell Studies to Define the Phenotype of Caudal Hindbrain Neurons Involved in Amylin Action

Based on the above-mentioned discussion, the exact nature of LPBN neurons mediating amylin's eating inhibitory (and probably weight-lowering) effect still remains unclear. Future studies, e.g., using single-cell and spatial transcriptomic analyses may better clarify the mode of action of amylin via this and other brain areas, and help to better differentiate neurons responsible for the mediation of physiological versus aversive effects on eating [117, 128, 129].

Single-cell sequencing studies indicated that amylin-responsive neurons in the AP seem to form a specific neuronal population, e.g., at least in part different from AP neurons being activated by GLP-1 or aversive stimuli like growth differentiation factor 15 (GDF-15); in the NTS, amylin- and GLP-1-sensitive neurons seem to overlap more [116, 117, 128]. Whether it is this population of NTS neurons that mediates the effects of CTR activation by sCT on eating and body weight remains to be investigated [84]; interestingly, the chemogenetic activation of these neurons activates a pathway involving non-CGRP LPBN neurons [84], similar to the amylin-responsive neurons in the AP that project to the LPBN [82]. This again highlights the need for a close characterization of LPBN neurons and their connections; in other words, it remains unclear whether similar to the stimulus-specific activation of certain neuronal populations in the AP [130], there may be selectivity at the level of CGRP-eric and non-CGRP LPBN neurons for their responsiveness to some stimuli. It will be important to define whether and how specific stimuli activate a certain subpopulation of neurons in the LPBN, where they receive input from, and where they project to.

Other Brain Areas Mediating the Actions of Amylin

Amylin binding sites are widely distributed throughout the brain [104], which is supported by the expression of all critical amylin receptor components in many brain areas, including data at the single-cell level [15, 26, 51, 105, 127, 131, 132].

Direct Amylin Action in the Hypothalamus

Soon after its discovery and based on direct amylin administration [11, 133, 134], various papers suggested that amylin may reduce eating by acting via the hypothalamus. At that time, it was not clear whether direct or indirect action through projections originating in the hindbrain [123, 135] would be responsible for the effect.

Since then, studies that peripheral amylin (or its analogs) reduces eating directly via the hypothalamus have still not been reported. Similar to effects in the AP [57], peripheral amylin has been shown to induce the phosphorylation of ERK (p-ERK) in the arcuate (ARC) and ventromedial (VMN) hypothalamic nuclei [93], and most p-ERK was found in proopiomelanocortin (POMC)-expressing neurons. Interestingly, the absence of hypothalamic CTR on POMC neurons resulted in an increase in body weight and ablated the thermogenic effect of sCT administration, but it did not block the acute anorectic effect of amylin [51]. It was also interesting to note that the amylin-induced p-ERK response in the hypothalamus did not require an intact AP, suggesting that amylin acts directly in those nuclei to activate ERK signaling [93]. Hence, the acute satiating effect of amylin may be unrelated to actions of amylin mediated by the activation of hypothalamic neurons, but the latter somehow may be involved in the control of body weight and perhaps amylin's thermogenic response [51]. Future experiments will need to define in detail the exact role and the functional relevance of amylin-activated neurons in the hypothalamus.

The specific effect of amylin-induced p-ERK in POMC, but not neuropeptide Y (NPY) neurons [93], seems to contradict findings that CTR-positive (and hence presumably amylin-sensitive) neurons colocalize with NPY rather than POMC in the ARC [136]. Genetic ablation of the leptin receptor (LepRb) specifically in CTR-positive neurons resulted in hyperphagic obesity, and cells expressing both the CTR and the LepRb receptors appeared to include NPY/AgRP cells, but not POMC-positive cells. Further, labeled sCT directly bound to and was taken up by neurons expressing NPY and Agouti-related peptide (AgRP), but not POMC neurons in the ARC [102]. Finally, amylin has recently been shown to directly suppress AgRP neurons based on a reduction of intracellular calcium signaling [137]. We are currently investigating whether direct action of amylin on AgRP neurons may be responsible for amylin's effect on glucose control [60], in particular to inhibit pancreatic glucagon secretion [138].

Overall, it seems safe to say that at least some effects of peripheral amylin in the hypothalamus seem to be independent of the AP [93]. It will therefore be important to determine whether peripheral amylin will actually be able to reach these sites. Amylin transport across the blood-brain barrier seems possible [100, 101, 139], but it is unknown whether this leads to biologically relevant concentrations at the receptor sites.

Central Reward Processing of Amylin in the Ventral Tegmental Area (VTA), the Nucleus Accumbens (NAc), the Dorsal Tegmental Area, and the Medial Prefrontal Cortex

Obesity results from a combination of causes, but it is well-established that palatable energy-dense food and its overconsumption are major factors [140]. Hence, when considering the overall control of eating, homeostatic and hedonic factors come into play [141]. Palatable foods are considered pleasurable and stimulate brain reward systems independent of their caloric value, which eventually contributes to overeating and ensuing increases in body weight and adiposity. One neurotransmitter system implicated in the rewarding and reinforcing effects of palatable food is the mesolimbic system, consisting of dopaminergic projections from the ventral tegmental area (VTA) to the nucleus accumbens (NAc) and other brain areas.

Amylin seems to affect the reward processing of eating, similar to other satiating hormones [15, 16, 142–144]. When given the choice, amylin-treated rats reduced the preference for high-fat diet relative to low-fat diet [74]. Further, local administration of sCT into the VTA reduced the release of dopamine into the NAc; this effect was counteracted by dopamine receptor activation in the NAc [16], and dopamine receptor antagonists administered into the NAc attenuated the inhibition of eating by sCT given into the VTA [16]. Another brain area implicated in the processing of reward stimuli, the lateral dorsal tegmental area (LDTg), also contains all amylin receptor components, and local amylin or sCT administration into the LDTg reduced eating by a meal-size effect, similar to the AP [13, 127].

Supporting the physiological relevance of these findings, local CTR knockdown in the VTA and the LDTg resulted in increased food intake and body weight gain in high-fat diet-fed rats [16, 17, 127]. However, subsequent studies showed that peripheral sCT also reduced NAc dopamine release [18], and the effect was absent in rats with AP or LPBN lesions [18], indicating that amylin's (or sCT's) effect on the reward system may at least in part be secondary to activation of the caudal hindbrain.

A recent study investigated further processing of reward-driven behaviors beyond the VTA as influenced by amylin [26]. Specifically, the authors tested the role of amylin on the dopaminergic pathway from the VTA to the medial prefrontal cortex (mPFC) to influence impulsive eating and the consumption of palatable foods. The mPFC is involved in the development of binge eating, and because the amylin agonist pramlintide is known to reduce binge-eating episodes in patients [145], this pathway seems of particular interest in amylin physiology. In this study [26], it was shown that intra-VTA administration of amylin reduced eating of a high-fat diet, attenuated the lipid-reward-mediated increase in neuronal activation in mPFC neurons, and reduced impulsive-like food-directed behavior. Further, the administration of dopamine agonists into the mPFC reduced the hyperphagic response to amylin [26].

Amylin's role in influencing reward-related behaviors may not be limited to food. Recent studies have shown that an amylin analog attenuated alcohol-related behaviors in alcohol use disorders and that sCT reduced the self-administration of alcohol. Interestingly, high-alcohol consumers have decreased CTR and increased RAMP1 expression in the NAc, indicating a potential causal role of disturbed amylin signaling in the development of such disorders [146, 147].

Altogether, these data indicate that amylin may influence various aspects of the reward system, probably by reducing VTA-mediated DA release. Important questions remain because it is still unclear whether amylin in fact reaches receptors in reward areas at biologically relevant concentrations after crossing the blood-brain barrier [100, 101]. Even though amylin is able to cross the blood-brain barrier, fluorescently labeled amylin analogs like sCT or cagrilintide seem to mainly reach circumventricular organs when injected peripherally in rats but they did not reach brain areas protected by the blood-brain barrier [102, 103]. Further, it must also be considered that the AMY1 also acts as a receptor for the neurotransmitter CGRP [148]. Hence, it is also plausible that the natural ligand to the CTR receptors in reward areas is not peripheral amylin but potentially locally released CGRP. Future studies will hopefully clarify whether peripheral amylin has single entry points for the mediation of specific actions (e.g., control of meal size, effect on the reward pathways, etc.) or whether these actions depend on the activation of a wider network throughout the brain [27, 149], including brain-endogenous neurotransmitters like CGRP.

Amylin–Leptin Interactions in the Regulation of Energy Homeostasis

Extensive research has been published reporting on the sensitizing action of amylin toward the metabolic effects of leptin. Importantly, a restoration of leptin sensitivity by amylin was also seen in clinical studies because the coadministration of leptin and amylin analogs, metreleptin and pramlintide, produced stronger weight reductions than either analog given alone [19]. The clinical studies have been stopped, not for the lack of efficacy but rather for the generation of neutralizing antibodies against the metreleptin compound.

Nonetheless, the concept of a leptin-sensitizing effect of amylin is of high interest, and a large number of studies shed light on how these two hormones act together. Animals with defective leptin signaling respond less to the administration of sCT [150, 151], and reexpression of leptin receptors in ventromedial hypothalamus (VMH) neurons in generally leptin receptor-deficient mice improved sensitivity to peripheral amylin [152]. Further, it was shown that peripheral amylin increased central leptin action to acutely reduce eating [24] by improving leptin sensitivity.

Hence, the interaction between amylin and leptin seems to be bidirectional because on one hand, amylin-deficient mice exhibited less hypothalamic LepRb, had a lower leptin-induced pSTAT3 expression in the ARC and VMN, and were less responsive to the weight-reducing effects of leptin [21], and on the other hand, animals with defective leptin signaling are less sensitive to amylin [22, 23, 150, 151]. A large series of experiments investigated the type of interaction, mode of interaction, and potential site(s) of interaction between amylin and leptin [19–21, 153–157], some of which will be summarized here.

For unknown reasons, extremely obese rats (and presumably humans [145]) may still react to amylin, but the synergizing effect of amylin on leptin action seems to be lost. This seems to involve long-term changes in leptin or amylin signaling because even when such extremely obese individuals lost weight by dietary restriction, the phenomenon was still observed meaning that leptin sensitization was not restored [157].

Amylin–Leptin Interactions in the AP and NTS

Individual AP neurons in the rat coexpress functional amylin and leptin receptors [50]. Interestingly, acute amylin administration increased the expression of the LepRb in AP neurons, which is consistent with increased leptin sensitivity [50]. Further, in vitro studies showed that LepRb-expressing AP neurons are coactivated by amylin and leptin, and the combined application produced a stronger response than individual stimuli [158]. The leptin-induced pSTAT3 response in the AP was enhanced in amylin-pretreated rats, and the leptin-induced pSTAT3 in the NTS was reduced in the absence of endogenous amylin [19, 21]. Similarly, leptin-receptor deficient db/db mice exhibited reduced amylin-induced satiation, paralleled by reduced amylin-induced Fos in the AP, and a lower expression of CTR. Surprisingly, even though leptin receptor-deficient ZDF rats also showed no reduction in food intake following amylin treatment, the amylin-induced Fos response and CTR expression in the AP were no different than WT rats. Hence, LepRb expression is required for the full anorexic effect of amylin, but there are some as yet unexplained differences in the neuronal activation in the AP depending on the type of LepRb mutation, which differs between db./db. mice and ZDF rats [151].

Amylin–Leptin Interactions in the VMH (ARC + VMN)

One of the earliest studies investigating hypothalamic amylin–leptin interactions [86] indicated that amylin reduced food intake and increased energy expenditure in leptin-resistant diet-induced obese (DIO) rats. DIO rats exhibit intrinsic leptin resistance already before the development of overt obesity [22, 159]. This phenomenon is characterized by reduced LepRb expression in the VMH [160, 161], reduced leptin receptor binding [162], reduced leptin-induced pSTAT3 [22, 163–165], and a reduced anorectic effect in response to leptin [159]. Amylin, on the other hand, increased leptin receptor activation in the VMN and leptin receptor binding in the ARC, VMN, and dorsomedial hypothalamic nucleus [21], and increased the expression of the POMC gene in the ARC of DIO rats [166]. Hence, the metabolic actions of leptin were restored by the action of amylin.

DIO rats also have reduced amylin binding in the dorsal VMN [165]. This may contribute to their reduced leptin sensitivity, because the depletion of CTR mRNA in the VMH in diet-resistant (DR) control rats reduced their leptin receptor binding and leptin-induced STAT3 phosphorylation. In other words, depletion of the CTR in the VMN rendered DR rats into a more DIO-like phenotype and led to increased adiposity [165].

The structural basis for a direct interaction of amylin and leptin is given by the codistribution of amylin receptor components and leptin receptors in many brain areas, including the hypothalamus [17, 104, 162, 165, 167], and it has been shown that the presence of the CTR in hypothalamic ARC neurons seems to be necessary for a full effect of leptin to control food intake [136].

One of the mechanistic links may depend on the action of interleukin-6 (IL-6) and its receptor. IL-6 activates STAT3 phosphorylation [168], and STAT3 controls the transcription of the LepRb and its transport to the cell surface [161]. Amylin, on the other hand, stimulated the production of IL-6 in hypothalamic microglia [23], and the amylin-induced effects on leptin signaling in the VMH were reduced in IL-6 knockout mice or in rats that had been pretreated with an IL-6 antibody [23]. Consistent with this potential mechanism, IL-6 increased the leptin response in dissociated VMN neurons [161]. VMN neurons from DIO rats also express less of the Bardet Biedl Syndrome-6 protein (BBS6) mRNA. Because BBS6 enhances the trafficking of the LepRb to the cell surface [169, 170], BBS6 deficiency may explain lower leptin receptor binding in DIO rats [162]. In support of our assumption, IL-6 was able to restore LepRb and BBS6 expression in VMN neurons from DIO rats to levels similar as in DR rats [161]. Together, these results implied that endogenous microglia-derived IL-6 (potentially via BBS6) may link amylin to enhanced VMH leptin signaling [23].

Amylin–Leptin Interactions in the VTA

The VTA, which is part of the reward pathway via dopaminergic projections to the NAc, not only expresses amylin (or CGRP) receptors but also leptin receptors [162, 171]; colocalization in the same cells has so far not been shown. Nonetheless, leptin and amylin reduce the intake of palatable food when given into the VTA [172, 173], and the coadministration of subthreshold doses of amylin and leptin produced a stronger suppression of eating and eventually also of body weight [172]. Interestingly, the local blockade of amylin receptors in the VTA reduced the ability of intra-VTA leptin to reduce eating [172]. Overall, these findings support the idea that leptin [174] and amylin [27, 149] act through a distributed network of neurons in the central nervous system, and that the same may be true for the specific sites of interaction between amylin and leptin.

Other Molecular Forms of Amylin and Their Potential Role in Physiology and Pathophysiology

Amylin Forms

The major source for circulating amylin is the pancreatic beta-cell where amylin is cosynthesized and cosecreted with insulin in response to eating [1]. Similar to other bioactive peptides, the mature 37-amino acid amylin peptide is derived from a larger precursor peptide which is processed by several sequential cleavage steps. This processing potentially results in numerous cellular products that may be released from the cells. The processing of the human amylin moiety, e.g., converts the pre-pro form via cleavage of the signal sequence to a 67 residue pro-amylin that differs from mature amylin by the presence of N- and C-terminal extensions. Further processing by prohormone convertases (PCs), carboxypeptidase E, and peptidyl glycine alpha-mandating monooxygenase lead to pro-amylin(1-51), pro-amylin(1-48) which contains the 11 residue N-terminal extension relative to mature amylin, and finally to the mature 37-amino acid peptide amylin(1-37) which includes the C-terminal amide and the disulfide bond between amino acids 2 and 7 [35, 175–177].

These processing steps for human amylin are of particular interest because mature human (and feline) amylin is prone to the formation of oligomers and amyloid fibrils that contribute to damaging pancreatic beta-cells in T2D [6, 8, 28, 36–40, 178–183]. Interestingly, however, not only mature amylin but also human pro-amylin(1-48) may lead to amyloid formation [184–188]. Mature amylin, pro-amylin(1-48), and other forms of amylin are found in the circulation, including amylin(17-37), amylin(24-37), and possibly amylin(12-37) [189–192]. It is unclear at present whether specific amylin forms may be more prevalent in health or in metabolic disease. Further, very little is known about the potential bioactivity of amylin processing intermediates and about their physiological or pathophysiological relevance.

Mature rodent and human amylin have similar pharmacology at the amylin receptor complexes [27, 33, 83], and human pro-amylin(1-48) and amylin similarly activate representative human amylin receptor subtypes AMY_1 and AMY_3 [83]. In fact, our recent data show that human pro-amylin(1-48), which is the peptide formed by the last step in the processing before "mature" amylin(1-37), is bioactive [41]. Human pro-amylin(1-48) was able to promote anorexia and to increase c-Fos, a marker of neuronal activation, in specific brain areas, similar to mature amylin.

Our results also showed that pro-amylin(1-48) exhibited similar in vitro toxicity to human mature amylin [41]. In early phases of T2D when insulin resistance increases amylin and insulin synthesis, the overexpression of pro-amylin(1-48) or amylin(1-37) may further lead to the formation of toxic oligomers, which exert toxicity by a variety of mechanisms [35, 193, 194].

In conclusion, our study highlighted that human pro-amylin(1-48) is a bioactive peptide that can activate amylin-responsive receptors and reduce eating. The same may be true for other amylin forms, but this still needs to be tested. Hence, with its N-terminal extension compared to mature amylin, amylin(1-48) was able to interact functionally with amylin receptors. This may also explain the bioactivity of recently developed long-acting amylin analogs that have large N-terminal extensions, such as the amylin analog cagrilintide [195].

Amylin Analogs Mimic Amylin's Effects on Eating

Based on amylin's and sCT's strong effects of eating under acute but also chronic conditions [68, 196], the development of amylin analogs and their potential use as anti-obesity drugs is not surprising [33], and many compounds are in clinical development. The receptor pharmacology of these agonists has not been determined in detail for all compounds; the best investigated and one of the most advanced agonists may be the CTR and AMY agonist cagrilintide which for many parameters seems to have similar in vitro receptor characteristics than sCT [55, 66, 195, 197–202]. It is important to note that receptor pharmacology has mainly been determined in cell culture and not in native tissue. Hence, reported results for the pharmacology of amylin agonists may differ depending on the cell type used [33, 43, 203].

The only amylin agonist in clinical use is pramlintide (Symlin®), which pharmacodynamically and pharmacokinetically is similar to native amylin [52, 145]. Due to its short biological half-life, which is similar to native amylin, it needs to be administered several times daily, i.e., typically with each individual meal [145]. The next-generation amylinomimetic davalintide was more efficacious, potent, and longer-lasting than amylin [75]; while it is still considered an amylin receptor agonist, its potency at the CTR is approx. 100 times higher than amylin. It is unclear at present whether it is for these characteristics that davalintide seems to decrease food intake, body weight, and fat mass to a greater extent than rat amylin in experimental obese rats. Importantly and similar to pramlintide, davalintide seemed to engage the same central pathways as rat amylin (see below; [75]).

To extend the half-life of amylin analogs and hence to increase the administration intervals, several strategies were followed, e.g., by the use of pegylated or glycosylated versions of amylin [204, 205]. To ease the administration of amylin analogs, orally available agonists, including preparations based on sCT and pramlintide (e.g., KBP compounds; [203, 206]), have also been tested [206–209].

More recently, several pharmaceutical companies started or extended their tests of long-acting injectable amylin analogs (e.g., [198, 210]; Astra Zeneca [https://www.astrazeneca.com/content/dam/az/Investor_Relations/events/ASCO-2024-IR-Presentation.pdf]; Guba [https://www.gubra.dk/mfn_news/gubra-announces-first-subject-dosed-in-phase-1-clinical-trial-of-amylin-agonist-gubamy-for-the-treatment-of-obesity/]; Lilly [https://www.lilly.com/discovery/clinical-development-pipeline#]; Nordic Bioscience [https://www.nordicbioscience.com/publications/kbp-066a-a-long-acting-dual-amylin-and-calcitonin-receptor-agonist-induces-weight-loss-and-improves-glycemic-control-in-obese-and-diabetic-rats]; Novo Nordisk [https://www.novonordisk.com/research-and-development/pipeline.html]; Structure Therapeutics [https://ir.structuretx.com/news-releases/news-release-details/structure-therapeutics-reports-positive-topline-data-its-phase]; Zealand [https://www.zealandpharma.com/pipeline/petrelintide/]), and many others.

Some compounds under development seem to be dual agonists at both the amylin and the calcitonin receptor, but the receptor pharmacology of many of these compounds has been insufficiently characterized [203]. Rather detailed data are available for cagrilintide, which is an acylated long-acting, nonselective human amylin receptor agonist [211]. The in vitro receptor activation profile of cagrilintide is similar to sCT as it does not differentiate between the CTR and AMY1 or AMY3, respectively (AMY2 has not been tested). Cagrilintide alone or in combination with the GLP-1 receptor agonist semaglutide has been shown to be highly effective in lowering body weight. Given the distribution of cagrilintide mainly in circumventricular organs after peripheral administration, cagrilintide most likely acts mainly via the caudal hindbrain [55, 65, 103, 195, 201, 202].

It is clear that the weight-lowering capacity of cagrilintide largely outweighs the weight-loss effects previously observed using pramlintide [202, 212–214]. Aside from obvious pharmacokinetic differences (the circulation half-life of cagrilintide is much longer than pramlintide [52, 215]), additional factors may be responsible for the enhanced effectiveness of cagrilintide. One possibility is the receptor activation profile because cagrilintide has a different receptor balance and is a rather unspecific CTR and AMY agonist while pramlintide is rather AMY specific [55, 66]. At present, however, it is unclear whether the activation of the CTR versus specific amylin receptor subtypes is critical for the enhanced clinical efficacy. Research in this respect has been hampered by the lack of receptor subtype-specific antagonists.

Another important difference between cagrilintide and pramlintide (or native amylin) is the receptor binding characteristics. Cagrilintide has a slower off-rate from the receptors, i.e., its residence time at the receptor is longer than that of amylin (but much shorter than of sCT). Finally, it is also possible that compared to amylin or pramlintide, amylin agonists like cagrilintide may reach CTR or AMY in different brain regions while (endogenous) amylin may mainly act via the AP.

In other words, activation of a wider range of receptor sites in a distributed network of neurons [27, 84, 149] may be associated with a stronger (pharmacological) effect.

Finally, recent studies also revealed some puzzling species differences in the action of amylin versus amylin agonists in rats and mice, in particular with respect to the role of RAMPs. sCT, similar to amylin, acutely reduces eating and chronically reduces eating and body weight gain, respectively, in rats [68, 69, 118, 196, 216–218]. However, an eating-inhibitory effect after sCT was only seen acutely in mice [53, 60, 108] while chronic administration of sCT in mice increased eating, and body weight increased more than in controls [53]. Even more puzzling was the finding that the absence of RAMP3 in RAMP3 knockout mice abolished the ability of NN1213, an AMY selective amylin agonist, to reduce eating and weight gain in mice, but it restored the ability of chronic sCT to reduce eating and body weight. In other words, chronic sCT was only effective as a weight-lowering drug in mice in the absence of RAMP3 [53]. The reason for these species differences is unknown at present. It is possible that the absence of one of the RAMPs is compensated by the upregulation of other RAMPs (or the CTR core protein), and such compensatory mechanisms may differ across species. In any event, such species differences in the role of RAMP and in the effects of amylin agonists need to be taken into account for the future developments of amylin-based drugs. The situation is somewhat reminiscent of the GLP-1/GIP coagonist tirzepatide, which seems to be a poor ligand at the mouse versus the human GIP receptor [219], again pointing to the importance of considering species differences.

Amyloid Formation in Pancreatic Islets

As mentioned earlier, amylin derived amyloid deposition is a typical pathyphysiological feature of T2D and probably contributes to progressive beta-cell destruction in T2D and in feline diabetes mellitus. Amylin from primates and felines is highly amyloidogenic, in particular under conditions of increased secretory demand [28]. Evidence for a pathophysiological role is multifold; amyloid severity inversely correlates with beta-cell area in pancreatic islets of T2D patients, some mutations of the amylin coding sequence increase amylin's propensity for aggregation and these mutations are associated with more severe T2D, and only cats and primates which produce amyloidogenic variants of amylin naturally develop signs of T2D. Finally, transgenic mice and rats expressing the amyloidogenic human IAPP (hIAPP) spontaneously develop a T2D phenotype characterized by islet amyloidosis and decreased beta-cell mass, and humanization of the nonamyloidogenic porcine amylin using CRISPR/Cas9 gene editing also leads to T2D in miniature pigs [8, 28, 35]

Mechanisms of Amyloid Genesis

Monomeric mature amylin consists of a 37-amino acid peptide [39] and its amylin amino acid sequence is generally highly conserved in mammals, but important differences occur in the "amyloidogenic region," mainly the amino acids 20–29. The amino acid sequence in this region is responsible for the highly amyloidogenic human or feline, but not of rodent amylin [220, 221]. Higher concentrations of amylin may favor its aggregation into oligomers and eventually into fibrils, at least under certain conditions, and this process may already start with pro-amylin or other intermediate molecules during the maturation of amylin [28, 41]. It is likely that abnormal processing of amylin then eventually leads to its deposition as amyloid in the islets, contributing to the progressive loss of pancreatic beta-cells. It is important to note that the beta-cell damage induced by amylin aggregation is more closely related with the early aggregation steps into amylin oligomers rather than with the amount of pancreatic amyloid visible by light microscopy (see below; and [28, 222]).

Pathological Effects of Amylin Deposits on Pancreatic β-Cells

Aggregated amylin leads to progressive beta-cell loss. The underlying events seem to be triggered by intracellular processes and may be aggravated by extracellular processes [28, 40]. Small intracellular aggregates of amylin (oligomers) lead to endoplasmic reticulum stress and the unfolded protein response [223], followed by damage to vesicular membranes and subsequent release of the fibrillary material into the cytosol. Reduced degradation of the misfolded proteins may then lead to intracellular toxicity [28, 40], accumulation of these aggregates, increased oxidative cellular stress through the formation of reactive oxygen species, and activation of inflammatory processes within beta-cells [224].

Therapeutic Approach to Reduce Amylin-Derived Fibrillogenic

Based on the current understanding that the most toxic entity triggering the pathophysiological events in pancreatic beta-cells is not mature fibrils but relatively small, prefibrillar oligomers [28, 225], several strategies have been developed trying to interfere with the toxicity of these early events and to preserve or restore functional beta-cell mass [226]. Early strategies were not always successful [227], but more recent studies provided promising results, both with "active" vaccination strategies against small oligomer aggregates [228, 229] and a "passive" vaccination strategy, i.e., the direct application of antibodies raised against amylin oligomers [8, 230].

One of the latter studies [8] provided important information about potential mechanisms of these strategies. Antibodies that were specifically directed against prefibrillar (human) amylin oligomers showed in vitro and in vivo bioactivity. The specific anti-oligomer antibodies reduced the islet amyloid content in isolated human islets and in cultured insulinoma (INS-1) cells. Under in vivo conditions, mainly using hIAPP transgenic rats and mice, chronic administration of the antibodies improved insulin secretion, reduced hyperglycemia, and slowed beta-cell failure. Further, treatment also prolonged the survival of human islets in engrafted mice. An interesting finding of that study was that the deposition of oligomers extracellularly could be directly demonstrated. Continued deposition of extracellular oligomers seemed to contribute to beta-cell pathogenesis and was in fact one of the probable targets for the beneficial action of antibodies. In other words, antibody treatment increased the phagocytic clearance of extracellular oligomers via macrophages. Finally, this study [8] also implied that oligomer removal may reduce the induction of the inflammasome, which is known to contribute to the beta-cell toxicity of amylin aggregation and amyloid deposition [231, 232]. Overall, it became clear that the removal of (extracellular) oligomers with the help of specific anti-oligomer antibodies preserved beta-cell function, slowed beta-cell exhaustion, and hence limited the progression of T2D in various disease models.

Conclusion

Our knowledge about amylin biology has increased dramatically in recent years. Shortly after the isolation and discovery of amylin from pancreatic islet amyloid deposits in type 2 diabetics and in diabetic cats, exciting data showed that amylin is also a "normal" secretory product of pancreatic beta-cells, being cosecreted with insulin. The best investigated metabolic action of amylin is its role to reduce eating and eventually to control body weight. The sites and mechanisms of action have been partly resolved and form the basis for the promising use of amylin receptor agonists as potent, efficacious, and safe anti-obesity and anti-diabetes treatments. At the same time, it is also clear that much remains to be learned, e.g., about the sites of action beyond the well-established caudal hindbrain (in particular the AP), about the role of the different amylin receptor subtypes, and about amylin's role to influence not only homeostatic controls of eating but also hedonic controls. Given the propensity of human (and feline) amylin to aggregate into oligomers and eventually insoluble fibrils, it is obvious that amylin mimetics for obesity and diabetes therapy are based on nonfibrillar forms of amylin, i.e., close to rodent amylin. Finally, recent data indicate that the "other face" of amylin, that of a fibril-forming molecule that potentially can damage pancreatic beta-cells and contribute to the pathophysiology of T2D, may also be an interesting target for treatment because strategies have been developed that reduce the toxicity of aggregated amylin molecules.

Acknowledgments and Disclosures

The continued financial support by the Swiss National Science Foundation is highly appreciated. Further substantial funding was obtained from the Novartis Foundation, the Olga Mayen Fisch Foundation, the Votable Foundation, and the University of Zurich (Forschungskredit and Zurich Center for Integrative Human Physiology). TAL has research collaborations and consults with Novo Nordisk, Structure Therapeutics, Zealand Pharma, Guba, AstraZeneca, Zealand Pharma, Roche, and Boehringer Ingelheim.

References

1 Cooper, G.J. (1994). Amylin compared with calcitonin gene-related peptide: structure, biology, and relevance to metabolic disease. *Endocr. Rev.* 15 (2): 163–201.

2 Johnson, K.H., Hayden, D.W., O'Brien, T.D., and Westermark, P. (1986). Spontaneous diabetes mellitus-islet amyloid complex in adult cats. *Am. J. Pathol.* 125 (2): 416–419.

3 Westermark, P., Wernstedt, C., Wilander, E., and Sletten, K. (1986). A novel peptide in the calcitonin gene related peptide family as an amyloid fibril protein in the endocrine pancreas. *Biochem. Biophys. Res. Commun.* 140 (3): 827–831.

4 Clark, A., Cooper, G.J., Lewis, C.E. et al. (1987). Islet amyloid formed from diabetes-associated peptide may be pathogenic in type-2 diabetes. *Lancet (London, England).* 2 (8553): 231–234.

5 Cooper, G.J., Willis, A.C., Clark, A. et al. (1987). Purification and characterization of a peptide from amyloid-rich pancreases of type 2 diabetic patients. *PNAS* 84 (23): 8628–8632.

6 Lutz, T.A. and Rand, J.S. (1995). Pathogenesis of feline diabetes mellitus. *Vet. Clin. North Am. Small Anim. Pract.* 25 (3): 527–552.

7 Lutz, T.A. and Rand, J.S. (1997). Detection of amyloid deposition in various regions of the feline pancreas by different staining techniques. *J. Comp. Pathol.* 116 (2): 157–170.

8 Wirth, F., Heitz, F.D., Seeger, C. et al. (2023). A human antibody against pathologic IAPP aggregates protects beta cells in type 2 diabetes models. *Nat. Commun.* 14 (1): 6294.

9 Balasubramaniam, A., Renugopalakrishnan, V., Stein, M. et al. (1991). Syntheses, structures and anorectic effects of human and rat amylin. *Peptides* 12 (5): 919–924.

10 Chance, W.T., Balasubramaniam, A., Stallion, A., and Fischer, J.E. (1993). Anorexia following the systemic injection of amylin. *Brain Res.* 607 (1–2): 185–188.

11 Chance, W.T., Balasubramaniam, A., Zhang, F.S. et al. (1991). Anorexia following the intrahypothalamic administration of amylin. *Brain Res.* 539 (2): 352–354.

12 Lutz, T.A., Del Prete, E., and Scharrer, E. (1994). Reduction of food intake in rats by intraperitoneal injection of low doses of amylin. *Physiol. Behav.* 55 (5): 891–895.

13 Lutz, T.A., Geary, N., Szabady, M.M. et al. (1995). Amylin decreases meal size in rats. *Physiol. Behav.* 58 (6): 1197–1202.

14 Baisley, S.K. and Baldo, B.A. (2014). Amylin receptor signaling in the nucleus accumbens negatively modulates mu-opioid-driven feeding. *Neuropsychopharmacology* 39 (13): 3009–3017.

15 Mietlicki-Baase, E.G., McGrath, L.E., Koch-Laskowski, K. et al. (2017). Amylin receptor activation in the ventral tegmental area reduces motivated ingestive behavior. *Neuropharmacology* 123: 67–79.

16 Mietlicki-Baase, E.G., Reiner, D.J., Cone, J.J. et al. (2015). Amylin modulates the mesolimbic dopamine system to control energy balance. *Neuropsychopharmacology* 40 (2): 372–385.

17 Mietlicki-Baase, E.G., Rupprecht, L.E., Olivos, D.R. et al. (2013). Amylin receptor signaling in the ventral tegmental area is physiologically relevant for the control of food intake. *Neuropsychopharmacology* 38: 1685–1697.

18 Whiting, L., McCutcheon, J.E., Boyle, C.N. et al. (2017). The area postrema (AP) and the parabrachial nucleus (PBN) are important sites for salmon calcitonin (sCT) to decrease evoked phasic dopamine release in the nucleus accumbens (NAc). *Physiol. Behav.* 176: 9–16.

19 Roth, J.D., Roland, B.L., Cole, R.L. et al. (2008). Leptin responsiveness restored by amylin agonism in diet-induced obesity: evidence from nonclinical and clinical studies. *PNAS* 105 (20): 7257–7262.

20 Trevaskis, J.L., Lei, C., Koda, J.E. et al. (2010). Interaction of leptin and amylin in the long-term maintenance of weight loss in diet-induced obese rats. *Obesity (Silver Spring)* 18 (1): 21–26.

21 Turek, V.F., Trevaskis, J.L., Levin, B.E. et al. (2010). Mechanisms of amylin/leptin synergy in rodent models. *Endocrinology* 151 (1): 143–152.

22 Johnson, M.D., Bouret, S.G., Dunn-Meynell, A.A. et al. (2016). Early postnatal amylin treatment enhances hypothalamic leptin signaling and neural development in the selectively bred diet-induced obese rat. *Am. J. Physiol. Regul. Integr. Comp. Physiol.* 311 (6): R1032–R1044.

23 Le Foll, C., Johnson, M.D., Dunn-Meynell, A.A. et al. (2015). Amylin-induced central IL-6 production enhances ventromedial hypothalamic leptin signaling. *Diabetes* 64 (5): 1621–1631.

24 Osto, M., Wielinga, P.Y., Alder, B. et al. (2007). Modulation of the satiating effect of amylin by central ghrelin, leptin and insulin. *Physiol. Behav.* 91 (5): 566–572.

25 Potes, C.S. and Lutz, T.A. (2010). Brainstem mechanisms of amylin-induced anorexia. *Physiol. Behav.* 100 (5): 511–518.

26 Geisler, C.E., Décarie-Spain, L., Loh, M.K. et al. (2024). Amylin modulates a ventral tegmental area-to-medial prefrontal cortex circuit to suppress food intake and impulsive food-directed behavior. *Biol. Psychiatry* 95: 938–950.

27 Mietlicki-Baase, E.G. and Hayes, M.R. (2014). Amylin activates distributed CNS nuclei to control energy balance. *Physiol. Behav.* 136: 39–46.

28 Westermark, P., Andersson, A., and Westermark, G.T. (2011). Islet amyloid polypeptide, islet amyloid, and diabetes mellitus. *Physiol. Rev.* 91 (3): 795–826.

29 Ogawa, A., Harris, V., McCorkle, S.K. et al. (1990). Amylin secretion from the rat pancreas and its selective loss after streptozotocin treatment. *J. Clin. Invest.* 85 (3): 973–976.

30 Boyle, C.N., Rossier, M.M., and Lutz, T.A. (2011). Influence of high-fat feeding, diet-induced obesity, and hyperamylinemia on the sensitivity to acute amylin. *Physiol. Behav.* 104 (1): 20–28.

31 Lutz, T.A. (2006). Amylinergic control of food intake. *Physiol. Behav.* 89 (4): 465–471.

32 Mulder, H., Leckstrom, A., Uddman, R. et al. (1995). Islet amyloid polypeptide (amylin) is expressed in sensory neurons. *J. Neuro-Oncol.* 15 (11): 7625–7632.

33 Hay, D.L., Chen, S., Lutz, T.A. et al. (2015). Amylin: pharmacology, physiology, and clinical potential. *Pharmacol. Rev.* 67 (3): 564–600.

34 Lutz, T.A. (2010). The role of amylin in the control of energy homeostasis. *Am. J. Physiol. Regul. Integr. Comp. Physiol.* 298 (6): R1475–R1484.

35 Raleigh, D., Zhang, X., Hastoy, B., and Clark, A. (2017). The β-cell assassin: IAPP cytotoxicity. *J. Mol. Endocrinol.* 59 (3): R121–r40.

36 Lutz, T.A., Ainscow, J., and Rand, J.S. (1994). Frequency of pancreatic amyloid deposition in cats from south-eastern Queensland. *Aust. Vet. J.* 71 (8): 254–256.

37 Arnelo, U., Blevins, J.E., Larsson, J. et al. (1996). Effects of acute and chronic infusion of islet amyloid polypeptide on food intake in rats. *Scand. J. Gastroenterol.* 31 (1): 83–89.

38 Paulsson, J.F. and Westermark, G.T. (2005). Aberrant processing of human proislet amyloid polypeptide results in increased amyloid formation. *Diabetes* 54 (7): 2117–2125.

39 Hoppener, J.W., Verbeek, J.S., de Koning, E.J. et al. (1993). Chronic overproduction of islet amyloid polypeptide/amylin in transgenic mice: lysosomal localization of human islet amyloid polypeptide and lack of marked hyperglycaemia or hyperinsulinaemia. *Diabetologia* 36 (12): 1258–1265.

40 Jurgens, C.A., Toukatly, M.N., Fligner, C.L. et al. (2011). beta-cell loss and beta-cell apoptosis in human type 2 diabetes are related to islet amyloid deposition. *Am. J. Pathol.* 178 (6): 2632–2640.

41 Mazzini, G., Le Foll, C., Boyle, C.N. et al. (2024). The processing intermediate of human amylin, pro-amylin(1–48), has in vivo and in vitro bioactivity. *Biophys. Chem.* 308: 107201.

42 Bower, R.L. and Hay, D.L. (2016). Amylin structure-function relationships and receptor pharmacology: implications for amylin mimetic drug development. *Br. J. Pharmacol.* 173 (12): 1883–1898.

43 Hay, D.L., Walker, C.S., Gingell, J.J. et al. (2016). Receptor activity-modifying proteins; multifunctional G protein-coupled receptor accessory proteins. *Biochem. Soc. Trans.* 44 (2): 568–573.

44 Bailey, R.J., Walker, C.S., Ferner, A.H. et al. (2012). Pharmacological characterization of rat amylin receptors: implications for the identification of amylin receptor subtypes. *Br. J. Pharmacol.* 166 (1): 151–167.

45 Christopoulos, G., Perry, K.J., Morfis, M. et al. (1999). Multiple amylin receptors arise from receptor activity-modifying protein interaction with the calcitonin receptor gene product. *Mol. Pharmacol.* 56 (1): 235–242.

46 McLatchie, L.M., Fraser, N.J., Main, M.J. et al. (1998). RAMPs regulate the transport and ligand specificity of the calcitonin-receptor-like receptor. *Nature* 393 (6683): 333–339.

47 Fischer, J.A., Muff, R., and Born, W. (2002). Functional relevance of G-protein-coupled-receptor-associated proteins, exemplified by receptor-activity-modifying proteins (RAMPs). *Biochem. Soc. Trans.* 30 (4): 455–460.

48 Muff, R., Buhlmann, N., Fischer, J.A., and Born, W. (1999). An amylin receptor is revealed following co-transfection of a calcitonin receptor with receptor activity modifying proteins-1 or −3. *Endocrinology* 140 (6): 2924–2927.

49 Tilakaratne, N., Christopoulos, G., Zumpe, E.T. et al. (2000). Amylin receptor phenotypes derived from human calcitonin receptor/RAMP coexpression exhibit pharmacological differences dependent on receptor isoform and host cell environment. *J. Pharmacol. Exp. Ther.* 294 (1): 61–72.

50 Liberini, C.G., Boyle, C.N., Cifani, C. et al. (2016). Amylin receptor components and the leptin receptor are co-expressed in single rat area postrema neurons. *Eur. J. Neurosci.* 43 (5): 653–661.

51 Coester, B., Koester-Hegmann, C., Lutz, T.A., and Le Foll, C. (2020). Amylin/calcitonin receptor-mediated signaling in POMC neurons influences energy balance and locomotor activity in chow-fed male mice. *Diabetes* 69 (6): 1110–1125.

52 Weyer, C., Maggs, D.G., Young, A.A., and Kolterman, O.G. (2001). Amylin replacement with pramlintide as an adjunct to insulin therapy in type 1 and type 2 diabetes mellitus: a physiological approach toward improved metabolic control. *Curr. Pharm. Des.* 7 (14): 1353–1373.

53 Arrigoni, S., Le Foll, C., Cabak, A. et al. (2021). A selective role for receptor activity-modifying proteins in subchronic action of the amylin selective receptor agonist NN1213 compared with salmon calcitonin on body weight and food intake in male mice. *Eur. J. Neurosci.* 54 (3): 4863–4876.

54 Cao, J., Belousoff, M.J., Liang, Y.L. et al. (2022). A structural basis for amylin receptor phenotype. *Science* 375: eabm9609.

55 Fletcher, M.M., Keov, P., Truong, T.T. et al. (2021). AM833 is a novel agonist of calcitonin family G protein-coupled receptors: pharmacological comparison with six selective and nonselective agonists. *J. Pharmacol. Exp. Ther.* 377 (3): 417–440.

56 Cao, J., Belousoff, M.J., Gerrard, E. et al. (2024). Structural insight into selectivity of amylin and calcitonin receptor agonists. *Nat. Chem. Biol.* 20 (2): 162–169.

57 Potes, C.S., Riediger, T., and Lutz, T.A. (2011). Amylin induced ERK1/2 phosphorylation may contribute to its eating inhibitory effect. *Appetite* 57: S34.

58 Mollet, A., Gilg, S., Riediger, T., and Lutz, T.A. (2004). Infusion of the amylin antagonist AC 187 into the area postrema increases food intake in rats. *Physiol. Behav.* 81 (1): 149–155.

59 Keov, P., Christopoulos, G., Hick, C.A. et al. (2024). Development of a novel assay for direct assessment of selective amylin receptor activation reveals novel differences in behavior of selective and nonselective peptide agonists. *Mol. Pharmacol.* 105 (5): 359–373.

60 Coester, B., Pence, S.W., Arrigoni, S. et al. (2020). RAMP1 and RAMP3 differentially control amylin's effects on food intake, glucose and energy balance in male and female mice. *Neuroscience* 447: 74–93.

61 Geary, N. (2005). A new way of looking at eating. *Am. J. Physiol. Regul. Integr. Comp. Physiol.* 288 (6): R1444–R1446.

62 Lutz, T.A. and Geary, N. (2008). Gastrointestinal factors in appetite and food research – animal research. In: *Appetite and Food Intake: Behavioral and Physiological Consideration* (ed. R. Harris and R. Mattes), 163–186. CRC Press.

63 Reidelberger, R.D., Haver, A.C., Arnelo, U. et al. (2004). Amylin receptor blockade stimulates food intake in rats. *Am. J. Physiol. Regul. Integr. Comp. Physiol.* 287 (3): R568–R574.

64 Roth, J.D., Trevaskis, J.L., Wilson, J. et al. (2008). Antiobesity effects of the beta-cell hormone amylin in combination with phentermine or sibutramine in diet-induced obese rats. *Int. J. Obes.* 32 (8): 1201–1210.

65 Kruse, T., Hansen, J.L., Dahl, K. et al. (2021). Development of Cagrilintide, a long-acting amylin analogue. *J. Med. Chem.* 64 (15): 11183–11194.

66 Larsen, A.T., Mohamed, K.E., Sonne, N. et al. (2022). Does receptor balance matter? – comparing the efficacies of the dual amylin and calcitonin receptor agonists cagrilintide and KBP-336 on metabolic parameters in preclinical models. *Biomed. Pharmacother.* 156: 113842.

67 Sun, X., Yang, D., Li, Y. et al. (2024). Identification and utility exploration of a highly potent and long-acting bullfrog GLP-1 analogue in GLP-1 and amylin combination therapy. *Peptides* 177: 171203.

68 Lutz, T.A., Mollet, A., Rushing, P.A. et al. (2001). The anorectic effect of a chronic peripheral infusion of amylin is abolished in area postrema/nucleus of the solitary tract (AP/NTS) lesioned rats. *Int. J. Obes. Relat. Metab. Disord.* 25 (7): 1005–1011.

69 Lutz, T.A., Tschudy, S., Rushing, P.A., and Scharrer, E. (2000). Amylin receptors mediate the anorectic action of salmon calcitonin (sCT). *Peptides* 21 (2): 233–238.

70 Young, A. (2005). Amylin and the integrated control of nutrient influx. *Adv. Pharmacol.* 52: 67–77.

71 Chance, W.T., Balasubramaniam, A., Chen, X., and Fischer, J.E. (1992). Tests of adipsia and conditioned taste aversion following the intrahypothalamic injection of amylin. *Peptides* 13 (5): 961–964.

72 Morley, J.E., Suarez, M.D., Mattamal, M., and Flood, J.F. (1997). Amylin and food intake in mice: effects on motivation to eat and mechanism of action. *Pharmacol. Biochem. Behav.* 56 (1): 123–129.

73 Rushing, P.A., Seeley, R.J., Air, E.L. et al. (2002). Acute 3rd-ventricular amylin infusion potently reduces food intake but does not produce aversive consequences. *Peptides* 23 (5): 985–988.

74 Mack, C., Wilson, J., Athanacio, J. et al. (2007). Pharmacological actions of the peptide hormone amylin in the long-term regulation of food intake, food preference, and body weight. *Am. J. Physiol. RegulIntegr. Comp. Physiol.* 293 (5): R1855–R1863.

75 Mack, C.M., Soares, C.J., Wilson, J.K. et al. (2010). Davalintide (AC2307), a novel amylin-mimetic peptide: enhanced pharmacological properties over native amylin to reduce food intake and body weight. *Int. J. Obes.* 34 (2): 385–395.

76 Thiele, T.E., Van, D.G., Campfield, L.A. et al. (1997). Central infusion of GLP-1, but not leptin, produces conditioned taste aversions in rats. *Am. J. Phys.* 272 (2 Pt 2): R726–R730.

77 Ervin, G.N., Mosher, J.T., Birkemo, L.S., and Johnson, M.F. (1995). Multiple, small doses of cholecystokinin octapeptide are more efficacious at inducing taste aversion conditioning than single, large doses. *Peptides* 16 (3): 539–545.

78 Berthoud, H.R., Sutton, G.M., Townsend, R.L. et al. (2006). Brainstem mechanisms integrating gut-derived satiety signals and descending forebrain information in the control of meal size. *Physiol. Behav.* 89 (4): 517–524.

79 Grill, H.J. and Hayes, M.R. (2009). The nucleus tractus solitarius: a portal for visceral afferent signal processing, energy status assessment and integration of their combined effects on food intake. *Int. J. Obes.* 33 (Suppl 1): S11–S15.

80 Campos, C.A., Bowen, A.J., Han, S. et al. (2017). Cancer-induced anorexia and malaise are mediated by CGRP neurons in the parabrachial nucleus. *Nat. Neurosci.* 20 (7): 934–942.

81 Campos, C.A., Bowen, A.J., Schwartz, M.W., and Palmiter, R.D. (2016). Parabrachial CGRP neurons control meal termination. *Cell Metab.* 23 (5): 811–820.

82 Boccia, L.B.T., Ghidewon, M.Y., Kulka, P. et al. (2022). Hypophagia induced by salmon calcitonin, but not by amylin, is partially driven by malaise and is mediated by CGRP neurons. *Mol. Metab.* 58: 101444.

83 Bower, R.L., Yule, L., Rees, T.A. et al. (2018). Molecular signature for receptor engagement in the metabolic peptide hormone amylin. *ACS Pharmacol. Transl. Sci.* 1 (1): 32–49.

84 Cheng, W., Gonzalez, I., Pan, W. et al. (2020). Calcitonin receptor neurons in the mouse nucleus tractus solitarius control energy balance via the non-aversive suppression of feeding. *Cell Metab.* 31 (2): 301–12.e5.

85 Huang, K.P., Acosta, A.A., Ghidewon, M.Y. et al. (2024). Dissociable hindbrain GLP1R circuits for satiety and aversion. *Nature* 632 (8025): 585–593.

86 Roth, J.D., Hughes, H., Kendall, E. et al. (2006). Antiobesity effects of the beta-cell hormone amylin in diet-induced obese rats: effects on food intake, body weight, composition, energy expenditure, and gene expression. *Endocrinology* 147 (12): 5855–5864.

87 Isaksson, B., Wang, F., Permert, J. et al. (2005). Chronically administered islet amyloid polypeptide in rats serves as an adiposity inhibitor and regulates energy homeostasis. *Pancreatology* 5 (1): 29–36.

88 Osaka, T., Tsukamoto, A., Koyama, Y., and Inoue, S. (2008). Central and peripheral administration of amylin induces energy expenditure in anesthetized rats. *Peptides* 29 (6): 1028–1035.

89 Wielinga, P.Y., Löwenstein, C., Alder, B., and Lutz, T.A. (2008). Effect of peripheral and central amylin on energy expenditure and body temperature. *Appetite* 51: 409.

90 Wielinga, P.Y., Lowenstein, C., Muff, S. et al. (2010). Central amylin acts as an adiposity signal to control body weight and energy expenditure. *Physiol. Behav.* 101 (1): 45–52.

91 Fernandes-Santos, C., Zhang, Z., Morgan, D.A. et al. (2013). Amylin acts in the central nervous system to increase sympathetic nerve activity. *Endocrinology* 154: 2481–2488.

92 Zhang, Z., Liu, X., Morgan, D.A. et al. (2011). Neuronal receptor activity modifying protein-1 promotes energy expenditure in mice. *Diabetes* 60: 1063–1071.

93 Lutz, T.A., Coester, B., Whiting, L. et al. (2018). Amylin selectively signals onto POMC neurons in the arcuate nucleus of the hypothalamus. *Diabetes* 67 (5): 805–817.

94 Roth, J.D., Hughes, H., Coffey, T. et al. (2007). Effects of prior or concurrent food restriction on amylin-induced changes in body weight and body composition in high-fat-fed female rats. *Am. J. Physiol. Endocrinol. Metab.* 293 (4): E1112–E1117.

95 Roth, J.D., D'Souza, L., Griffin, P.S. et al. (2012). Interactions of amylinergic and melanocortinergic systems in the control of food intake and body weight in rodents. *Diabetes Obes. Metab.* 14: 608–615.

96 Trevaskis, J.L., Turek, V.F., Wittmer, C. et al. (2010). Enhanced amylin-mediated body weight loss in estradiol-deficient diet-induced obese rats. *Endocrinology* 151 (12): 5657–5668.

97 Asarian, L., Boyle, C.N., and Lutz, T.A. (2011). Estradiol (E2) increases the acute eating-inhibitory effect of amylin in ovariectomized (OVX) rats. *Appetite* 57: S2.

98 Lutz, T.A., Senn, M., Althaus, J. et al. (1998). Lesion of the area postrema/nucleus of the solitary tract (AP/NTS) attenuates the anorectic effects of amylin and calcitonin gene-related peptide (CGRP) in rats. *Peptides* 19 (2): 309–317.

99 Watanabe, H., Takahashi, E., Kobayashi, M. et al. (2006). The estrogen-responsive adrenomedullin and receptor-modifying protein 3 gene identified by DNA microarray analysis are directly regulated by estrogen receptor. *J. Mol. Endocrinol.* 36 (1): 81–89.

100 Banks, W.A. and Kastin, A.J. (1998). Differential permeability of the blood-brain barrier to two pancreatic peptides: insulin and amylin. *Peptides* 19 (5): 883–889.

101 Banks, W.A., Kastin, A.J., Maness, L.M. et al. (1995). Permeability of the blood-brain barrier to amylin. *Life Sci.* 57 (22): 1993–2001.

102 Zakariassen, H.L., John, L.M., Lykkesfeldt, J. et al. (2020). Salmon calcitonin distributes into the arcuate nucleus to a subset of NPY neurons in mice. *Neuropharmacology* 167: 107987.

103 Secher, A., Lundh, S., Gerstenberg, M. et al. (2022). Cagrilintide and semaglutide target both the hypothalamic and brainstem neurons in the rodent brain. *Obesity (Silver Spring, Md.).* 30 (suppl 1): 126.

104 Sexton, P.M., Paxinos, G., Kenney, M.A. et al. (1994). in vitro autoradiographic localization of amylin binding sites in rat brain. *Neuroscience* 62 (2): 553–567.

105 Becskei, C., Riediger, T., Zund, D. et al. (2004). Immunohistochemical mapping of calcitonin receptors in the adult rat brain. *Brain Res.* 1030 (2): 221–233.

106 Edwards, G.L., BRCJ, G., RPCCM, D., and Young, A. (1998). Area postrem (AP)-lesions block the regulation of gastric emptying by amylin. *Neurogastroenterol. Motil.* 114 (26): A748.

107 Fukuda, T., Hirai, Y., Maezawa, H. et al. (2013). Electrophysiologically identified presynaptic mechanisms underlying amylinergic modulation of area postrema neuronal excitability in rat brain slices. *Brain Res.* 1494: 9–16.

108 Abegg, K., Hermann, A., Boyle, C.N. et al. (2017). Involvement of amylin and leptin in the development of projections from the area postrema to the nucleus of the solitary tract. *Front. Endocrinol.* 8: 324.

109 Lutz, T.A., Althaus, J., Rossi, R., and Scharrer, E. (1998). Anorectic effect of amylin is not transmitted by capsaicin-sensitive nerve fibers. *Am. J. Phys.* 274 (6 Pt 2): R1777–R1782.

110 Lutz, T.A., Del Prete, E., and Scharrer, E. (1995). Subdiaphragmatic vagotomy does not influence the anorectic effect of amylin. *Peptides* 16 (3): 457–462.

111 Morley, J.E., Flood, J.F., Horowitz, M. et al. (1994). Modulation of food intake by peripherally administered amylin. *Am. J. Phys.* 267 (1 Pt 2): R178–R184.

112 Wickbom, J., Herrington, M.K., Permert, J. et al. (2008). Gastric emptying in response to IAPP and CCK in rats with subdiaphragmatic afferent vagotomy. *Regul. Pept.* 148 (1–3): 21–25.

113 Coester, B., Foll, C.L., and Lutz, T.A. (2020). Viral depletion of calcitonin receptors in the area postrema: a proof-of-concept study. *Physiol. Behav.* 223: 112992.

114 Potes, C.S., Turek, V.F., Cole, R.L. et al. (2010). Noradrenergic neurons of the area postrema mediate amylin's hypophagic action. *Am. J. Physiol. Regul. Integr. Comp. Physiol.* 299 (2): R623–R631.

115 Lutz, T.A. (2012). Control of energy homeostasis by amylin. *Cell. Mol. Life Sci.* 69: 1947–1965.

116 Zuger, D., Forster, K., Lutz, T.A., and Riediger, T. (2013). Amylin and GLP-1 target different populations of area postrema neurons that are both modulated by nutrient stimuli. *Physiol. Behav.* 112–113: 61–69.

117 Ludwig, M.Q., Cheng, W., Gordian, D. et al. (2021). A genetic map of the mouse dorsal vagal complex and its role in obesity. *Nat. Metab.* 3 (4): 530–545.

118 Braegger, F.E., Asarian, L., Dahl, K. et al. (2014). The role of the area postrema in the anorectic effects of amylin and salmon calcitonin: behavioral and neuronal phenotyping. *Eur. J. Neurosci.* 40 (7): 3055–3066.

119 Riediger, T., Schmid, H.A., Lutz, T., and Simon, E. (2001). Amylin potently activates AP neurons possibly via formation of the excitatory second messenger cGMP. *Am. J. Physiol. Regul. Integr. Comp. Physiol.* 281 (6): R1833–R1843.

120 Boccia, L., Le Foll, C., and Lutz, T.A. (2020). Noradrenaline signaling in the LPBN mediates amylin's and salmon calcitonin's hypophagic effect in male rats. *FASEB J.* 34 (11): 15448–15461.

121 Becskei, C., Grabler, V., Edwards, G.L. et al. (2007). Lesion of the lateral parabrachial nucleus attenuates the anorectic effect of peripheral amylin and CCK. *Brain Res.* 1162: 76–84.
122 Riediger, T., Zuend, D., Becskei, C., and Lutz, T.A. (2004). The anorectic hormone amylin contributes to feeding-related changes of neuronal activity in key structures of the gut-brain axis. *Am. J. Physiol. Regul. Integr. Comp. Physiol.* 286 (1): R114–R122.
123 Potes, C.S., Lutz, T.A., and Riediger, T. (2010). Identification of central projections from amylin-activated neurons to the lateral hypothalamus. *Brain Res.* 1334: 31–44.
124 Carter, M.E., Soden, M.E., Zweifel, L.S., and Palmiter, R.D. (2013). Genetic identification of a neural circuit that suppresses appetite. *Nature* 503 (7474): 111–114.
125 Schwaber, J.S., Sternini, C., Brecha, N.C. et al. (1988). Neurons containing calcitonin gene-related peptide in the parabrachial nucleus project to the central nucleus of the amygdala. *J. Comp. Neurol.* 270 (3): 416–426, 398–399.
126 Carter, M.E., Han, S., and Palmiter, R.D. (2015). Parabrachial calcitonin gene-related peptide neurons mediate conditioned taste aversion. *J. Neurosci.* 35 (11): 4582–4586.
127 Reiner, D.J., Mietlicki-Baase, E.G., Olivos, D.R. et al. (2017). Amylin acts in the lateral dorsal tegmental nucleus to regulate energy balance through gamma-aminobutyric acid signaling. *Biol. Psychiatry* 82: 828–838.
128 Zhang, C., Kaye, J.A., Cai, Z. et al. (2021). Area postrema cell types that mediate nausea-associated behaviors. *Neuron* 109 (3): 461–72.e5.
129 Nardone, S., De Luca, R., Zito, A. et al. (2024). A spatially-resolved transcriptional atlas of the murine dorsal pons at single-cell resolution. *Nat. Commun.* 15 (1): 1966.
130 Michel, S., Becskei, C., Erguven, E. et al. (2007). Diet-derived nutrients modulate the effects of amylin on c-Fos expression in the area postrema and on food intake. *Neuroendocrinology* 86 (2): 124–135.
131 Ueda, T., Ugawa, S., Saishin, Y., and Shimada, S. (2001). Expression of receptor-activity modifying protein (RAMP) mRNAs in the mouse brain. *Brain Res. Mol. Brain Res.* 93 (1): 36–45.
132 Liberini, C., Cifani, C., Boyle, C. et al. (2013). Gene expression profiling of single amylin- activated neuron in the rat area postrema. *Proceedings, Society for Neuroscience Meeting*.
133 Skofitsch, G., Wimalawansa, S.J., Jacobowitz, D.M., and Gubisch, W. (1995). Comparative immunohistochemical distribution of amylin-like and calcitonin gene related peptide like immunoreactivity in the rat central nervous system. *Can. J. Physiol. Pharmacol.* 73 (7): 945–956.
134 Davidowa, H. (2007). Histamine H1-receptors differentially mediate the action of amylin on hypothalamic neurons in control and in overweight rats. *Behav. Brain Res.* 182 (1): 28–35.
135 Barth, S.W., Riediger, T., Lutz, T.A., and Rechkemmer, G. (2003). Differential effects of amylin and salmon calcitonin on neuropeptide gene expression in

the lateral hypothalamic area and the arcuate nucleus of the rat. *Neurosci. Lett.* 341 (2): 131–134.

136 Pan, W., Adams, J.M., Allison, M.B. et al. (2018). Essential role for hypothalamic calcitonin receptor expressing neurons in the control of food intake by leptin. *Endocrinology* 159 (4): 1860–1872.

137 Su, Z., Alhadeff, A.L., and Betley, J.N. (2017). Nutritive, post-ingestive signals are the primary regulators of AgRP neuron activity. *Cell Rep.* 21 (10): 2724–2736.

138 Gedulin, B.R., Rink, T.J., and Young, A.A. (1997). Dose-response for glucagonostatic effect of amylin in rats. *Metab. Clin. Exp.* 46 (1): 67–70.

139 Kastin, A.J. and Pan, W. (2016). Involvement of the blood-brain barrier in metabolic regulation. *CNS Neurol. Disord. Drug Targets* 15 (9): 1118–1128.

140 Volkow, N.D., Wang, G.J., and Baler, R.D. (2011). Reward, dopamine and the control of food intake: implications for obesity. *Trends Cogn. Sci.* 15 (1): 37–46.

141 Munzberg, H., Qualls-Creekmore, E., Yu, S. et al. (2016). Hedonics act in unison with the homeostatic system to unconsciously control body weight. *Front. Nutr.* 3: 6.

142 Dickson, S.L., Shirazi, R.H., Hansson, C. et al. (2012). The glucagon-like peptide 1 (GLP-1) analogue, exendin-4, decreases the rewarding value of food: a new role for mesolimbic GLP-1 receptors. *J. Neurosci.* 32 (14): 4812–4820.

143 Mietlicki-Baase, E.G., Ortinski, P.I., Rupprecht, L.E. et al. (2013). The food intake-suppressive effects of glucagon-like peptide-1 receptor signaling in the ventral tegmental area are mediated by AMPA/kainate receptors. *Am. J. Physiol. Endocrinol. Metab.* 305 (11): E1367–E1374.

144 Skibicka, K.P. (2013). The central GLP-1: implications for food and drug reward. *Front. Neurosci.* 7: 181.

145 Smith, S.R., Blundell, J.E., Burns, C. et al. (2007). Pramlintide treatment reduces 24-h caloric intake and meal sizes and improves control of eating in obese subjects: a 6-wk translational research study. *Am. J. Physiol. Endocrinol. Metab.* 293 (2): E620–E627.

146 Kalafateli, A.L., Vallof, D., Colombo, G. et al. (2019). An amylin analogue attenuates alcohol-related behaviours in various animal models of alcohol use disorder. *Neuropsychopharmacology* 44 (6): 1093–1102.

147 Kalafateli, A.L., Vallof, D., and Jerlhag, E. (2019). Activation of amylin receptors attenuates alcohol-mediated behaviours in rodents. *Addict. Biol.* 24 (3): 388–402.

148 Le Foll, C. and Lutz, T.A. (2020). Systemic and central amylin, amylin receptor signaling, and their physiological and pathophysiological roles in metabolism. *Compr. Physiol.* 10 (3): 811–837.

149 Boccia, L., Gamakharia, S., Coester, B. et al. (2020). Amylin brain circuitry. *Peptides* 132: 170366.

150 Eiden, S., Daniel, C., Steinbrueck, A. et al. (2002). Salmon calcitonin – a potent inhibitor of food intake in states of impaired leptin signalling in laboratory rodents. *J. Physiol.* 541 (Pt 3): 1041–1048.

151 Duffy, S., Lutz, T.A., and Boyle, C.N. (2018). Rodent models of leptin receptor deficiency are less sensitive to amylin. *Am. J. Physiol. Regul. Integr. Comp. Physiol.* 315 (4): R856–R865.

152 Senn, S.S., Le Foll, C., Whiting, L. et al. (2019). Unsilencing of native leptin receptors (LepR) in hypothalamic SF1 neurons does not rescue obese phenotype in LepR-deficient mice. *Am. J. Physiol. Regul. Integr. Comp. Physiol.* 317: R451–R460.

153 Chan, J.L., Roth, J.D., and Weyer, C. (2009). It takes two to tango: combined amylin/leptin agonism as a potential approach to obesity drug development. *J. Investig. Med.* 57 (7): 777–783.

154 Roth, J.D., Trevaskis, J.L., Turek, V.F., and Parkes, D.G. (2010). "Weighing in" on synergy: preclinical research on neurohormonal anti-obesity combinations. *Brain Res.* 1350: 86–94.

155 Trevaskis, J.L., Coffey, T., Cole, R. et al. (2008). Amylin-mediated restoration of leptin responsiveness in diet-induced obesity: magnitude and mechanisms. *Endocrinology* 149 (11): 5679–5687.

156 Trevaskis, J.L., Parkes, D.G., and Roth, J.D. (2010). Insights into amylin-leptin synergy. *Trends Endocrinol. Metab.* 21 (8): 473–479.

157 Trevaskis, J.L., Wittmer, C., Athanacio, J.R. et al. (2016). Amylin/leptin synergy is absent in extreme obesity and not restored by calorie restriction-induced weight loss in rats. *Obes. Sci. Pract.* 2 (4): 385–391, http://onlinelibrary.wiley.com/doi/10.1002/osp4.62/pdf.

158 Smith, P.M., Brzezinska, P., Hubert, F. et al. (2016). Leptin influences the excitability of area postrema neurons. *Am. J. Physiol. Regul. Integr. Comp. Physiol.* 310 (5): R440–R448.

159 Gorski, J.N., Dunn-Meynell, A.A., and Levin, B.E. (2007). Maternal obesity increases hypothalamic leptin receptor expression and sensitivity in juvenile obesity-prone rats. *Am. J. Physiol. Regul. Integr. Comp. Physiol.* 292 (5): R1782–R1791.

160 Levin, B.E., Dunn-Meynell, A.A., Ricci, M.R., and Cummings, D.E. (2003). Abnormalities of leptin and ghrelin regulation in obesity-prone juvenile rats. *Am. J. Physiol. Endocrinol. Metab.* 285 (5): E949–E957.

161 Larsen, L., Le Foll, C., Dunn-Meynell, A.A., and Levin, B.E. (2016). IL-6 ameliorates defective leptin sensitivity in DIO ventromedial hypothalamic nucleus neurons. *Am. J. Physiol. Regul. Integr. Comp. Physiol.*; In Press.

162 Irani, B.G., Dunn-Meynell, A.A., and Levin, B.E. (2007). Altered hypothalamic leptin, insulin and melanocortin binding associated with moderate fat diet and predisposition to obesity. *Endocrinology* 148 (1): 310–316.

163 Levin, B.E., Dunn-Meynell, A.A., and Banks, W.A. (2004). Obesity-prone rats have normal blood-brain barrier transport but defective central leptin signaling prior to obesity onset. *Am. J. Phys.* 286: R143–R150.

164 Bouret, S.G., Gorski, J.N., Patterson, C.M. et al. (2008). Hypothalamic neural projections are permanently disrupted in diet-induced obese rats. *Cell Metab.* 7 (2): 179–185.

165 Dunn-Meynell, A.A., Le Foll, C., Johnson, M.D. et al. (2016). Endogenous VMH amylin signaling is required for full leptin signaling and protection from diet-induced obesity. *Am. J. Physiol. Regul. Integr. Comp. Physiol.* 310 (4): R355–R365.

166 Levin, B.E., Dunn-Meynell, A.A., Balkan, B., and Keesey, R.E. (1997). Selective breeding for diet-induced obesity and resistance in Sprague-Dawley rats. *Am. J. Phys.* 273: R725–R730.

167 Christopoulos, G., Paxinos, G., Huang, X.F. et al. (1995). Comparative distribution of receptors for amylin and the related peptides calcitonin gene related peptide and calcitonin in rat and monkey brain. *Can. J. Physiol. Pharmacol.* 73 (7): 1037–1041.

168 Auernhammer, C.J., Kopp, F.B., Vlotides, G. et al. (2004). Comparative study of gp130 cytokine effects on corticotroph AtT-20 cells – redundancy or specificity of neuroimmunoendocrine modulators? *Neuroimmunomodulation* 11 (4): 224–232.

169 Rahmouni, K., Fath, M.A., Seo, S. et al. (2008). Leptin resistance contributes to obesity and hypertension in mouse models of Bardet-Biedl syndrome. *J. Clin. Invest.* 118 (4): 1458–1467.

170 Seo, S., Guo, D.F., Bugge, K. et al. (2009). Requirement of Bardet-Biedl syndrome proteins for leptin receptor signaling. *Hum. Mol. Genet.* 18 (7): 1323–1331.

171 Figlewicz, D.P., Evans, S.B., Murphy, J. et al. (2003). Expression of receptors for insulin and leptin in the ventral tegmental area/substantia nigra (VTA/SN) of the rat. *Brain Res.* 964 (1): 107–115.

172 Mietlicki-Baase, E.G., Olivos, D.R., Jeffrey, B.A., and Hayes, M.R. (2015). Cooperative interaction between leptin and amylin signaling in the ventral tegmental area for the control of food intake. *Am. J. Physiol. Endocrinol. Metab.* 308 (12): E1116–E1122.

173 Hommel, J.D., Trinko, R., Sears, R.M. et al. (2006). Leptin receptor signaling in midbrain dopamine neurons regulates feeding. *Neuron* 51 (6): 801–810.

174 Myers, M.G. Jr., Munzberg, H., Leinninger, G.M., and Leshan, R.L. (2009). The geometry of leptin action in the brain: more complicated than a simple ARC. *Cell Metab.* 9 (2): 117–123.

175 Tu, L.H., Serrano, A.L., Zanni, M.T., and Raleigh, D.P. (2014). Mutational analysis of preamyloid intermediates: the role of his-tyr interactions in islet amyloid formation. *Biophys. J.* 106 (7): 1520–1527.

176 Chen, Y.C., Taylor, A.J., and Verchere, C.B. (2018). Islet prohormone processing in health and disease. *Diabetes Obes. Metab.* 20 (Suppl 2): 64–76.

177 Wang, J., Xu, J., Finnerty, J. et al. (2001). The prohormone convertase enzyme 2 (PC2) is essential for processing pro-islet amyloid polypeptide at the NH2-terminal cleavage site. *Diabetes* 50 (3): 534–539.

178 Westermark, G.T., Krogvold, L., Dahl-Jørgensen, K., and Ludvigsson, J. (2017). Islet amyloid in recent-onset type 1 diabetes-the DiViD study. *Ups. J. Med. Sci.* 122 (3): 201–203.

179 Westermark, G.T., Westermark, P., Berne, C. et al. (2008). Widespread amyloid deposition in transplanted human pancreatic islets. *N. Engl. J. Med.* 359 (9): 977–979.

180 Kahn, S.E., Templin, A.T., Hull, R.L., and Verchere, C.B. (2019). Probing the meaning of persistent propeptide release in type 1 diabetes. *Diabetes Care* 42 (2): 183–185.

181 Udayasankar, J., Kodama, K., Hull, R.L. et al. (2009). Amyloid formation results in recurrence of hyperglycaemia following transplantation of human IAPP transgenic mouse islets. *Diabetologia* 52 (1): 145–153.

182 Potter, K.J., Abedini, A., Marek, P. et al. (2010). Islet amyloid deposition limits the viability of human islet grafts but not porcine islet grafts. *PNAS* 107 (9): 4305–4310.

183 Beery, M.L., Jacobsen, L.M., Atkinson, M.A. et al. (2019). Islet amyloidosis in a child with type 1 diabetes. *Islets* 11 (2): 44–49.

184 Meng, F. and Raleigh, D.P. (2011). Inhibition of glycosaminoglycan-mediated amyloid formation by islet amyloid polypeptide and proIAPP processing intermediates. *J. Mol. Biol.* 406 (3): 491–502.

185 Abedini, A. and Raleigh, D.P. (2009). A critical assessment of the role of helical intermediates in amyloid formation by natively unfolded proteins and polypeptides. *Protein Eng. Des. Sel.* 22 (8): 453–459.

186 Marzban, L., Rhodes, C.J., Steiner, D.F. et al. (2006). Impaired NH2-terminal processing of human proislet amyloid polypeptide by the prohormone convertase PC2 leads to amyloid formation and cell death. *Diabetes* 55 (8): 2192–2201.

187 Paulsson, J.F., Andersson, A., Westermark, P., and Westermark, G.T. (2006). Intracellular amyloid-like deposits contain unprocessed pro-islet amyloid polypeptide (proIAPP) in beta cells of transgenic mice overexpressing the gene for human IAPP and transplanted human islets. *Diabetologia* 49 (6): 1237–1246.

188 Shih, A.Z.L., Chen, Y.C., Speckmann, T. et al. (2022). SORLA mediates endocytic uptake of proIAPP and protects against islet amyloid deposition. *Mol. Metab.* 65: 101585.

189 Miyazato, M., Nakazato, M., Shiomi, K. et al. (1992). Molecular forms of islet amyloid polypeptide (IAPP/amylin) in four mammals. *Diabetes Res. Clin. Pract.* 15 (1): 31–36.

190 Esser, N., Hogan, M.F., Aplin, A. et al. (2019). 2124-P: the tissue plasminogen activator (tPA)/plasmin system reduces amyloid formation by cleaving human islet amyloid polypeptide (hIAPP). *Diabetes (New York, NY)* 68 (Supplement 1): 2124.

191 Esser, N., Hogan, M.F., Templin, A.T. et al. (2020). Plasmin-mediated cleavage of human islet amyloid polypeptide (hIAPP) protects beta-cells from amyloid-induced toxicity. *Diabetes* 69: 2039.

192 Esser, N., Hogan, M.F., Templin, A.T. et al. (2020). 2039-P: Plasmin-mediated cleavage of human islet amyloid polypeptide (hIAPP) protects ß-cells from amyloid-induced toxicity. *Diabetes (New York, NY).* 69 (Supplement_1): 2039.

193 Abedini, A., Plesner, A., Cao, P. et al. (2016). Time-resolved studies define the nature of toxic IAPP intermediates, providing insight for anti-amyloidosis therapeutics. *elife* 5: e12977.

194 Munhoz, A.C., Riva, P., Simões, D. et al. (2016). Control of insulin secretion by production of reactive oxygen species: study performed in pancreatic islets from fed and 48-hour fasted wistar rats. *PLoS One* 11 (6): e0158166.

195 Frias, J.P., Deenadayalan, S., Erichsen, L. et al. (2023). Efficacy and safety of co-administered once-weekly cagrilintide 2.4 mg with once-weekly semaglutide 2.4 mg in type 2 diabetes: a multicentre, randomised, double-blind, active-controlled, phase 2 trial. *Lancet* 402 (10403): 720–730.

196 Reidelberger, R.D., Kelsey, L., and Heimann, D. (2002). Effects of amylin-related peptides on food intake, meal patterns, and gastric emptying in rats. *Am. J. Physiol. Regul. Integr. Comp. Physiol.* 282 (5): R1395–R1404.

197 David, J.M., Lau, C.W., McFarlane, J. et al. (2020). Efficacy and safety of AM833 for weight loss: a dose-finding trial in adults with overweight/obesity, *Proceedings, The Obesity Week: Oral Presentation 043.*

198 Dehestani, B., Stratford, N.R., and le Roux, C.W. (2021). Amylin as a future obesity treatment. *J. Obes. Metab. Syndr.* 30 (4): 320–325.

199 Dahl, K.J.L.H., Skyggebjerg, R.B., John, L.M. et al. (2020). Preclinical weight loss efficacy of AM833 in animal models of obesity, *Proceedings, The Obesity Week: Poster 330.*

200 Thomas, K.K.D., Schäffer, L., Jakob, L. et al. (2020). AM833 – development of a long-acting amylin analogue, *Proceedings, The Obesity Week, Poster 028.*

201 Becerril, S. and Frühbeck, G. (2021). Cagrilintide plus semaglutide for obesity management. *Lancet (London, England).* 397 (10286): 1687–1689.

202 Enebo, L.B., Berthelsen, K.K., Kankam, M. et al. (2021). Safety, tolerability, pharmacokinetics, and pharmacodynamics of concomitant administration of multiple doses of cagrilintide with semaglutide 2·4 mg for weight management: a randomised, controlled, phase 1b trial. *Lancet (London, England).* 397 (10286): 1736–1748.

203 Hay, D.L., Garelja, M.L., Poyner, D.R., and Walker, C.S. (2018). Update on the pharmacology of calcitonin/CGRP family of peptides: IUPHAR review 25. *Br. J. Pharmacol.* 175 (1): 3–17.

204 Guerreiro, L.H., Guterres, M.F., Melo-Ferreira, B. et al. (2013). Preparation and characterization of PEGylated amylin. *AAPS Pharm. Sci. Tech.* 14 (3): 1083–1097.

205 Kowalczyk, R., Brimble, M.A., Tomabechi, Y. et al. (2014). Convergent chemoenzymatic synthesis of a library of glycosylated analogues of pramlintide: structure-activity relationships for amylin receptor agonism. *Org. Biomol. Chem.* 12 (41): 8142–8151.

206 Andreassen, K.V., Feigh, M., Hjuler, S.T. et al. (2014). A novel oral dual amylin and calcitonin receptor agonist (KBP-042) exerts antiobesity and antidiabetic effects in rats. *Am. J. Physiol. Endocrinol. Metab.* 307 (1): E24–E33.

207 Feigh, M., Andreassen, K.V., Hjuler, S.T. et al. (2013). Oral salmon calcitonin protects against impaired fasting glycemia, glucose intolerance, and obesity induced by high-fat diet and ovariectomy in rats. *Menopause* 20: 785–794.

208 Feigh, M., Nielsen, R.H., Hansen, C. et al. (2012). Oral salmon calcitonin improves fasting and postprandial glycemic control in lean healthy rats. *Horm. Metab. Res.* 44 (2): 130–134.

209 Leinung, M.C. and Grasso, P. (2012). [D-Leu-4]-OB3, a synthetic peptide amide with leptin-like activity, augments the effects of orally delivered exenatide and pramlintide acetate on energy balance and glycemic control in insulin-resistant male C57BLK/6-m db/db mice. *Regul. Pept.* 179 (1–3): 33–38.

210 Brings, A., Borghardt, J.M., Skarbaliene, J. et al. (2018). Modeling energy intake and body weight effects of a long-acting amylin analogue. *J. Pharmacokinet. Pharmacodyn.* 45 (2): 215–233.

211 Fletcher, M.M., Keov, P., Truong, T.T. et al. (2021). AM833 is a novel agonist of calcitonin family G protein-coupled receptors: pharmacological comparison to six selective and non-selective agonists. *J. Pharmacol. Exp. Ther.* 377: 417–440.

212 Adler, B.L., Yarchoan, M., Hwang, H.M. et al. (2014). Neuroprotective effects of the amylin analogue pramlintide on Alzheimer's disease pathogenesis and cognition. *Neurobiol. Aging* 35 (4): 793–801.

213 Chapman, I., Parker, B., Doran, S. et al. (2005). Effect of pramlintide on satiety and food intake in obese subjects and subjects with type 2 diabetes. *Diabetologia* 48 (5): 838–848.

214 Hollander, P., Maggs, D.G., Ruggles, J.A. et al. (2004). Effect of pramlintide on weight in overweight and obese insulin-treated type 2 diabetes patients. *Obes. Res.* 12 (4): 661–668.

215 Boyle, C.N., Lutz, T.A., and Le Foll, C. (2018). Amylin – Its role in the homeostatic and hedonic control of eating and recent developments of amylin analogs to treat obesity. *Mol. Metab.* 8: 203–210.

216 Grabler, V. and Lutz, T.A. (2004). Chronic infusion of the amylin antagonist AC 187 increases feeding in Zucker fa/fa rats but not in lean controls. *Physiol. Behav.* 81 (3): 481–488.

217 Arnelo, U., Permert, J., Larsson, J. et al. (1997). Chronic low dose islet amyloid polypeptide infusion reduces food intake, but does not influence glucose metabolism, in unrestrained conscious rats: studies using a novel aortic catheterization technique. *Endocrinology* 138 (10): 4081–4085.

218 Chelikani, P.K., Haver, A.C., and Reidelberger, R.D. (2007). Effects of intermittent intraperitoneal infusion of salmon calcitonin on food intake and adiposity in obese rats. *Am. J. Physiol. Regul. Integr. Comp. Physiol.* 293 (5): R1798–R1808.

219 El, K., Douros, J.D., Willard, F.S. et al. (2023). The incretin co-agonist tirzepatide requires GIPR for hormone secretion from human islets. *Nat. Metab.* 5 (6): 945–954.

220 Betsholtz, C., Johnson, K.H., and Westermark, P. (1989). "Amylin" hormone. *Nature* 338: 211.

221 Matveyenko, A.V. and Butler, P.C. (2006). Islet amyloid polypeptide (IAPP) transgenic rodents as models for type 2 diabetes. *ILAR J.* 47 (3): 225–233.

222 Zini, E., Lunardi, F., Zanetti, R. et al. (2016). Endocrine pancreas in cats with diabetes mellitus. *Vet. Pathol.* 53 (1): 136–144.

223 Preston, A.M., Gurisik, E., Bartley, C. et al. (2009). Reduced endoplasmic reticulum (ER)-to-Golgi protein trafficking contributes to ER stress in lipotoxic mouse beta cells by promoting protein overload. *Diabetologia* 52 (11): 2369–2373.

224 Donath, M.Y., Dalmas, E., Sauter, N.S., and Boni-Schnetzler, M. (2013). Inflammation in obesity and diabetes: islet dysfunction and therapeutic opportunity. *Cell Metab.* 17 (6): 860–872.

225 Lorenzo, A., Razzaboni, B., Weir, G.C., and Yankner, B.A. (1994). Pancreatic islet cell toxicity of amylin associated with type-2 diabetes mellitus. *Nature* 368 (6473): 756–760.

226 Potter, K.J., Scrocchi, L.A., Warnock, G.L. et al. (2009). Amyloid inhibitors enhance survival of cultured human islets. *Biochim. Biophys. Acta* 1790 (6): 566–574.

227 Lin, C.Y., Gurlo, T., Kayed, R. et al. (2007). Toxic human islet amyloid polypeptide (h-IAPP) oligomers are intracellular, and vaccination to induce anti-toxic oligomer antibodies does not prevent h-IAPP-induced beta-cell apoptosis in h-IAPP transgenic mice. *Diabetes* 56 (5): 1324–1332.

228 Vogt, A.S., Roesti, E.S., Mohsen, M.O. et al. (2021). Anti-IAPP monoclonal antibody improves clinical symptoms in a mouse model of type 2 diabetes. *Vaccines (Basel).* 9 (11).

229 Roesti, E.S., Boyle, C.N., Zeman, D.T. et al. (2020). Vaccination against amyloidogenic aggregates in pancreatic islets prevents development of type 2 diabetes mellitus. *Vaccines (Basel).* 8 (1): 116.

230 Bortoletto, A.S., Graham, W.V., Trout, G. et al. (2022). Human islet amyloid polypeptide (hIAPP) protofibril-specific antibodies for detection and treatment of type 2 diabetes. *Adv Sci (Weinh).* 9 (34): e2202342.

231 Denroche, H.C. and Verchere, C.B. (2018). IAPP and type 1 diabetes: implications for immunity, metabolism and islet transplants. *J. Mol. Endocrinol.* 60 (2): R57–r75.

232 Donath, M.Y. (2013). When metabolism met immunology. *Nat. Immunol.* 14 (5): 421–422.

4

Peptide-Based GLP-1 Receptor Agonists for the Treatment of Type 2 Diabetes and Obesity

János T. Kodra[1], Lars Linderoth[1], Steffen Reedtz-Runge[2], Thomas Kruse[1], and Jacob C. Kofoed[1]

[1] *Novo Nordisk A/S, Peptide Research, Novo Nordisk Park, 2760 Måløv, Denmark*
[2] *Novo Nordisk A/S, Structure and Interactions, Novo Nordisk Park, 2760 Måløv, Denmark*

Introduction

In 1921, the discovery of insulin by Banting and Best paved the way for life-saving treatment for people living with type 1 diabetes mellitus (T1DM) [1]. Blood glucose could now be controlled by chronic administration of exogenous insulin. The discovery of insulin led to tremendous efforts in engineering the insulin molecule for better and more convenient treatments for people living with both type 1 and type 2 diabetes mellitus (T2DM). Nevertheless, insulin-based therapies continue to have two disadvantages: risk of hypoglycemia and weight gain. Consequently, many alternative treatment options have emerged, mainly within the field of T2DM.

One particular endogenous peptide hormone, glucagon-like peptide-1 (GLP-1), has been intensively studied and engineered for better treatments not only for people with T2DM but also for people with obesity. This chapter provides an overview of the background, developments, and future outlook of GLP-1 peptide receptor agonists for the treatment of T2DM and obesity.

GLP-1 is part of the incretin hormone family, which is secreted from the gastrointestinal tract in response to nutrient ingestion. The phenomenon, known as the incretin effect, explains how oral glucose administration leads to notably higher plasma insulin levels compared to intravenous glucose administration. While the first incretin, glucose-dependent insulinotropic polypeptide (GIP), was discovered in the 1970s, GLP-1 was not identified until the 1980s following the cloning and sequencing of mammalian proglucagon genes and complementary DNAs [2, 3]. It was found that the proglucagon gene encodes for glucagon and two other peptide hormones that share 50% homology with glucagon (Figure 4.1). As a result, these peptides were named GLP-1 and glucagon-like peptide 2 (GLP-2) [3, 4]. Both GLP-1 and GLP-2 were examined for their insulinotropic activity due to their similarity to glucagon, and it was determined that only GLP-1 could stimulate insulin secretion (for a more comprehensive review of the discovery of GLP-1, see [2]).

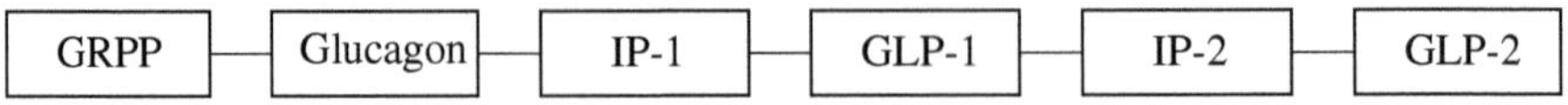

Figure 4.1 Human proglucagon as encoded on complementary DNA. Glicentin-related pancreatic polypeptide (GRPP), intervening peptide (IP) [2, 3].

```
hGLP-1(1-37)   HDEFERHAEGTFTSDVSSYLEGQAAKEFIAWLVKGRG--------
hGLP-1(7-37)   ------HAEGTFTSDVSSYLEGQAAKEFIAWLVKGRG--------
Exendin-4      ------HGEGTFTSDLSKQMEEEAVRLFIEWLKNGGPSSGAPPPS
                     * ******* *   *  *   ** **  *
```

Figure 4.2 Sequence alignment of GLP-1(1–37), GLP-1(7–37), and exendin-4 (C-terminally amidated).

The bioactive sequence of GLP-1 was not initially identified from the proglucagon gene, as early studies suggested that the bioactive GLP-1 consists of 37 amino acids when cleaved from proglucagon. However, another cleavage of proglucagon results in a shorter version of GLP-1 with six fewer amino acids, known as GLP-1(7–37) (Figure 4.2). This shorter version, along with a one amino acid truncated form called GLP-1(7–36)-amide, resulting from the enzymatic cleavage of the C-terminal glycine by peptidylglycine α-amidating monooxygenase, was identified as the biologically active GLP-1 hormone [2, 5]. Both of these peptides exhibit equal potency [6]; consequently, GLP-1 is often used as a generic term encompassing these two forms of GLP-1.

Another prominent member of the GLP-1 family is exendin-4 (Ex4), which was isolated from the saliva of *Heloderma suspectrum* [7]. Ex4 exhibits similar biological properties to GLP-1, and with a 53% sequence homology between the two, they are believed to share a common ancestor [8–10]. It is worth noting that the peptide sequence numbering for Ex4 begins at 1, unlike the active hormone GLP-1s, which starts at 7 (Figure 4.2).

GLP-1 Biology

GLP-1 is secreted from intestinal endocrine L-cells found in both the small and large intestines upon nutrient ingestion. GLP-1 has various physiological effects, including enhancing the synthesis and release of insulin from pancreatic β-cells in a glucose-dependent manner and suppressing glucagon release from pancreatic α-cells [11]. Additionally, GLP-1 promotes satiety, reduces energy intake, and inhibits gastric emptying. More recently, some GLP-1 analogs have been found to exhibit cardiovascular protective effects [12, 13]. It is, however, essential to note that common side effects associated with GLP-1 analogs include nausea and vomiting, though these effects can be significantly reduced through gradual dosing adjustments [2].

Due to GLP-1 effects on lowering glucose levels and inhibiting food intake, substantial efforts have been directed toward developing GLP-1-based therapies for treating T2DM and obesity. However, a key challenge with using GLP-1 as a therapeutic agent is its short half-life in the human bloodstream, which is only a few minutes. The short half-life is due to kidney glomerular filtration and the action of the enzyme dipeptidyl peptidase-IV (DPP-IV), which cleaves the first two amino acids from the N-terminal of GLP-1, rendering the peptide hormone unable to activate its receptor. Some treatments of T2DM involve the use of oral small molecule agents such as sitagliptin, developed by Merck, which inhibit DPP-IV activity [14] (see other chapter of this book).

GLP-1 Receptor Binding and Activation

The activity of GLP-1 is facilitated through its binding to and activation of the GLP-1 receptor (GLP-1R), which belongs to the class B G-protein-coupled receptor family. When bound to the receptor, GLP-1 adopts an α-helical conformation. The proposed two-domain binding mechanism (binding and activation) has been validated by the 3D structures of active-state GLP-1R/Gs complexes with GLP-1 and semaglutide (see section titled "Semaglutide") determined by cryo-electron microscopy (cryo-EM) (Figure 4.3) [15, 16]. In the binding process, the C-terminal portion of GLP-1 interacts with the extracellular domain (ECD) of the GLP-1R. At the same time, the N-terminal part binds to the transmembrane domain (TMD) of the GLP-1R, ultimately leading to receptor activation. The C-terminal segment of GLP-1 is sufficient for binding to the receptor ECD, as demonstrated by the

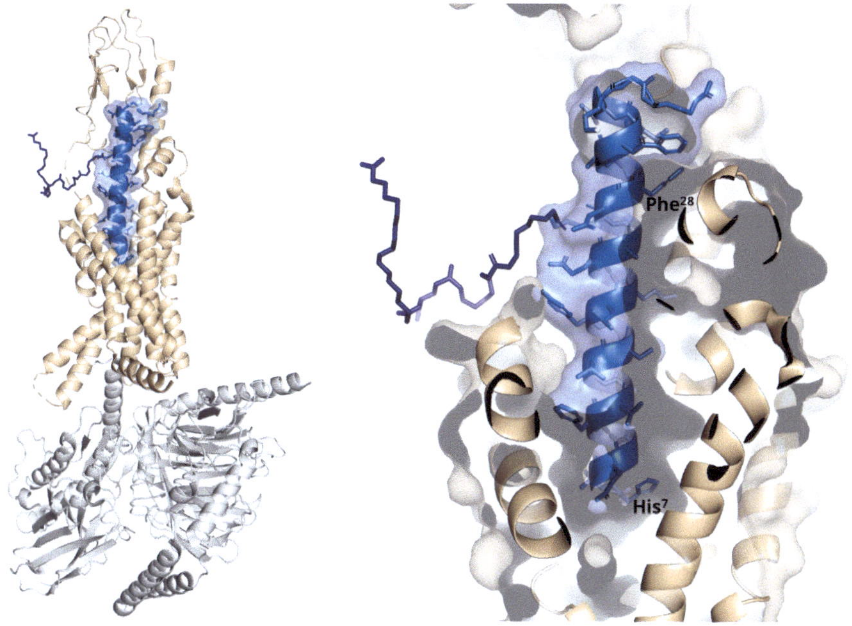

Figure 4.3 Cryo-EM structure of semaglutide bound to the GLP-1 receptor/Gs complex showing the molecular details His7 interaction with the TMD and Phe28 interaction with the ECD/ECL1.

crystal structure of GLP-1 in complex with the isolated ECD. On the other hand, the N-terminal segment of GLP-1 is crucial for receptor activation, as evidenced by the N-terminal truncation of Ex4, which results in the competitive antagonist exendin(9–39) [17]. This antagonist maintains binding to the receptor ECD but fails to initiate signaling through the receptor TMD.

Since its discovery in the 1980s, extensive research has been conducted on the sequence of human GLP-1. In 1993, a study used alanine scanning (replacement of each amino acid with L-alanine) to investigate each amino acid's relative importance for binding and activating the GLP-1 receptor [18]. This study revealed that the N-terminal segment spanning residues 7–15 was crucial for receptor activation. Cryo-EM structures further elucidated these early findings, which demonstrated that residues 7–15 penetrate deeply into the TMD of GLP-1R [15]. In contrast, the central and C-terminal segments were less affected by alanine substitutions, with the notable exceptions being Phe28 and Ile29. The substitution of Phe28 with alanine had the most significant impact on receptor binding compared to all other alanine substitutions throughout the GLP-1 sequence. This finding is consistent with the crystal and cryo-EM structures of GLP-1R, which illustrate that position 26 is accessible for the acylation of semaglutide (see section titled "Semaglutide"), whereas Phe28 and Ile29 are nestled within a hydrophobic binding site provided by the receptor ECD and ECL1 [16]. The role of the residues in the central and C-terminal segments of GLP-1 primarily involves supporting a helical structure and interacting in a specific manner with extracellular loops and the ECD of the GLP-1R.

Clinical Relevant Peptide GLP-1 Receptor Agonists

From its initial discovery in the 1980s, several decades passed before the launch of the first therapy based on GLP-1 receptor agonists, which benefited diabetes patients. Subsequent pharmaceutical developments progressed rapidly, leading to the launch of several new products in the past 10 years, both for diabetes and obesity. Despite the long history of GLP-1 discovery, ongoing research unveils more insights into this fascinating hormone class from biological and structural perspectives. The field is expanding continuously with even a peptide oral tablet-based treatment utilizing a GLP-1R agonist approved by the American Food and Drug Administration (FDA). An overview of the FDA-approved GLP-1R agonist-based therapies is shown in Table 4.1.

The following chapters cover peptide GLP-1 receptor agonists that have been FDA-approved or advanced to the clinic.

Exendin-4-Based Analogs

Exenatide

Exenatide (exendin-4, Figure 4.4) was the first GLP-1R agonist to become available for treating T2DM. It was approved by the FDA in 2005. Amylin initially brought it into the clinic and later codeveloped with Eli Lilly. Exenatide was originally isolated

Table 4.1 Timeline for American Food and Drug Administration (FDA)-approved peptide GLP-1 receptor agonists.

Year	GLP-1 receptor mono agonist	Administration route	Main indication
2005	Exenatide	Once- or twice-daily subcutaneous	Diabetes
2010	Liraglutide	Once-daily subcutaneous	Diabetes
2010	Exenatide LAR	Once-weekly subcutaneous	Diabetes
2014	Dulaglutide	Once-weekly subcutaneous	Diabetes
2014	Albiglutide	Once-weekly subcutaneous	Diabetes
2014	Liraglutide	Once-weekly subcutaneous	Obesity
2016	Lixisenatide	Once- or twice-daily subcutaneous	Obesity
2017	Semaglutide	Once-weekly subcutaneous	Diabetes
2019	Semaglutide	Once-daily oral	Obesity
2021	Semaglutide	Once-weekly subcutaneous	Obesity

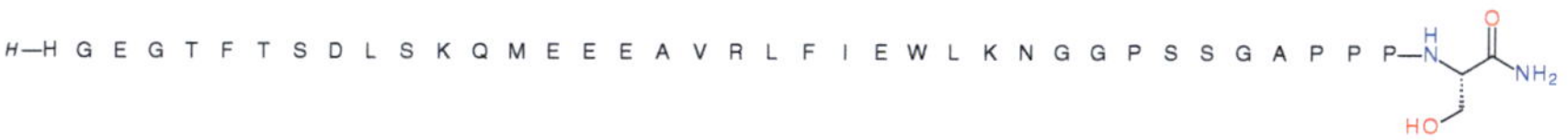

Figure 4.4 Chemical structure of exendin-4.

from the salivary secretions of the Gila monster [7, 19], but the marketed version is made synthetically. Exendin-4 is an ortholog of mammalian GLP-1 and shares around 50% similarity to the human GLP-1 (Figure 4.2). The evolutionary origin of exendin genes (exendins 1–4) has not been fully resolved, but it has been suggested that exendins evolved by duplication from a glucagon-like peptide gene precursor [8–10].

Exendin-4 binds to the intact human glucagon-like peptide-1 receptor (GLP-1R) similarly to GLP-1. Unlike GLP-1, it is stable toward degradation by DPP-IV and shows increased stability toward other peptidases such as the neutral endopeptidase (NEP) [20]. It is cleared by renal extraction [21] and has a longer half-life in vivo than GLP-1 [22]. The marketed formulation of exenatide is dosed subcutaneously twice a day, generally before the first and last meals of the day. The reported glycemic effect of exenatide is around 0.5–1% decrease in HbA1c [23].

Exenatide Long-Acting Release (LAR)

Exenatide LAR was the first GLP-1 receptor agonist on the market suitable for once-weekly dosing. Exenatide LAR is based on a sustained drug release technology where the active ingredient is encapsulated in dissolvable poly-(D,L-lactide-co-glycolide) (PLG) microspheres. Following subcutaneous once-weekly injection, exenatide microspheres remain in place under the skin and slowly degrade, releasing active exenatide continuously into circulation [24]. The reported glycemic effect of the marketed exenatide LAR formulation is around a 1.5% reduction in

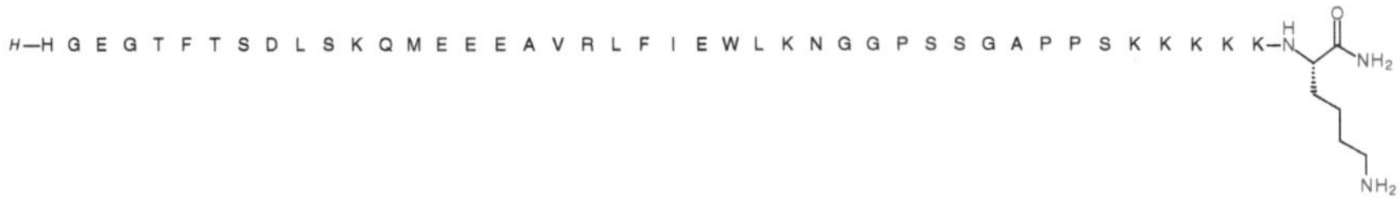

Figure 4.5 Chemical structure of lixisenatide.

HbA1c along with a bodyweight reduction of around 2 kg [25, 26]. A phase 3 study on the potential effect of exenatide-LAR in Parkinson patients found no evidence to support exenatide as a disease-modifying treatment for people with Parkinson's disease [27].

Lixisenatide

Lixisenatide is an analog of exendin-4 where the C-terminus has been modified; the C-terminus has been shortened with one proline residue, and then six lysines (Figure 4.5) have been added. A modification that makes it suitable for once-daily injections [28]. It was created by Zealand Pharma in 2003 and later licensed to Sanofi, which developed the drug. It was approved in 2013 by the European Medicines Agency (EMEA) for treating type II diabetes and by the FDA in 2016 for the same indication.

In CHO-K1 cells expressing human GLP-1R, lixisenatide was reported to have a fourfold greater affinity to GLP-1R ($IC_{50} = 1.4 \pm 0.2$ nM) compared to with native GLP-1 (7–36 amide) ($IC_{50} = 5.5 \pm 1.3$ nM) [29]. In the clinical phase 3 GetGoal program, dosing 20 μg once daily of lixisenatide resulted in HbA1c reduction of 0.79% and bodyweight reduction of 2.96 ± 0.23 kg was reported [30, 31]. In addition to using lixisenatide alone, a fixed-dose combination of lixisenatide and insulin glargine has been developed to treat T2DM [32]. On January 1, 2023, Sanofi announced that lixisenatide would no longer be available in the US market. The discontinuation was a business decision and was not due to safety or efficacy issues [33]. In late August 2023, it was reported that lixisenatide improves Parkinson's disease symptoms in early disease [34].

Efpeglenatide

Efpeglenatide has been developed by Hanmi Pharmaceuticals and is based on a single amino acid-modified Ex4 analog coupled to a human immunoglobulin G molecule IgG4 Fc fragment via a flexible linker [35] (see Figure 4.6). In contrast to dulaglutide (see section titled "Dulaglutide"), only one Ex4 peptide is fused to the Fc. Fusion to an Fc results in a slow clearance that permits once-weekly dosing, and even a less frequent dosing is under investigation. Efpeglenatide given once weekly in T2DM has been shown to lower HbA1c by approximately 1% when given at a 6 mg dose [36].

In a cardiovascular outcome trial among patients with T2DM followed over 1.8 years, efpeglenatide has been shown to reduce overall major adverse cardiovascular events (MACE) as well as the patients in the treatment groups demonstrated improved kidney function [37].

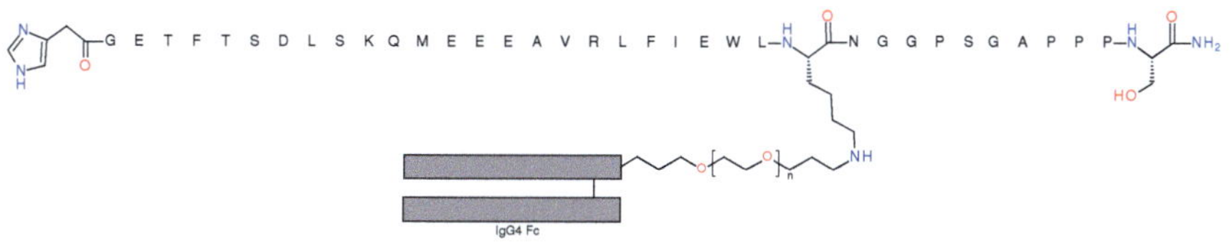

Figure 4.6 Chemical structure of efpeglenatide.

Loxenatide

Another Ex4-based analog is loxenatide, a pegylated version of Ex4 for once-weekly dosing. It has been approved in China for treating T2DM and is undergoing further clinical studies. Compared to Ex4, four substitutions in the peptide backbone ([dAla2, Nle14, Gln28, Cys39]-Ex4) [35] has been introduced in addition, it has been pegylated via maleimide chemistry (see Figure 4.7). Pegylated exenatide is designed for once-weekly dosing, and it seems potent as the doses in clinical trials for clinically relevant reductions in HbA1c are relatively low, 0.1 or 0.2 mg [38]. A recent study on weight management in overweight and obese patients with T2DM demonstrated a weight loss of 8.37% when dosing pegylated loxenatide at 0.3 mg once-weekly subcutaneously [39].

Noiiglutide

Noiiglutide (HS-2004, SHR-2042), under clinical investigation by Jiangsu Hengrui Pharmaceuticals, is hGLP-1 (8Aib, 36G) fused to the C-terminal nine distal residues of exendin-4 linked to the epsilon-amino group of an alpha-palmitoylated lysine (see Figure 4.8) [40]. The palmitoyl moiety of noiiglutide allows for once daily dosing, and in phase 2 clinical trials Chinese adults with obesity achieved a weight loss of up to 9.8% after 24 weeks of treatment (daily sc 0.12 → 0.36 mg).

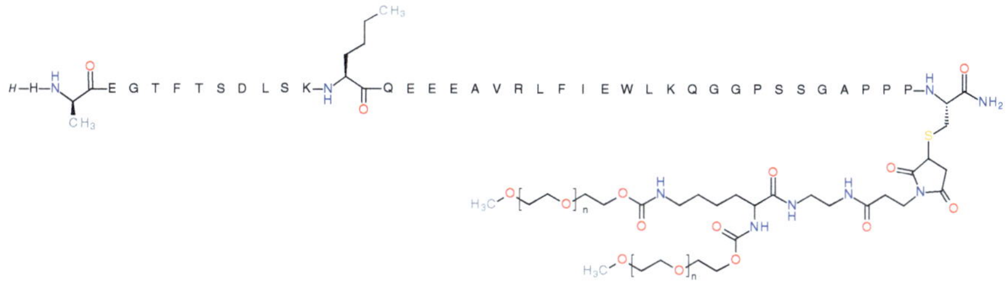

Figure 4.7 Chemical structure of loxenatide.

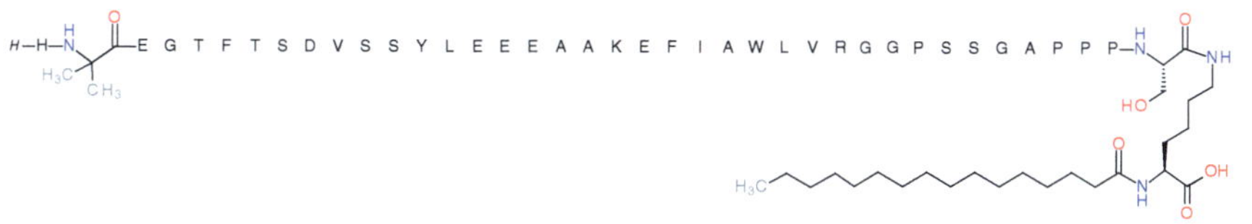

Figure 4.8 Chemical structure of noiiglutide.

Visepegenatide

Visepegenatide (PB-119) [41, 42], under clinical development by PegBio, is a polyethylene glycolated exendin-4 obtained by modification of a single amino acid in exenatide, replacing Ser39 with Cys similar to loxenatide.

The pharmacokinetics of visepegenatide showed slow absorption and a mean elimination half-life of 51–64 h. In phase 3 clinical trials in T2DM patients, once-weekly 150 μg visepegenatide injection gave significant HbA1c reduction (−1.36%) after 24 weeks of treatment [43].

GLP-1-Based Analogs

Liraglutide

Liraglutide, commercialized by Novo Nordisk, was the first human-based GLP-1 analog to obtain regulatory approval in the European Union in 2009 and the United States in 2010. It is dosed once daily by subcutaneous administration. The prolongation of the in vivo half-life of human GLP-1 was obtained by attachment of palmitic acid and a γ-glutamic acid (γ-Glu) linker.

The introduction of fatty acid "protractors" was a field that was pioneered at Novo Nordisk in the early 1990s [44, 45] when myristic acid was attached covalently to insulin (insulin detemir). Once in circulation, the fatty acid binds reversibly to albumin in plasma and eventually to cell surfaces, reducing kidney clearance. Albumin is the most abundant circulating protein found in plasma.

In liraglutide, the palmitic acid is attached to the form of a γ-Glu moiety, which functions as a "linker" (see Figure 4.9) for the fatty acid moiety and the peptide backbone. GLP-1 has two free lysines in positions 26 and 34, which are suitable for attachment of a fatty acid. It is conceivable that using position 26 as the attachment point for the fatty acid sidechain offers increased protection due to the channel-like structure of the DPP-4 enzyme [46]. The peptide backbone of liraglutide is produced by fermentation. To achieve selective acylation of the lysine in position 26, the other lysine in position 34 of liraglutide was substituted with an arginine. In neutral formulation, liraglutide exists primarily as heptamers [47]. This causes slow absorption from the injection site, combined with systemic albumin binding, which enables once-day dosing. Liraglutide has been marketed worldwide since 2009 for T2DM and since 2014 for obesity. In 2018, it was published that liraglutide added to the standard of care reduced the risk for major cardiovascular events and all-cause mortality in patients with type 2 diabetes mellitus and chronic kidney disease [48].

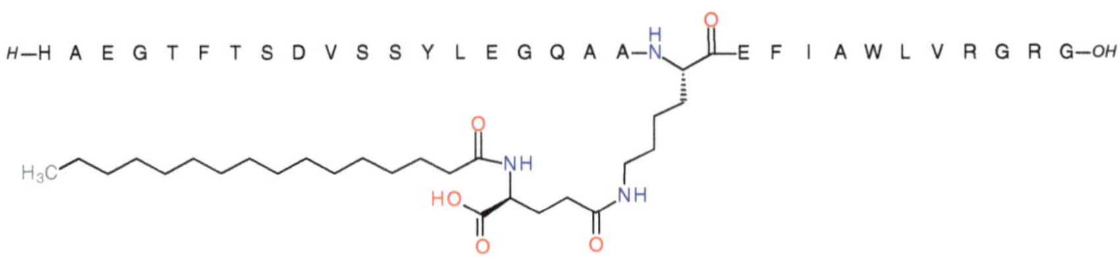

Figure 4.9 Chemical structure of liraglutide.

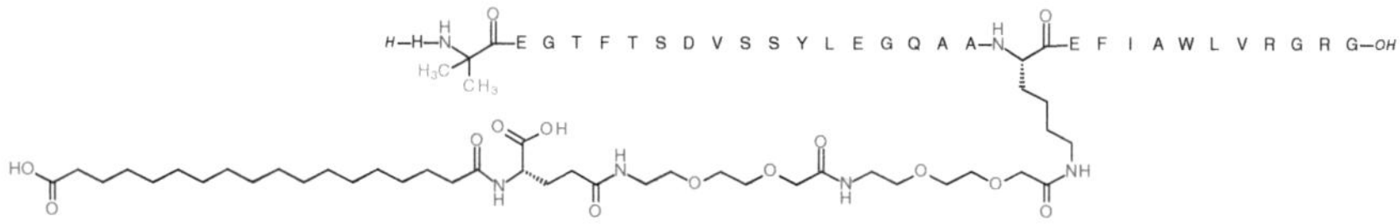

Figure 4.10 Chemical structure of semaglutide.

Semaglutide

Liraglutide is approved for once-daily dosing, and the molecule has been further developed to suit a once-weekly dosing regimen by Novo Nordisk, and that molecule is named semaglutide. The structure is illustrated in Figure 4.10. Semaglutide differs in three essential structural elements from liraglutide: an unnatural amino acid in position 8, a spacer element, and a modified fatty acid. Amino-isobutyric acid (Aib) in position 8 is introduced to avoid DPP-4 cleavage without loss of potency. The fatty di-acid provides stronger albumin binding than the C16 mono acid used in liraglutide and two amino-diethoxy-acetyl units as spacer appeared optimal for potency [49]. The resulting semaglutide molecule was marketed in 2017 to treat T2DM and in 2022 for obesity. The weekly subcutaneous dose is 0.5 or 1.0 mg for T2DM and 2.4 mg for the treatment of obesity. The mean weight loss reported for obesity was 14.9% in the clinical trials using a 2.4 mg weekly subcutaneous dose [12]. In the SELECT trial (semaglutide's Effects on Cardiovascular Outcomes in People with Overweight or Obesity), 17,604 patients with a body mass index (BMI) of 27 or greater and preexisting cardiovascular disease but without diabetes, treatment with once-weekly subcutaneous semaglutide at a dose of 2.4 mg for a mean duration of 33 months reduced the risk of a composite of death from cardiovascular causes, nonfatal myocardial infarction, or nonfatal stroke by 20% [50].

The high potency of semaglutide has also been pivotal for the subsequent advancement aiming for oral dosing of semaglutide. Oral administration of peptides is hindered through extensive degradation by proteolytic enzymes and poor absorption from the gastrointestinal barrier into the bloodstream due to the high molecular weight, hydrophilicity, and low permeability [51, 52]. To increase the oral absorption of semaglutide, a coformulation with the absorption enhancer sodium N-[8(2-hydroxybenzoyl)amino]caprylate (SNAC) (developed by Emisphere Technologies) has been developed. This has shown auspicious results in clinical trials [53] and has been approved by the FDA for treating T2DM with tablets containing 7 or 14 mg of semaglutide taken orally once daily.

Taspoglutide

Taspoglutide is a GLP-1 analog codeveloped by Roche and Ipsen with >90% sequence identity to human GLP-1(7–36)-amide. Taspoglutide was modified in the N-terminus with an 8Aib to stabilize against DPP-IV cleavage. Since further enzymatic C-terminal cleavage products of [Aib8] hGLP-1(7–36)-amide was found in plasma, an additional Aib was introduced in position 35 to generate [Aib8, Aib35] human GLP-1(7–36)-amide (see Figure 4.11).

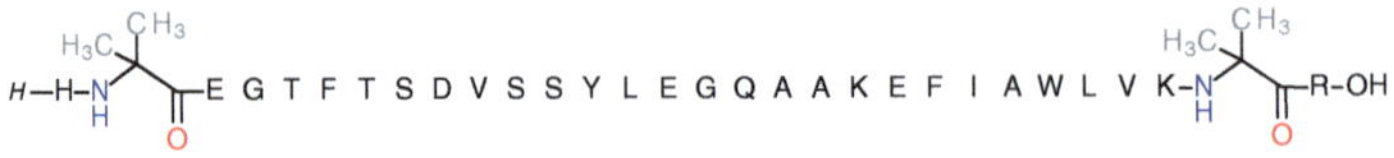

Figure 4.11 Chemical structure of taspoglutide.

Receptor binding and activation experiments revealed that the amino acid substitutions introduced in taspoglutide did not compromise the interaction with GLP-1 receptor [54, 55]. Compared to human GLP-1, taspoglutide was more stable in rat plasma, and first-order disappearance kinetics showed a half-life approximately 10 times longer than native human GLP-1. In clinical trials, taspoglutide was produced as a sustained-release formulation, giving maximum exposure at 24 h and sustained plasma levels for two weeks following subcutaneous injection. In the 24-week T-emerge 2 trial, subjects treated with 20 mg taspoglutide achieved an HbA1c lowering of −1.24% from baseline and a change in body weight of −2.3 kg [56]. A high number of adverse events in phase 3 trials, including gastrointestinal symptoms and local injection site reactions, triggered Roche to withdraw taspoglutide before release. The development of anti-drug antibodies was identified as the root cause for the injection site reactions [57].

Albiglutide and Albenatide

GLP-1 agonists conjugated to albumin through direct covalent conjugation have also been pursued to obtain long-circulating half-lives.

Albiglutide is a once-weekly GLP-1 receptor agonist approved in 2014 and marketed by GlaxoSmithKline (GSK). Albiglutide is a fusion of a GLP-1 dimer to human albumin (see Figure 4.12). Protection against DPP-IV was accomplished by replacing the natural Ala8 residue at the DPP-IV cleavage site with a Gly8 [58, 59]. Albumin has a remarkably long serum half-life (approximately 19 days in humans) due to its recycling via the neonatal Fc receptor (FcRn) [60] and the albiglutide GLP-1-albumin fusion protein consequently has a half-life of 6–8 days in humans with maximum plasma concentration at 2–4 days making it suitable for once-weekly dosing [61]. In the HARMONY 7 32-week clinical trial, subjects treated with albiglutide 30 mg once weekly titrated to 50 mg at week six achieved a model-adjusted change in HbA1c from baseline to week 32 of approximately −0.8% and a change in bodyweight of approximately −0.6 kg [62]. In July 2017, GSK announced that the company was discontinuing the manufacturing and sale of albiglutide worldwide due to limited prescribing of the drug and declining sales.

Another example of albumin conjugation is albenatide (CJC-1134-PC) developed by Conjuchem where the surface-exposed free cysteine on human serum albumin (HSA) is coupled to the C-terminal part of Ex4 via maleimide chemistry. Preliminary results from clinical trials indicate a half-life in humans of approximately

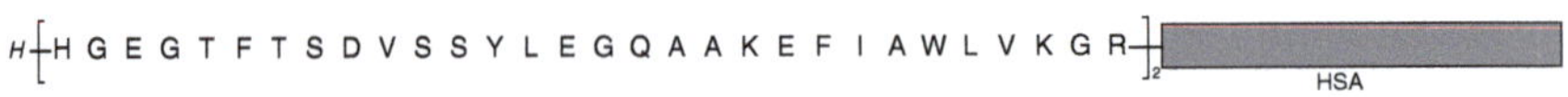

Figure 4.12 Chemical structure of albiglutide.

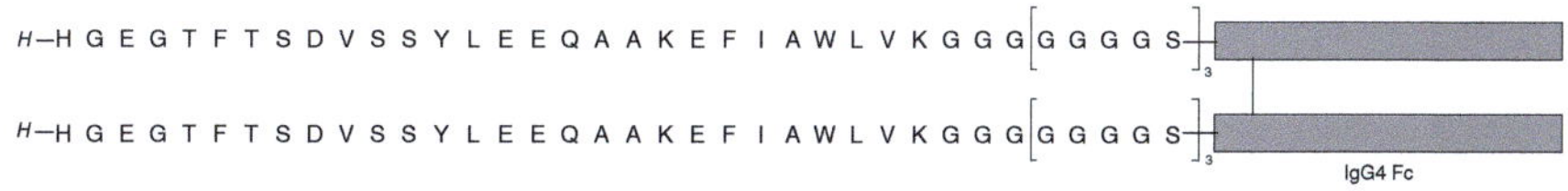

Figure 4.13 Chemical structure of dulaglutide.

eight days, whereby CJC-1134 is suitable for once-weekly dosing [63]. Furthermore, a reduction of HbA1c of 1.4% together with a moderate weight loss has been observed with CJC-1134-PC in clinical phase II trials [64].

Dulaglutide

Dulaglutide was marketed by Eli Lilly in 2014. It is a dimeric GLP-1 analog fused to an engineered Fc fragment via a linker: [Gly8, Glu22, Gly36] GLP-1(7–37)-(Gly4Ser)3Ala-[Ala234, Ala235, Pro228]-IgG4-Fc. The GLP-1 part is DPP-IV protected using Gly8, and to improve in vitro potency, the Gly in position 22 was replaced by Glu (a substitution also found in Ex4). Gly36 was introduced to de-immunize the fusion protein. The immunoglobulin is a modified IgG4 isotype optimized at two selected positions (F234A and L235A) to reduce interaction with high-affinity Fc receptors, which significantly reduced dose-dependent cytotoxicity over the IgG1 version. Finally, S228 was mutated to proline to eliminate half-antibody formation (see Figure 4.13) [65].

In humans, dulaglutide has a half-life of approximately 3.75 days due to its recycling via FcRn, making it suitable for once-weekly dosing. In the AWARD-6 trial, subjects treated with dulaglutide 1.5 mg once-weekly achieved a change in HbA1c from baseline to week 24 of approximately −1.4% and a change in body weight of approximately −2.9 kg [13].

In the "The Researching Cardiovascular Events With a Weekly Incretin in Diabetes" (REWIND) study, dulaglutide was associated with a 9% reduced index of atherosclerosis in patients with type 2 diabetes and established CV disease or various levels of CV risk [66].

Ecnoglutide

Ecnoglutide (XW-003), under clinical investigation by Sciwind Biosciences, is structurally closely related to semaglutide being an analog of human GLP-1(7–37) featuring a valine in position 8 for DDP-IV protection, a glutamic acid in position 22, and an acylated lysine in position 30 with the semaglutide C18 fatty diacid albumin binder attached via the amino-diethoxyacetyl linker (see Figure 4.14) [67]. in vitro, ecnoglutide is on par with semaglutide regarding cAMP induction

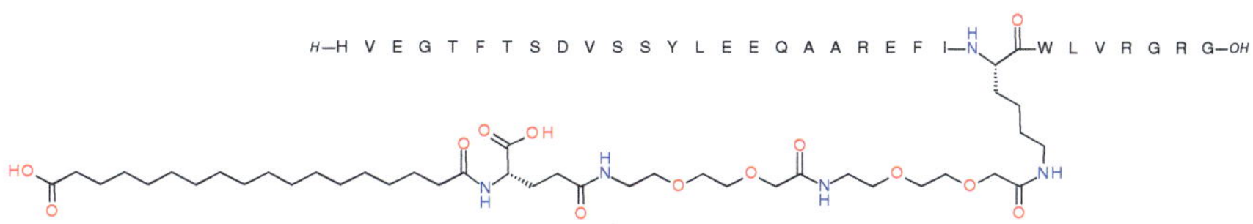

Figure 4.14 Chemical structure of ecnoglutide.

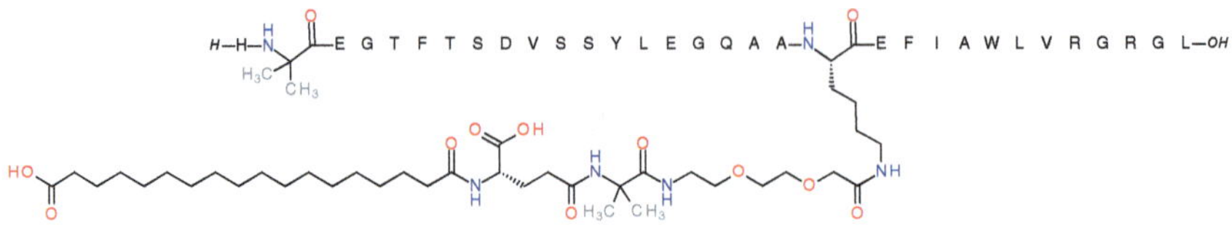

Figure 4.15 Chemical structure of utreglutide.

potency but shows markedly decreased GLP-1 receptor beta-arrestin signaling and internalization.

In humans, the half-life at steady state ranged from 124 to 138 h, supporting once-weekly dosing. Adverse events included decreased appetite, nausea, and headache. In phase 2 clinical trials, patients with T2DM given 0.4, 0.8, and 1.2 mg encoglutide once weekly had statistically significant HbA1c reductions from baseline of −1.81, −1.90, and −2.39%, respectively.

In phase 2 clinical trials in adults with obesity, once-weekly dosing of ecnoglutide (2.4 mg) resulted in a weight loss of approximately 15% at week 26. Phase 3 clinical trials with ecnoglutide are in progress.

Utreglutide

Utreglutide (GL0034), under clinical investigation by Sun Pharma, is structurally closely related to semaglutide, being an analog of human GLP-1(7–37) featuring an Aib in position 8 for DDP-IV protection, a C-terminal leucine extension, and an acylated lysine in position 26 with a C18 fatty diacid via amino-diethoxyacetyl-amino isobutyric acid linker (see Figure 4.15) [68]. Preclinically, the C-terminal leucine was found to have beneficial effects on antidiabetic and weight loss efficacy in db/db mice. The Aib unit in the linker was reported to provide stability toward peptidases and to balance hydrogen bond donor and acceptor properties.

In humans, utreglutide has a half-life of approximately 113 h, making it suitable for once-weekly dosing. In phase 1 clinical trials, multiple-ascending once-weekly subcutaneous doses of utreglutide for up to eight weeks were well tolerated in individuals with normal body weight. Dose-dependent reductions in body weight of up to −10.7% were observed following treatment (0.45 → 1.5 mg) for four to eight weeks [69]. Phase 2 clinical trials are expected to commence in the second half of 2024 [70].

HyGlutide

HyGlutide (GX-G6, TG103) [71, 72], under clinical investigation by Genexine, Inc., and developed by CSPC Zhongqi Pharmaceutical Technology, is a fusion protein comprising two molecules of GLP-1 fused to the hinge with natural glycosylated regions and N-terminal region of CH2 domain of IgD, which is in turn fused to the C-terminal region of CH2 domain and the entire CH3 region of human IgG, aiming to extend the duration of action and reduce the immunotoxicity [71, 72]. In the GLP-1 part of the molecule, alanine 8 was substituted for glycine to render the molecule DPP-IV stable.

In vitro, GX-G6 has GLP-1R potency on par with dulaglutide. In humans, the half-life was about 165 h, making it suitable for once-weekly or twice-monthly dosing. GX-G6 is in phase 2 clinical trials.

ZT002

ZT002, under clinical development of QL Biopharm, is a semaglutide-like double fatty acid-modified C-terminally extended human GLP-1 in which the second fatty acid is positioned in the C-terminal extension [73].

In humans, ZT002 has a half-life of approximately 13 days, potentially supporting monthly administration. In multiple-ascending dose phase 1 clinical studies, the mean percent change in body weight from baseline to week 12 was −9.6 and −13.1% in week 14 for 40 mg ZT002 and 80 mg ZT002 biweekly. Phase 2 initiation is anticipated in Q3 2024 (Figure 4.16) [74].

Bofanglutide

Bofanglutide (GZR18), under clinical investigation by Gan and Lee Pharmaceuticals, is structurally closely related to semaglutide, being an analog of human GLP-1(7–37) featuring a glycine in position 8 for DDP-IV protection, and an acylated lysine in position 26 with a C22 fatty diacid (see Figure 4.17). in vitro, GZR18 has approximately 10-fold lower GLP-1R potency in the absence and presence of HSA compared to semaglutide [75]. Bofanglutide has a long half-life supporting bi-weekly injection or once daily oral dosing in SNAC formulation.

In the phase 2 clinical trial, obese and overweight participants receiving bi-weekly injections of bofanglutide had a significant reduction in the percent change in body weight from baseline. The highest dose of 48 mg bi-weekly −17.29% weight loss was

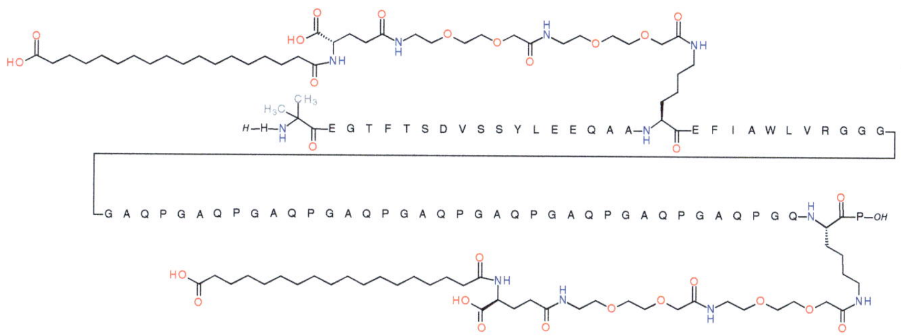

Figure 4.16 Chemical structure of ZT002.

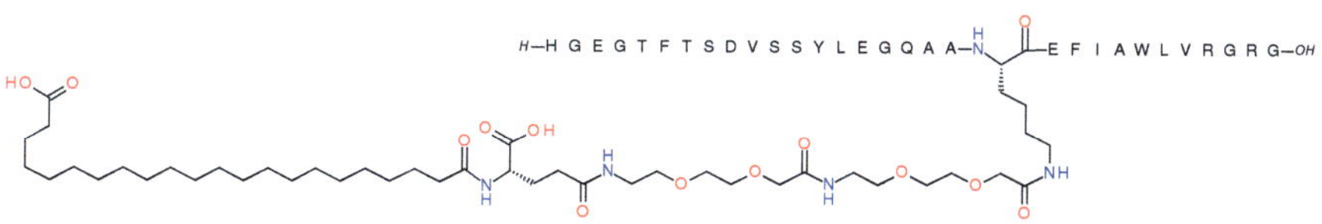

Figure 4.17 Chemical structure of bofanglutide.

achieved [76]. In phase 1 clinical trial, healthy participants were treated with 60 mg bofanglutide daily for two weeks, achieving an average weight reduction of −4.16% from baseline [77].

Summary and Outlook

The advancement of diabetes treatment has come a long way since the discovery of insulin. While insulin therapy has played a pivotal role in managing type 1 and type 2 diabetes, its limitations, such as hypoglycemia and weight gain, have spurred the development of alternative therapies. Among these, glucagon-like peptide-1 receptor agonists (GLP-1RAs) have emerged as a promising class of medications, offering effective glycemic control with additional cardiovascular and weight management benefits. Furthermore, semaglutide has advanced to oral formulations, improving accessibility and convenience for patients. Through various studies and trials, GLP-1RAs have shown their potential in providing flexible and patient-friendly treatment options for type 2 diabetes. The continued development and refinement of GLP-1RAs hold significant promise in the diabetes management landscape. Future research should focus on enhancing their efficacy, understanding their long-term effects, and exploring their applications beyond diabetes. The integration of advanced drug delivery methods could further improve the patient experience, especially in terms of dosing convenience and adherence. As our understanding of the biological pathways involved deepens, there may be opportunities to customize these therapies for individual patient profiles, paving the way for personalized medicine in diabetes care. Thus, GLP-1RAs are poised to play a vital role in the future of diabetes treatment and management.

References

1 Frederick, G. *Banting – Nobel Lecture*, NobelPrize.org. Nobel Prize Outreach 2026. Fri. 15 May 2026. https://www.nobelprize.org/prizes/medicine/1923/banting/lecture/.

2 Drucker, D.J., Habener, J.F., and Holst, J.J. (2017). Discovery, characterization, and clinical development of the glucagon-like peptides. *J. Clin. Invest.* 127 (12): 4217–4227.

3 Baggio, L.L. and Drucker, D.J. (2007). Biology of incretins: GLP-1 and GIP. *Gastroenterology* 132 (6): 2131–2157.

4 Drucker, D.J. (1998). Glucagon-like peptides. *Diabetes* 47 (2): 159–169.

5 Mojsov, S., Heinrich, G., Wilson, I.B. et al. (1986). Preproglucagon gene expression in pancreas and intestine diversifies at the level of post-translational processing. *J. Biol. Chem.* 261 (25): 11880–11889.

6 Orskov, C., Wettergren, A., and Holst, J.J. (1993). Biological effects and metabolic rates of glucagonlike peptide-1 7–36 amide and glucagonlike peptide-1 7–37 in healthy subjects are indistinguishable. *Diabetes* 42 (5): 658–661.

7 Eng, J., Kleinman, W.A., Singh, L. et al. (1992). Isolation and characterization of exendin-4, an exendin-3 analogue, from Heloderma suspectum venom. Further evidence for an exendin receptor on dispersed acini from guinea pig pancreas. *J. Biol. Chem.* 267 (11): 7402–7405.

8 Fry, B.G., Roelants, K., Winter, K. et al. (2010). Novel venom proteins produced by differential domain-expression strategies in beaded lizards and gila monsters (genus Heloderma). *Mol. Biol. Evol.* 27 (2): 395–407.

9 Kodra, J.T., Skovgaard, M., Madsen, D., and Liberles, D.A. (2007). Linking sequence to function in drug design with ancestral sequence reconstruction. In: *Ancestral Sequence Reconstruction* (Oxford, 2007; online edn, Oxford Academic, 1 Sept. 2008) (ed. D.A. Liberles). Oxford University Press. https://doi.org/10.1093/acprof:oso/9780199299188.003.0003. eprint: https://academic.oup.com/book/0/chapter/146487957/chapter-ag-pdf/45002224/book\LY1\textbackslash_4459\LY1\textbackslash_section\LY1\textbackslash_146487957.ag.pdf (accessed 15 May 2026).

10 Skovgaard, M., Kodra, J.T., Gram, D.X. et al. (2006). Using evolutionary information and ancestral sequences to understand the sequence-function relationship in GLP-1 agonists. *J. Mol. Biol.* 363 (5): 977–988.

11 Meier, J.J. (2012). GLP-1 receptor agonists for individualized treatment of type 2 diabetes mellitus. *Nat. Rev. Endocrinol.* 8 (12): 728–742.

12 Wilding, J.P.H., Batterham, R.L., Calanna, S. et al. (2021). Once-weekly semaglutide in adults with overweight or obesity. *N. Engl. J. Med.* 384 (11): 989–1002. https://doi.org/10.1056/nejmoa2032183.

13 Dungan, K.M., Povedano, S.T., Forst, T. et al. (2014). Once-weekly dulaglutide versus once-daily liraglutide in metformin-treated patients with type 2 diabetes (AWARD-6): a randomised, open-label, phase 3, non-inferiority trial. *Lancet* 384 (9951): 1349–1357.

14 Hoare, S.R.J. (2005). Mechanisms of peptide and nonpeptide ligand binding to Class B G-protein-coupled receptors. *Drug Discov. Today* 10 (6): 417–427.

15 Zhang, Y., Sun, B., Feng, D. et al. (2017). Cryo-EM structure of the activated GLP-1 receptor in complex with a G protein. *Nature* 546 (7657): 248–253.

16 Zhang, X., Belousoff, M.J., Liang, Y.-L. et al. (2021). Structure and dynamics of semaglutide- and taspoglutide-bound GLP-1R-Gs complexes. *Cell Rep.* 36 (2): 109374. https://doi.org/10.1016/j.celrep.2021.109374.

17 Thorens, B., Porret, A., Bühler, L. et al. (1993). Cloning and functional expression of the human islet GLP-1 receptor: demonstration that exendin-4 is an agonist and exendin-(9–39) an antagonist of the receptor. *Diabetes* 42 (11): 1678–1682. https://doi.org/10.2337/diab.42.11.1678.

18 Adelhorst, K., Hedegaard, B.B., Knudsen, L.B., and Kirk, O. (1994). Structure-activity studies of glucagon-like peptide-1. *J. Biol. Chem.* 269 (9): 6275–6278.

19 Göke, R., Fehmann, H.C., Linn, T. et al. (1993). Exendin-4 is a high potency agonist and truncated exendin-(9–39)-amide an antagonist at the glucagon-like peptide 1-(7–36)-amide receptor of insulin-secreting beta-cells. *J. Biol. Chem.* 268 (26): 19650–19655.

20 Thum, A., Hupe-Sodmann, K., Göke, R. et al. (2002). Endoproteolysis by isolated membrane peptidases reveal metabolic stability of glucagon-like peptide-1 analogs, exendins-3 and -4. *Exp. Clin. Endocrinol. Diabetes* 110 (3): 113–118. https://doi.org/10.1055/s-2002-29087.

21 Simonsen, L., Holst, J.J., and Deacon, C.F. (2006). Exendin-4, but not glucagon-like peptide-1, is cleared exclusively by glomerular filtration in anaesthetised pigs. *Diabetologia* 49 (4): 706–712.

22 Parkes, D.G., Pittner, R., Jodka, C. et al. (2001). Insulinotropic actions of exendin-4 and glucagon-like peptide-1 in vivo and in vitro. *Metabolism* 50 (5): 583–589.

23 Gentilella, R., Bianchi, C., Rossi, A., and Rotella, C.M. (2009). Exenatide: a review from pharmacology to clinical practice. *Diabetes Obes. Metab.* 11 (6): 544–556.

24 DeYoung, M.B., MacConell, L., Sarin, V. et al. (2011). Encapsulation of exenatide in poly-(D,L-lactide-co-glycolide) microspheres produced an investigational long-acting once-weekly formulation for type 2 diabetes. *Diabetes Technol. Ther.* 13 (11): 1145–1154.

25 L. MacConell, D. Maggs, Y. Li, P. Griffin, C. Wysham Abstracts of the 49th annual meeting of the EASD *Diabetologia* 56 (Suppl 1), 1–566 (2013). https://doi.org/10.1007/s00125-013-3012-z.

26 Wysham, C., Grimm, M., and Chen, S. (2013). Once weekly exenatide: efficacy, tolerability and place in therapy. *Diabetes Obes. Metab.* 15 (10): 871–881.

27 Vijiaratnam, N., Girges, C., Auld, G. et al. (2025). Exenatide once a week versus placebo as a potential disease-modifying treatment for people with Parkinson's disease in the UK: a phase 3, multicentre, double-blind, parallel-group, randomised, placebo-controlled trial. *Lancet* 405 (10479): 627–636. https://doi.org/10.1016/s0140-6736(24)02808-3.

28 Christensen, M., Knop, F.K., Holst, J.J., and Vilsboll, T. (2009). Lixisenatide, a novel GLP-1 receptor agonist for the treatment of type 2 diabetes mellitus. *IDrugs* 12 (8): 503–513.

29 Thorkildsen, C., Neve, S., Larsen, B.D. et al. (2003). Glucagon-like peptide 1 receptor agonist ZP10A increases insulin mRNA expression and prevents diabetic progression in db/db mice. *J. Pharmacol. Exp. Ther.* 307 (2): 490–496.

30 Rosenstock, J., Raccah, D., Korányi, L. et al. (2013). Efficacy and safety of lixisenatide once daily versus exenatide twice daily in type 2 diabetes inadequately controlled on metformin: a 24-week, randomized, open-label, active-controlled study (GetGoal-X). *Diabetes Care* 36 (10): 2945–2951.

31 Bain, S.C. (2014). The clinical development program of lixisenatide: a once-daily glucagon-like peptide-1 receptor agonist. *Diabetes Ther.* 5 (2): 367–383.

32 Rosenstock, J., Aronson, R., Grunberger, G. et al. (2016). Benefits of LixiLan, a titratable fixed-ratio combination of insulin glargine plus lixisenatide, versus insulin glargine and lixisenatide monocomponents in type 2 diabetes inadequately controlled on oral agents: the LixiLan-O randomized trial. *Diabetes Care* 39 (11): 2026–2035. https://doi.org/10.2337/dc16-0917. eprint: https://diabetesjournals.org/care/article-pdf/39/11/2026/544198/dc160917.pdf.

33 Optumrx (2023). Sanofi – discontinuation of Adlyxin® (lixisenatide). https://professionals.optumrx.com/publications/library/drugwithdrawal_adlyxin_2023-0117.html (online; accessed 10 December 2024).

34 Meissner, W.G. (2023). GLP1-R agonist improves Parkinson disease symptoms in early disease. https://www.ccjm.org/page/mds-2023/glp1-r-agonist-parkinson (online; accessed 10 December 2024).

35 Chen, X., Lv, X., Yang, G. et al. (2017). Polyethylene glycol loxenatide injections added to metformin effectively improve glycemic control and exhibit favorable safety in type 2 diabetic patients. *J. Diabetes* 9 (2): 158–167.

36 Frias, J.P., Choi, J.D., Rosenstock, J. et al. (2022). Efficacy and safety of once-weekly efpeglenatide monotherapy versus placebo in type 2 diabetes: the AMPLITUDE-M randomized controlled trial. *Diabetes Care* 45 (7): 1592–1600. https://doi.org/10.2337/dc21-2656. eprint: https://diabetesjournals.org/care/article-pdf/45/7/1592/715989/dc212656.pdf.

37 Gerstein, H.C., Sattar, N., Rosenstock, J. et al. (2021). Cardiovascular and renal outcomes with efpeglenatide in type 2 diabetes. *N. Engl. J. Med.* 385: 896–810, 907. https://doi.org/10.1056/NEJMoa2108269. eprint: https://www.nejm.org/doi/pdf/10.1056/NEJMoa2108269.

38 Salamah, H.M., Marey, A., Elsayed, E. et al. (2023). Efficacy and safety of polyethylene glycol loxenatide in type 2 diabetic patients: a systematic review and meta-analysis of randomized controlled trials. *Sci. Rep.* 13 (1): https://doi.org/10.1038/s41598-023-46274-x.

39 Cai, H., Chen, Q., Duan, Y. et al. (2023). Short-term effect of polyethylene glycol loxenatide on weight loss in overweight or obese patients with type 2 diabetes: an open-label, parallel-arm, randomized, metformin-controlled trial. *Front. Endocrinol.* 14: 1106868. https://doi.org/10.3389/fendo.2023.1106868.

40 Yang, Z., Jiang, F., Sun, C. et al. (2024). Safety, pharmacokinetics and pharmacodynamics of multipledose noiiglutide (SHR20004), a novel GLP/-1 receptor agonist, in Chinese obese subjects without diabetes mellitus. *Diabetes. Obes. Metab.* https://doi.org/10.1111/dom.16080.

41 Cui, H., Zhao, C.-Y., Lv, Y. et al. (2020). Safety, tolerability and pharmacokinetics of single dose polyethylene glycolated exenatide injection (PB-119) in healthy volunteers. *Eur. J. Drug Metab. Pharmacokinet.* 45 (3): 361–369. https://doi.org/10.1007/s13318-020-00605-9.

42 Ji, L., Du, Y., Xu, M. et al. (2021). Efficacy and safety of PEGylated exenatide injection (PB-119) in treatment-naive type 2 diabetes mellitus patients: a phase II randomised, double-blind, parallel, placebo-controlled study. *Diabetologia* 64 (5): 1066–1078. https://doi.org/10.1007/s00125-021-05392-9.

43 Yan, X., Ma, J., Liu, Y. et al. (2024). Efficacy and safety of visepegenatide, a long-acting weekly GLP-1 receptor agonist as monotherapy in type 2 diabetes mellitus: a randomised, double-blind, parallel, placebo-controlled phase 3 trial. *Lancet Reg. Health West. Pac.* 47: 101101. https://doi.org/10.1016/j.lanwpc.2024.101101.

44 Kurtzhals, P., Havelund, S., Jonassen, I. et al. (1995). Albumin binding of insulins acylated with fatty acids: characterization of the ligand-protein interaction and correlation between binding affinity and timing of the insulin effect in vivo. *Biochem. J.* 312 (3): 725–731.

45 Kurtzhals, P., Havelund, S., Jonassen, I., and Markussen, J. (1997). Effect of fatty acids and selected drugs on the albumin binding of a long-acting, acylated insulin analogue. *J. Pharm. Sci.* 86 (12): 1365–1368.

46 Aertgeerts, K., Ye, S., Tennant, M.G. et al. (2004). Crystal structure of human dipeptidyl peptidase IV in complex with a decapeptide reveals details on substrate specificity and tetrahedral intermediate formation. *Protein Sci.* 13 (2): 412–421.

47 Frederiksen, T.M., Sønderby, P., Ryberg, L.A. et al. (2015). Oligomerization of a glucagon-like peptide 1 analog: bridging experiment and simulations. *Biophys. J.* 109 (6): 1202–1213. https://doi.org/10.1016/j.bpj.2015.07.051.

48 Mann, J.F.E., Fonseca, V., Mosenzon, O. et al. (2018). Effects of liraglutide versus placebo on cardiovascular events in patients with type 2 diabetes mellitus and chronic kidney disease: results from the LEADER trial. *Circulation* 138 (25): 2908–2918. https://doi.org/10.1161/circulationaha.118.036418.

49 Lau, J., Bloch, P., Schäffer, L. et al. (2015). Discovery of the once-weekly glucagon-like peptide-1 (GLP-1) analogue semaglutide. *J. Med. Chem.* 58 (18): 7370–7380.

50 Lincoff, A.M., Brown-Frandsen, K., Colhoun, H.M. et al. (2023). Semaglutide and cardiovascular outcomes in obesity without diabetes. *N. Engl. J. Med.* 389 (24): 2221–2232. https://doi.org/10.1056/nejmoa2307563.

51 Aguirre, T.A.S., Teijeiro-Osorio, D., Rosa, M. et al. (2016). Current status of selected oral peptide technologies in advanced preclinical development and in clinical trials. *Adv. Drug Deliv. Rev.* 106: 223–241. https://doi.org/10.1016/j.addr.2016.02.004.

52 Drucker, D.J. (Dec. 2019). Advances in oral peptide therapeutics. *Nat. Rev. Drug Discov.* 19 (4): 277–289. https://doi.org/10.1038/s41573-019-0053-0.

53 Davies, M., Pieber, T.R., Hartoft-Nielsen, M.-L. et al. (2017). Effect of oral semaglutide compared with placebo and subcutaneous semaglutide on glycemic control in patients with type 2 diabetes. *JAMA* 318 (15): 1460.

54 Dong, J.Z., Shen, Y., Zhang, J. et al. (2011). Discovery and characterization of taspoglutide, a novel analogue of human glucagon-like peptide-1, engineered for sustained therapeutic activity in type 2 diabetes. *Diabetes Obes. Metab.* 13 (1): 19–25.

55 Sebokova, E., Christ, A.D., Wang, H. et al. (2010). Taspoglutide, an analog of human glucagon-like Peptide-1 with enhanced stability and in vivo potency. *Endocrinology* 151 (6): 2474–2482.

56 Rosenstock, J., Balas, B., Charbonnel, B. et al. (2013). The fate of taspoglutide, a weekly GLP-1 receptor agonist, versus twice-daily exenatide for type 2 diabetes: the T-emerge 2 trial. *Diabetes Care* 36 (3): 498–504.

57 Kueh, C.J.L. and Fisher, M. (2014). Taspoglutide. *Pract. Diab.* 31 (9): 393.

58 Trujillo, J.M. and Nuffer, W. (2014). Albiglutide: a new GLP-1 receptor agonist for the treatment of type 2 diabetes. *Ann. Pharmacother.* 48 (11): 1494–1501.

59 Onge, E.L.S. and Miller, S.A. (2010). Albiglutide: a new GLP-1 analog for the treatment of type 2 diabetes. *Expert. Opin. Biol. Ther.* 10 (5): 801–806.
60 Chaudhury, C., Mehnaz, S., Robinson, J.M. et al. (2003). The major histocompatibility complex-related Fc receptor for IgG (FcRn) binds albumin and prolongs its lifespan. *J. Exp. Med.* 197 (3): 315–322.
61 Bush, M.A., Matthews, J.E., De Boever, E.H. et al. (2009). Safety, tolerability, pharmacodynamics and pharmacokinetics of albiglutide, a long-acting glucagon-like peptide-1 mimetic, in healthy subjects. *Diabetes Obes. Metab.* 11 (5): 498–505.
62 Pratley, R.E., Nauck, M.A., Barnett, A.H. et al. (2014). Once-weekly albiglutide versus once-daily liraglutide in patients with type 2 diabetes inadequately controlled on oral drugs (HARMONY 7): a randomised, open-label, multicentre, non-inferiority phase 3 study. *Lancet Diabetes Endocrinol.* 2 (4): 289–297.
63 Baggio, L.L., Huang, Q., Cao, X., and Drucker, D.J. (2008). An albumin-exendin-4 conjugate engages central and peripheral circuits regulating murine energy and glucose homeostasis. *Gastroenterology* 134 (4): 1137–1147.
64 Wang, M., Kipnes, M. S., Matheson, S., & Wen, S. (2009, June). *PC-DAC(TM):Exendin-4 (CJC-1134-PC) Significantly Reduces HbA1c and Body Weight as an Adjunct Therapy to Metformin: Two Randomized, Double-Blind, Placebo-Controlled, 12 Week, Phase II Studies in Patients with Type 2 Diabetes Mellitus.* Poster presented at the 69th Scientific Sessions of the American Diabetes Association (ADA), New Orleans, LA.
65 Glaesner, W., Vick, A.M., Millican, R. et al. (2010). Engineering and characterization of the long-acting glucagon-like peptide-1 analogue LY2189265, an Fc fusion protein. *Diabetes Metab. Res. Rev.* 26 (4): 287–296.
66 Ferrannini, G., Mellbin, L.G., Kirabo, F. et al. (Aug. 2022). Dulaglutide and a domposite outcome reflecting atherosclerosis in the REWIND trial: a post Hoc analysis. *Diabetes Care* 45 (10): e146–e147. https://doi.org/10.2337/dc22-0903.
67 Guo, W., Xu, Z., Zou, H. et al. (2023). Discovery of ecnoglutide – a novel, long-acting, cAMP-biased glucagon-like peptide-1 (GLP-1) analog. *Mol. Metab.* 75: 101762. https://doi.org/10.1016/j.molmet.2023.101762.
68 Jones, B., Burade, V., Akalestou, E. et al. (2022). in vivo and in vitro characterization of GL0034, a novel long-acting glucagonlike peptide-1 receptor agonist. *Diabetes. Obes. Metab.* 24 (11): 2090–2101. https://doi.org/10.1111/dom.14794.
69 Thennati (2023). 766-P: safety and tolerability of once-weekly GL0034 (utreglutide) in healthy individuals – a multiple ascending dose study. *Diabetes* 72: 766. https://doi.org/10.2337/db23-766-P.
70 Sun Pharma (2024). Sun pharma reports Q3FY24 results. https://sunpharma.com/wp-content/uploads/2024/01/Press-Release-Sun-Pharma-Q3FY24-Financial-Result.pdf (online; accessed 10 December 2024).
71 Jin, J., Cui, G., Mi, N. et al. (2023). Safety, pharmacokinetics, and pharmacodynamics of TG103, a novel long-acting GLP-1/Fc fusion protein after a single ascending dose in Chinese healthy subjects. *Eur. J. Pharm. Sci.* 185: 106448. https://doi.org/10.1016/j.ejps.2023.106448.

72 Byun, M., Seo, C., Woo, J., and Sung, Y. (2019). 114-LB: GX-G6, a novel long-acting glucagon-like peptide receptor agonist: result of phase I study in healthy volunteers. *Diabetes* 68 (Supplement 1): 114 LB. https://doi.org/10.2337/db19-114-lb.

73 Zhang, Y., Wu, X., Zou, H., et al. (2021). Polypeptide conjugates and methods of uses, U.S. Patent 11529394B2, December 2021.

74 Zhou, H., Ji, L., Song, X. et al. (2024). ZT002, a novel ultra long-acting GLP-1 receptor agonist in adults with overweight or obesity: a randomised, placebo-controlled, multiple ascending dose phase 1c study. *Diabetologia* 67 (Suppl 1): Abstract 147. https://doi.org/10.1007/s00125-025-06581-6.

75 Zhang, M., Zhang, Y., Peng, X. et al. (2022). GZR18, a novel long-acting GLP-1 analog, demonstrated positive in vitro and in vivo pharmacokinetic and pharmacodynamic characteristics in animal models. *Eur. J. Pharmacol.* 928: 175107. https://doi.org/10.1016/j.ejphar.2022.175107.

76 Gan and Lee Pharmaceuticals (2024). Gan and Lee pharmaceuticals bi-weekly (twice a month) GLP-1 receptor agonist GZR18 injection achieved 17.29 pct weight loss at 30 weeks in a phase iib clinical trial. https://www.ganlee.com/detail/751.html (online; accessed 12 December 2024).

77 Gan and Lee Pharmaceuticals (2024). Gan and Lee pharmaceuticals announced positive phase 1 results for its oral GLP-1 receptor agonist GZR18 tablet in healthy participants, demonstrating 4.16 pct weight reduction in two weeks. https://www.ganlee.com/detail/764.html (online; accessed 12 December 2024).

5

Oral Agents Used to Treat Type 2 Diabetes and Obesity

John Liddle[1], Ekaterina Ratkova[1], Cátia A. Bonito[1], Christopher J. Rhodes[2], and Sarah Will[2]

[1]*AstraZeneca, Biopharmaceuticals R&D, Early Cardiovascular, Renal and Metabolism, Pepparedsleden 1, 431 83 Mölndal, Sweden*
[2]*AstraZeneca, Biopharmaceuticals R&D, Early Cardiovascular, Renal and Metabolism, One Medimmune Way, Gaithersburg, MD 20878, USA*

Introduction

Depending on how one looks at it, there has been quite a long history for the use of oral agents for the treatment of type 2 diabetes (T2D) or obesity. Arguably, this could go back a few thousand years where the ancient Greeks (Socrates and Hippocrates included) were aware of the unhealthy effects associated with obesity prescribing diet and exercise regimes, and, for presumably more severe cases, the use of emetics and cathartics for weight loss [1]. For the latter, the actual active ingredient was probably unknown but, nonetheless, it illustrates the concept of oral agents to treat obesity and associated metabolic disease is not new. Here, we review the more recent history of known oral agent small molecules used to treat T2D *or* obesity, a timeline is shown in Figure 5.1. This is now leading to the future therapeutic approaches that will treat both T2D *and* obesity, most likely with small molecule GLP-1 receptor agonists leading the way.

Type 2 Diabetes Oral Agents

We appreciate that there are many agents used to treat T2D, both oral and injectable (insulin included) therapeutics, as well as certain surgical procedures. In this chapter, the focus is entirely on oral agents that tend to be more acceptable to patients, where trypanophobia can still be an issue for many [2]. Over the past 75 years, there have been >10 classes of oral agents used to treat T2D (Table 5.1 and Figure 5.1).

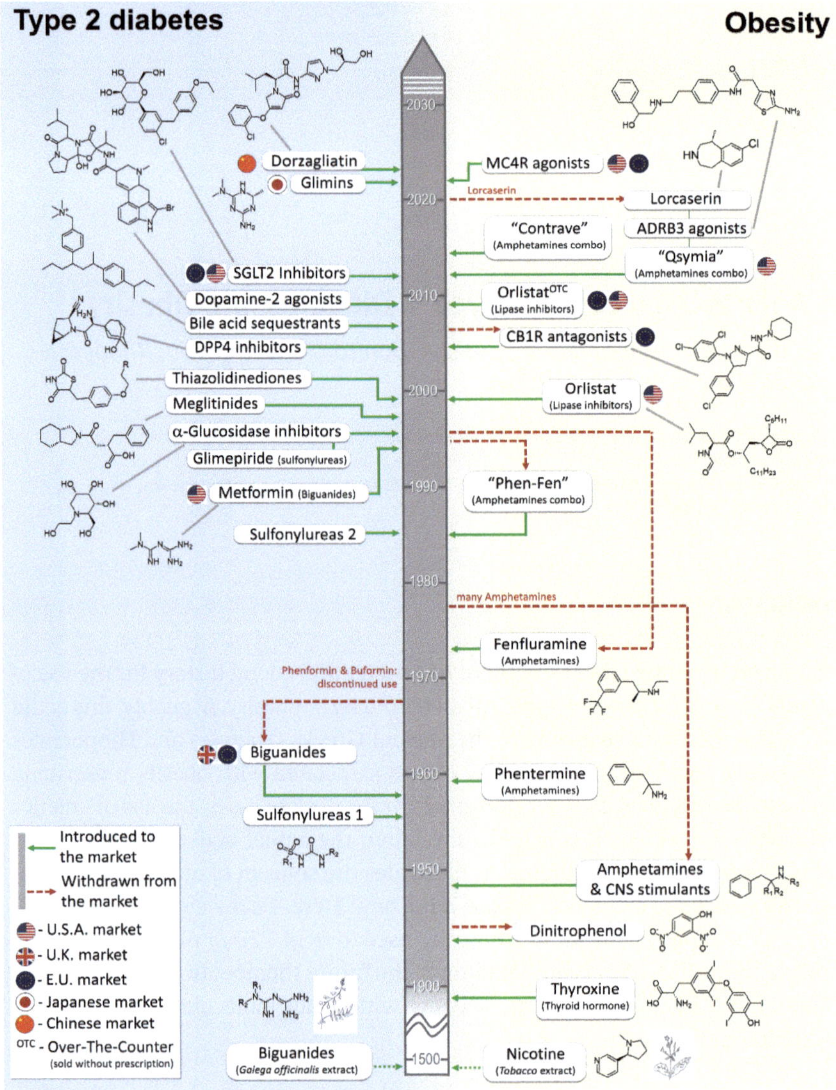

Figure 5.1 Timeline of history of known oral agent small molecules used to treat T2D or obesity.

Table 5.1 Type 2 diabetes (T2D) oral drugs.

Drug class	Drug name(s)	Date introduced	Mechanism of action
Biguanides	• Phenformin • Buformin • Metformin (Glucophage)	• 1400–1450: *Galega officinalis* extract • 1958 (parts of Europe/UK), but Phenformin and Buformin withdrawn in late 1970 (lactic acidosis) • 1994 (USA) for T2D	Not well defined. Effects include improving insulin resistance and inhibition of hepatic glucose production.
Sulfonylureas. (1st generation)	• Tolbutamide • Chlorpropamide • Acetohexamide • Carbutamide • Glycyclamide (Tolcyclamide) • Metahexamide • Tolazumdie	1956	Increases insulin secretion in a non-glucose dependent manner via depolarization of pancreatic β-cells.
Sulfonylureas. (2nd generation)	• Glibenclamide (Glyburide) • Glibornuride • Gliclazide • Glipizide • Gliquidone • Glisoxepide • Glyclopyramide • Glimepiride	1984 1995 (Glimepiride)	
α-Glucosidase inhibitors	• Acarbose • Miglitol • Voglibose	1995	Competitive inhibitors of enzymes that digest carbohydrates in the gut allowing for less glucose absorption.
Meglitinides (Glinides)	• Repaglinide (Prandin) • Nateglinide (Starlix) • Mitiglinide (Glufast)	1997	Similar to sulfonylureas except shorter acting.
Thiazolidinediones (Glitazones)	• Troglitazone • Pioglitazone • Rosiglitazone • Lobeglitazone	1999	• Increases preadipocyte differentiation to increase adipocyte mass and appropriate endogenous lipid storage. • Decreases ectopic fat to improve insulin sensitivity and glucose homeostasis.

(Continued)

Table 5.1 (Continued)

Drug class	Drug name(s)	Date introduced	Mechanism of action
Dipeptidyl peptidase-4 (DPP4) inhibitors	• Sitagliptin • Vildagliptin • Saxagliptin • Linagliptin • Gemigliptin • Anagliptin • Teneligliptin • Alogliptin • Trelagliptin • Omarigliptin • Evogliptin • Gosogliptin • Dutogliptin • Neogliptin • Retagliptin • Denagliptin • Cofrogliptin	2006	Inhibition of DPP4, leading to increase of active GLP-1 and GIP in circulation.
Bile acid sequestrants	• Colesevelam • Cholestyramine • Colestipol	2008	Not well defined. May reduce insulin resistance and improve glucose clearance without affecting hepatic glucose production.
Dopamine-2 agonists	• Bromocriptine • Cabergoline	2009	Not well defined. Improvements in glucose homeostasis thought to be mediated via improving dopaminergic/sympathetic tone in CNS.
Sodium-glucose co-transporter-2 (SGLT2) inhibitors	• Canagliflozin • Dapagliflozin • Empagliflozin • Ertugliflozin • Ipragliflozin • Luseogliflozin • Remogliflozin etabonate • Tofogliflozin	2012 (EU) 2013 (USA)	Inhibit sodium-glucose transport in kidney tubules (SGTL2) to reduce reabsorption of glucose, leading to glucosuria and therefore lower blood glucose.
Glimins	• Imeglimin	2021 (Japan)	Not well defined – believed to act via enhanced insulin action.
Glucokinase activator (GKA)	• Dorzagliatin	2022 (China)	Activation of hepatic and pancreatic glucokinase in presence of glucose, leading to increased insulin secretion and decreased hepatic glucose production.

Sulfonylureas

The first-generation class of sulfonylureas were introduced in the 1950s and may be considered the first *bone fide* small molecule "chemical" used as an oral medication to treat T2D [3]. They are insulin secretagogues that boost endogenous insulin secretion and thus lower hyperglycemia. A second generation of sulfonylureas was introduced in the 1980s, that were more potent enabling a lower and once-daily dosing, as well as less hepatic toxicity [4]. As sulfonylureas boost secretion of the prime anabolic hormone, insulin, their use in diabetes treatment is associated with body weight gain [5].

Sulfonylureas bind to the "SulfonylUrea Receptor, SUR1, subunit of the ATP-sensitive K^+-channel on pancreatic islet β-cells" plasma membrane to close the channel and prevent K^+ efflux, thus depolarizing the cell (Figure 5.2). This then opens voltage-sensitive Ca^{2+}-channels to rapidly elevate cytosolic $[Ca^{2+}]_i$ flux which is a prerequisite to stimulate insulin secretion [6]. As this mechanism bypasses the need for β-cell metabolism to increase the intracellular ATP:ADP ratio that physiologically closes the ATP-sensitive K^+-channel, the action of sulfonylureas are glucose-independent [6]. This glucose-independent aspect of sulfonylureas results in two significant adverse issues: a higher instance of hypoglycemia [7, 8]; and a chronic decrease in the endogenous insulin secretory pool since (pro)insulin biosynthesis is not regulated in parallel [9]. Therefore, sulfonylureas have short-term (≤6 months) benefits for glucose homeostasis in T2D, however, in the long-run they are detrimental to the β-cell functional mass and the diabetes condition progressively worsens [7, 10, 11]. Interestingly, certain sulfonylurea compounds are

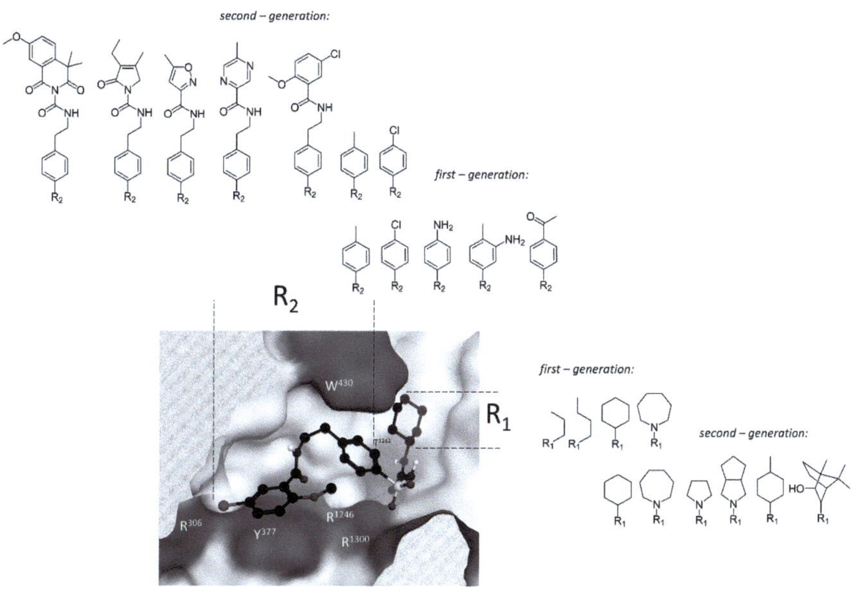

Figure 5.2 Overview of chemical structures for 1st and 2nd -generations of sulfonylureas. R-group analysis is mapped on active conformation of Glibenclamide (2nd -generation of sulfonylureas) bound to human pancreatic ATP-sensitive potassium channel (PDB ID: 5YKE).

used in agriculture, mostly as herbicides, and have been linked to lean forms of T2D [12].

Nonetheless, this class of oral diabetes drug is still used to date, especially as a second-line therapy for treating T2D, usually in combination with another oral agent [13, 14]. Furthermore, sulfonylureas are also quite effective as a monotherapy in treating certain rare forms of monogenic diabetes, especially those that are variant in the ATP-sensitive K^+-channel subunits [15, 16].

Biguanides

This class of drugs have actually been used to treat symptoms of T2D since Medieval times, if one considers that they are the "active ingredient" in extracts of French Lilac (*Galega officinalis*) (Figure 5.3) [17]. Biguanides, essentially two linked guanidine core structures, were synthesized in 1879 [18]. In the 1950s, three biguanides – phenformin, buformin, and metformin were used for diabetes therapy in Europe [17, 19], but phenformin and buformin were generally discontinued in the 1970s mostly due to high incidence of lactic acidosis [19]. However, metformin gradually continued use in Europe as it had less risk of lactic acidosis, with an ability to counter insulin resistance without weight gain and less chance of hypoglycemia [19]. In 1994, metformin was approved for treatment of T2D in the USA and, today, metformin is the most commonly prescribed drug to improve glucose homeostasis, on the World Health Organization's essential medicine list [20], and is the recommended first option for the treatment of common T2D [21–23]. Longer-term metformin treatment for T2D is also associated with a reduced cardiovascular disease risk [24].

Metformin improves glucose homeostasis in T2D by decreasing insulin resistance and hepatic glucose production. However, the mechanism by which it improves insulin sensitivity remains essentially unclear, although several have been suggested [22, 25]. Most commonly mentioned, is metformin being an activator of AMP-activated protein kinase (AMPK) an enzyme that plays a role in regulating

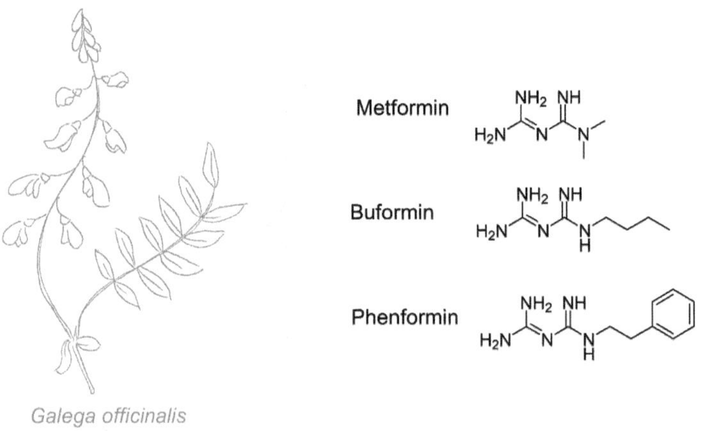

Figure 5.3 Chemical structures of biguanides.

cellular energy homeostasis [26], particularly in hepatocytes. However, this association is only realized at very high concentrations of metformin [22] and not seen in AMPK *null* mice [27]. Other potential mechanisms including metformin, affecting cellular redox via inhibiting mitochondrial complex-I in oxidative phosphorylation/electron transport that may inhibit hepatic gluconeogenesis [22, 25]; inhibition of the mitochondrial glycerol phosphate shuttle to also affect cellular redox [22, 25]; interference of glucagon signaling by dampening [cAMP] generation [28]; modulation of the gut microbiome, and potential anti-inflammatory effects [25] – to mention but a few. Metformin has also been touted to have positive effects on longevity [29, 30].

Alpha-Glucosidase Inhibitors

These are saccharide compounds that when taken orally, competitively inhibit digestive enzymes in the family of glucosidases (Figure 5.4), which, in the gut breakdown complex carbohydrates and lower the availability of glucose monomers from a meal [31, 32]. This in return can improve glucose homeostasis in T2D. However, since there is an increase in undigested carbohydrate remaining in the gut lumen the gut microbiome propagates causing uncomfortable gastrointestinal adverse effects, such as abdominal cramping, flatulence and diarrhea, that is both dependent on the dose and meal content [33]. There is also a stringent time-dependent dosing required prior to each meal [33]. Although α-glucosidase inhibitors can improve glycemic control, other therapeutics appear more effective [32]. For these collective reasons, patient compliance with this class of oral therapeutics to treat T2D has been relatively low [32].

Meglitinides (Glinides)

This class of drug was first approved for treatment of T2D in 1997, and act like the sulfonylureas. They are insulinotropic and indeed have a similar mechanism of action

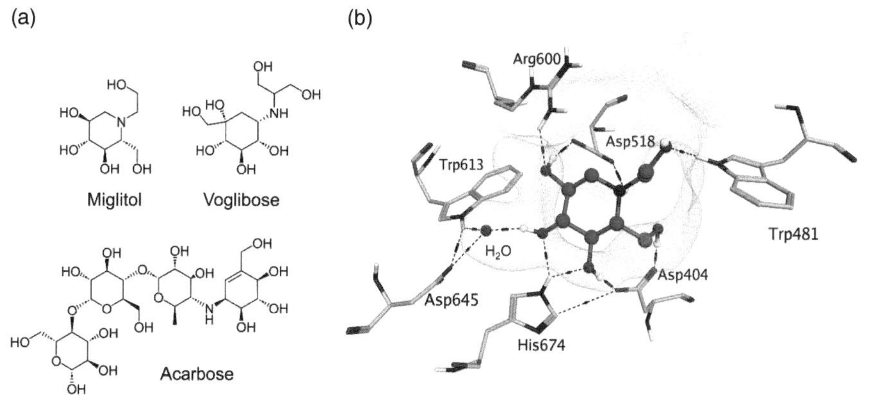

Figure 5.4 (a) Chemical structures of α-glucosidase inhibitors in clinical practice; (b) Miglitol bound to human α-glucosidase (PDB ID: 5NN6).

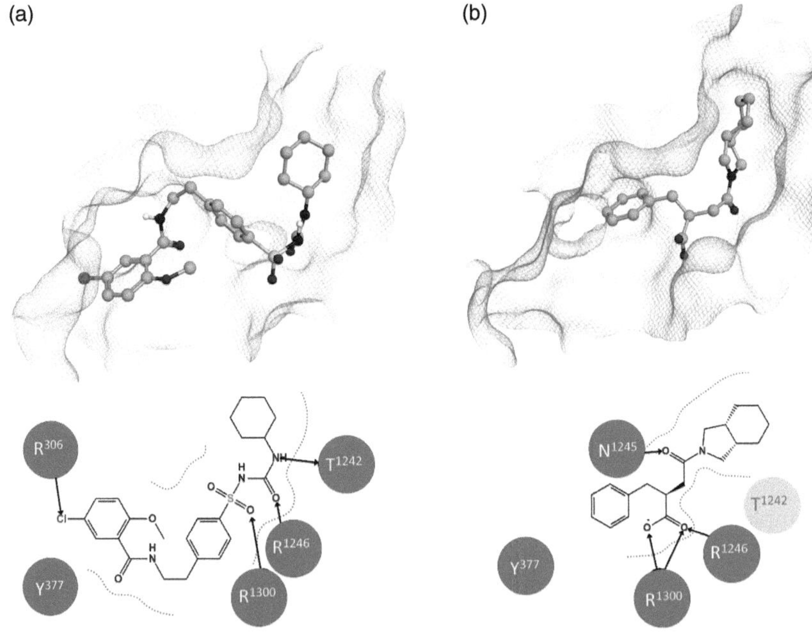

Figure 5.5 Comparison of binding modes of sulfonylurea, Glibenclamide (a) and glinide, Mitiglinide (b) in complex with SUR1 subunit of the human pancreatic ATP-sensitive potassium channel (PDB IDs: 5YKE & 7WIT, correspondently).

by binding to the SUR1 subunit and activating the ATP-sensitive K^+-channel on pancreatic endocrine β-cells (Figure 5.5). However, they have lower binding affinity and faster dissociation from SUR1, which is intended to lower the risk of hypoglycemia, but requires more frequent dosing (with each meal) compared with daily dosing of 2nd generation sulfonylureas. Notwithstanding, the adverse side effects of meglitinides are similar to those aforementioned for sulfonylureas [34, 35]. The meglitinides are mostly used in combination with metformin and do not adversely affect cardiovascular benefit [34, 36].

Thiazolidinediones

This class of compounds act as nuclear receptor agonists for the gamma member of the Peroxisome Proliferator-Activated Receptor family – PPARγ (Figure 5.6). They mimic the effect of the endogenous ligands, prostaglandins and eicosanoids, which are unsaturated fatty acids [37]. As an oral T2D therapeutic, thiazolidinediones (TZDs) act to improve insulin sensitivity and glucose homeostasis [38]. The principal mechanism of action for TZDs is to increase preadipocyte differentiation which expands the adipocyte mass and creates a larger appropriate storage place for endogenous triglyceride [39]. Storing lipid where it is meant to be in adipose

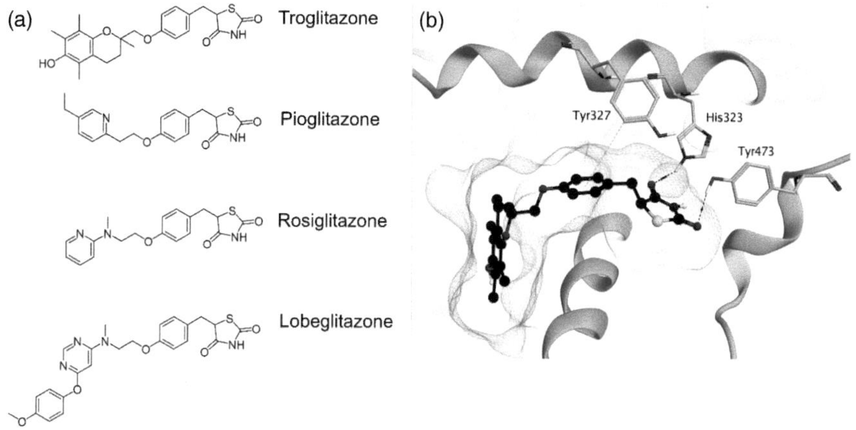

Figure 5.6 (a) Chemical structures of thiazolidinediones; (b) Troglitazone bound to human PPARγ (PDB ID: 6DGO).

tissue, can decrease ectopic fat which improves insulin sensitivity and consequently lowers glucose levels [40]. TZDs also increase adiponectin levels and may have anti-inflammatory effects, that adds to improving insulin sensitivity [41, 42]. In addition, it has been reported that TZDs can slow mitochondrial pyruvate transport to increase fatty acid oxidation which also contributes to lowering ectopic fat deposition and improving insulin sensitivity [41].

The early versions of TZDs (e.g., troglitazone), were approved (in 1997) for improving glycemic control in adjunct to diet and exercise in T2D but withdrawn for liver toxicity (in 2000). However, later versions (e.g., rosiglitazone) showed fewer hepatic effects. Although quite good at reducing insulin resistance in T2D, TZDs have common side effects of edema and body weight gain, the latter symptomatic of PPARγ -induced increased in adipose and improved insulin sensitivity [43]. There is also an increased risk of bone fractures with TZDs [10, 44], most likely as preadipocytes and preosteoblasts share the same precursor cell lineage in early differentiation and PPARγ signaling biases toward preadipocyte differentiation [45]. The most contentiously debated side effect of TZDs, however, was a perceived increased risk of cardiovascular events that arose in 2007 [38, 46]. Extensive press coverage between 2007 and 2013 resulted in the USA Food and Drug Administration (FDA) restricting TZD use in 2008 and the European Medicines Agency (EMA) suspending TZD use in Europe (2010). Since then, revised meta-analyses, clinical trials (e.g., RECORD [47]) and other approaches have indicated no overall morbidity or mortality for cardiovascular risk with TZD use compared to other glucose lowering drugs [47, 48] and now it is thought that TZDs might even be cardioprotective [49]. Nonetheless, the perception of this cardiovascular risk remains resulting in relatively low usage of TZDs as an insulin sensitizing treatment. Moreover, in the aftermath of the original suggestion [46], since 2008 cardiovascular outcomes trial are recommended for all diabetes drug development [50]. This certainly benefits the treatment of T2D and comorbidities, but it also markedly increases the cost of developing new T2D therapeutics.

Dipeptidyl Peptidase-4 (DPP4) Inhibitors

Incretins, such as Glucagon-Like Peptide 1 (GLP-1) and Glucose-dependent Insulinotropic Polypeptide (GIP), potentiate glucose-induced insulin secretion and peptide mimetics of these have been used to treat T2D [51, 52]. However, the endogenous incretins are rapidly inactivated by N-terminal proteolytic cleavage by dipeptidyl peptidase-4 (DPP4) [53], and lack sustained effect. By inhibiting DPP4, this prevents the exopeptidase N-terminal cleavage of the active incretins to their inactive forms, thereby keeping a higher proportion of circulating active incretins for a more robust potentiation of endogenous glucose-induced insulin secretion and thus better control of glucose homeostasis [54, 55]. They are relatively safe and tolerable, and because incretins only potentiate glucose-induced insulin secretion, having no insulinotropic effect on their own, the incidence of hypoglycemia is low [54, 55]. DPP4 inhibition can improve glycemic control in T2D alone, but they are more effective in combination with other T2D therapies such a metformin [46, 55].

DPP4 inhibitors (Figure 5.7) were approved in 2006 and began their use to treat T2D at a moment in time where TZDs were being questioned for increased cardiovascular risk [46, 55] (see above). Despite their modest efficacy, with few other oral T2D treatment options at the time beyond metformin and considering the hypoglycemic risk for sulfonylureas, they became widely used early on. This may illustrate a patient preference for oral versus injectable T2D medications [56].

Bile Acid Sequestrants

This class of drug is primarily used to treat hyperlipidemia and lower cholesterol, although they do have some glucose lowering activity and hence occasionally are used to treat T2D [57]. Bile acid sequestrants interrupt enterohepatic circulation of bile acids to reduce circulating cholesterol (Figure 5.8) and then, as a consequence, may reduce insulin resistance and improve glucose clearance without affecting hepatic glucose production. The mechanism at the molecular level for glucose lowering needs better definition, but it has been speculated to be based on increased engagement of certain bile acids with nuclear receptors [57]. In this regard, it has been suggested some bile acid sequestrants decrease glucose by enhancing GLP-1 secretion in the gut via certain G-protein coupled receptors [58].

As bile acid sequestrants are not absorbed from the gastrointestinal tract adverse effects are mostly limited to be gastrointestinal including constipation, nausea, bloating, flatulence, diarrhea, and heartburn. They also interfere with vitamin absorption, so vitamin supplementation is recommended with their use [59].

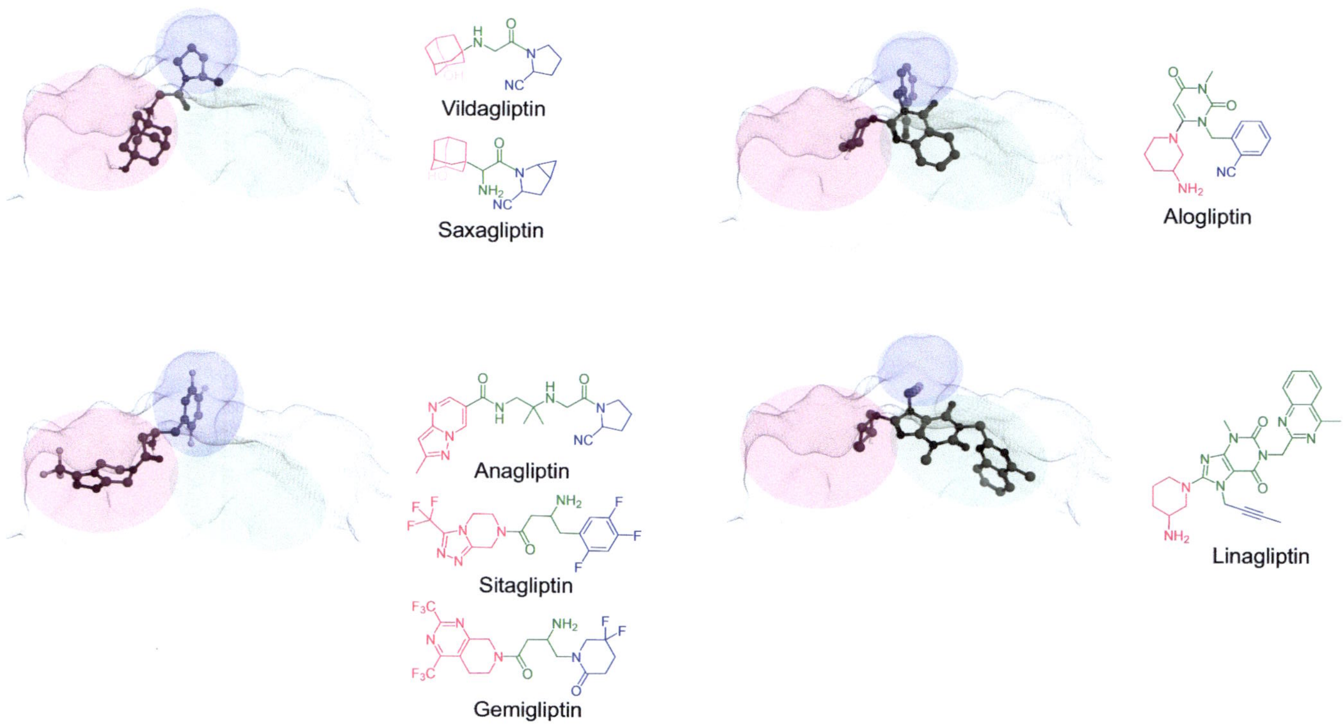

Figure 5.7 Overview of chemical structures and binding modes of DPP4 inhibitors. The receptor contains three binding areas: S1-pocket (blue), S2-pocket (pink), and S3-pocket (green). Moieties of small molecule inhibitors binding in corresponding pocket are highlighted accordingly.

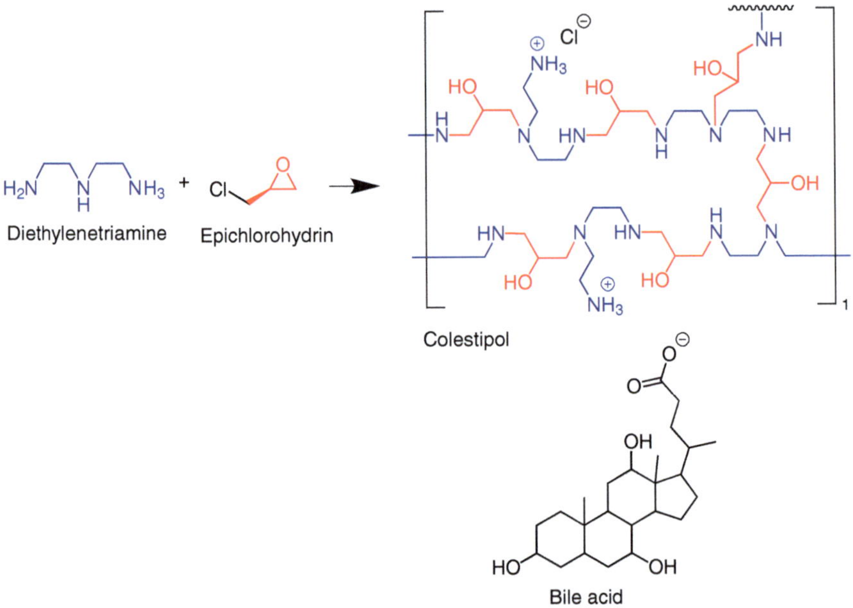

Figure 5.8 An approximate structure of a bile acid sequestrant, Colestipol, which is a hydrochloride of the product of copolymerization of epichlorohydrin with diethylenetriamine. Colestipol works as an ion exchange resin trapping bile acid (i.e. exchanges chloride ions for bile acids), thus preventing their reabsorption and circulation.

Dopamine-2 Agonists

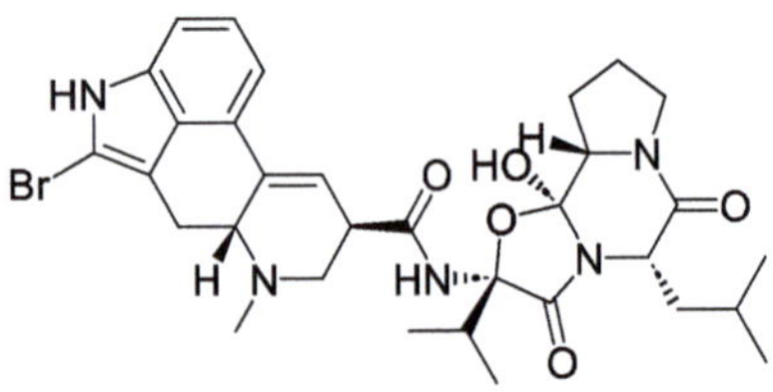

Bromocriptine

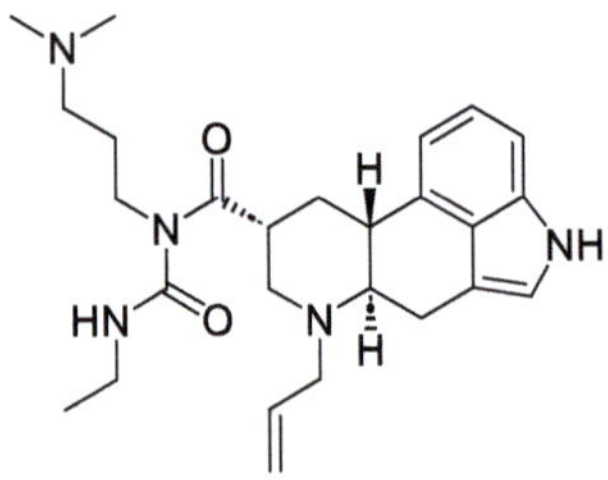

Cabergoline

These reagents were originally meant to treat pituitary tumors, but were also found to have some effect on improving glucose homeostasis [60]. Indeed, impaired glucose tolerance and insulin secretory dysfunction is observed in mice where the dopamine (D2)-receptor is disrupted [61]. A quick release formulation of bromocriptine was approved for the treatment of T2D in 2009 and cabergoline is also used [62]. They are effective at lowering fasting blood glucose and HbA1c, and may indicate some cardioprotective effects [63], but the mechanism of action is not well defined. There are no direct effects on insulin sensitivity, insulin secretion or glucose and lipid metabolism. Effects on improving glucose homeostasis is thought to be mediated via improving dopaminergic/sympathetic tone in central nervous system (CNS), that may partly involve resetting the circadian clock. Despite adverse effects being relatively mild and transient [60], they are not widely used to treat T2D.

Sodium-Glucose Transporter-2 (SGLT2) Inhibitors

These compounds specifically inhibit the sodium-glucose transport in kidney tubules (SGTL2) to reduce reabsorption of glucose in the kidney and thereby lower blood glucose. This is a mechanism that has been known for quite a while since a related compound Phlorozin, an extract of apple tree bark that inhibits both intestinal SGLT1 and renal SGLT2, was shown to increase glucosuria by von Mering in 1886 [64] and subsequently to reduce glycemia in T2D preclinical models [65]. But, Phlorozin was never used clinically as its oral bioavailability was low (<5%). However, beginning in 2012 a new generation of SGLT2 specific inhibitors were approved to treat T2D [66, 67], including dapagliflozin, empaglifozin and canagliflozin [68] (Figure 5.9). They are relatively effective at improving glucose homeostasis in T2D and improving β-cell function [66, 67, 69]. Side-effects, including increased urinary tract infections, occasional instances of normoglycemic ketoacidosis, and osmotic diuresis, are relatively mild and manageable [66, 67]. SGLT2 inhibition is relatively neutral for body weight loss in T2D treatment [70].

More recently, beyond being an effective T2D therapy, SGLT2 inhibition has also shown efficacy for cardiovascular disease and, heart failure in particular [71–73], along with protection against chronic kidney disease progression [74, 75] with or without T2D. Consequently, SGLT2 inhibitors are now on the World Health Organization's essential medicine list [20], and recently recommended as a first line pharmacological therapy for T2D, specifically for patients with cardiovascular disease, heart failure, or chronic kidney disease, usually in combination with metformin [76].

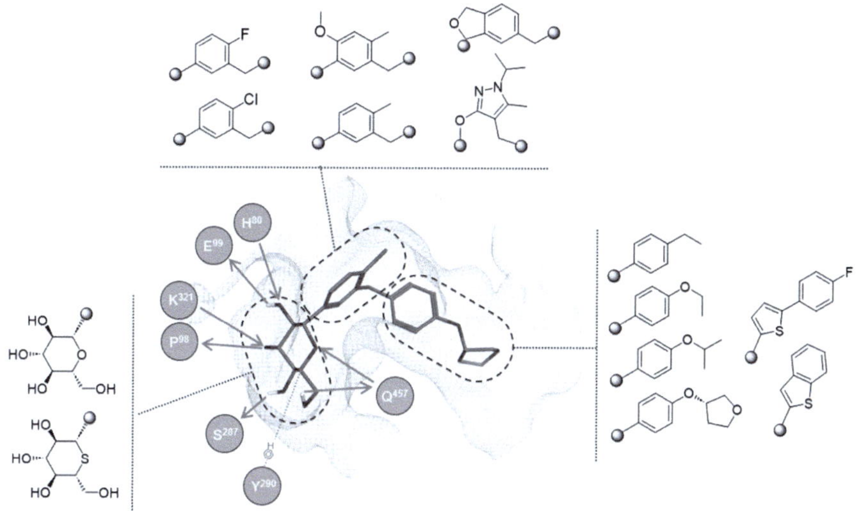

Figure 5.9 Overview of chemical structures of SGLT2 inhibitors. R-group analysis is mapped on active conformation of Empagliflozin bound to human SGLT2 (PDB ID: 7VSI).

Glimins

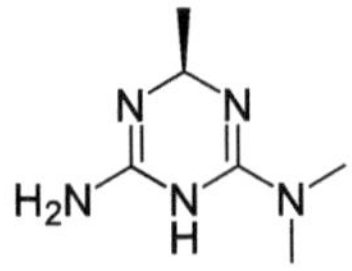

Imeglimin

Imeglimin is a first in class "oxidative phosphorylation blocker" approved in Japan in 2021 as an oral agent for the treatment of T2D [77]. It is believed to act via enhanced insulin action (inhibition of hepatic gluconeogenesis and increased muscle glucose uptake), and restoration of normal endogenous insulin secretion. Its mechanism of action is unknown, although it is speculated to enhance β-oxidation to reduce excessive fuel accumulation along with less reactive oxygen species (ROS) production [77]. The dose is quite high (≥1000 mg) and effects on glycemia are relatively modest, but more effective when used in combination [78]. Furthermore, imeglimin is relatively well tolerated and most side effects are limited to gastrointestinal issues and hypoglycemia [79].

Other (Non-Approved) Small Molecule T2D Treatments

Driven by the type 2 diabetes pandemic there has been much activity to develop additional and better small molecules to treat the disease, but none yet approved by the FDA or EMA, either due to lack of efficacy and or safety concerns. Among these are – glucagon receptor antagonists to prevent hepatic glucose production [80]; small molecule insulin receptor agonists and sensitizers [81]; GPR-40 agonists that mimic fatty acids to stimulate endogenous insulin secretion [82]; GPR-119 agonists that stimulate endogenous incretin secretion to then potentiate glucose-induced insulin secretion [83]; protein-tyrosine phosphatase 1b (PTP1B) inhibitors to improve insulin signaling via sustained insulin receptor tyrosine phosphorylation [84], and 11β-Hydroxysteroid dehydrogenase type 1 (11β-HSD1) inhibitors to reduce cortisol and improve insulin sensitivity [85]. Additionally, glucokinase activators promote both hepatic glucose uptake and endogenous insulin secretion to reduce glycemia [86], and in 2022 the first glucokinase activator, dorzagliatin, was approved for T2D treatment in China [87] (Figure 5.1).

Obesity Oral Agents

As previously mentioned, treatments for obesity can be traced back to Ancient Greece and the medical problems associated with being overweight have been appreciated since then. We do appreciate that there are many fads, "fat-burning" devices, surgical procedures, and injectable (GLP-1 analogs included) therapeutics to promote body weight loss in obesity. But in this chapter, as with the prior T2D

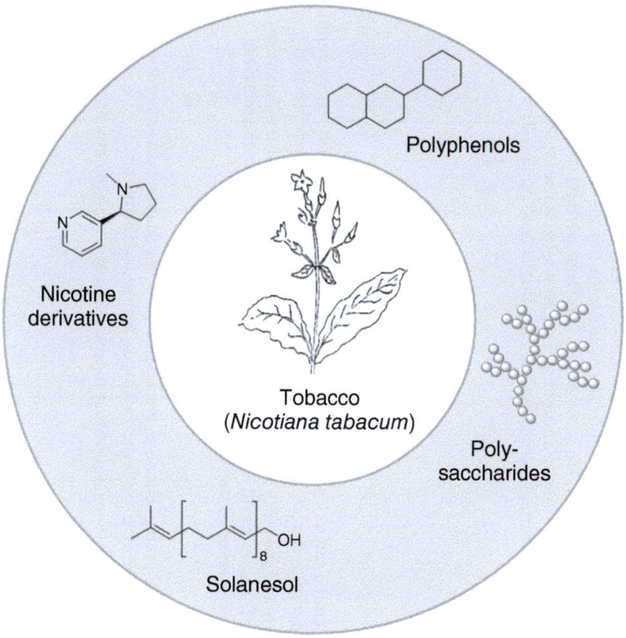

Figure 5.10 Main components of *Tabacco* extract.

section, the focus will be on ~15 classes of *bone fide* identifiable small molecule agents used to treat obesity over the last 150 years or so (Figure 5.1 and Table 5.2).

Nicotine

Since the late 1400s it has been known that extracts of tobacco leaves (*Nicotiana tabacum*) can attenuate body weight gain among early use for several other medical conditions [88]. Nicotine, being the active ingredient (Figure 5.10), suppresses appetite, and may also activate adipose metabolism [89]. While pure nicotine may have beneficial effects [90], these are far outweighed by its downside of numerous side effects [91] and oncogenic potential [92]. It is not commonly used for obesity, as it is not particularly effective, and today there are much better options.

Thyroxine

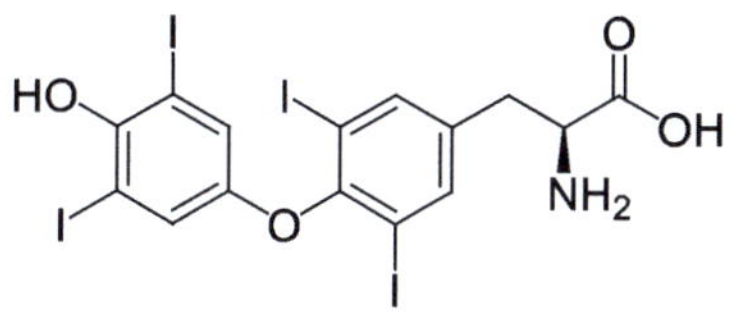

Thyroxine (T4)

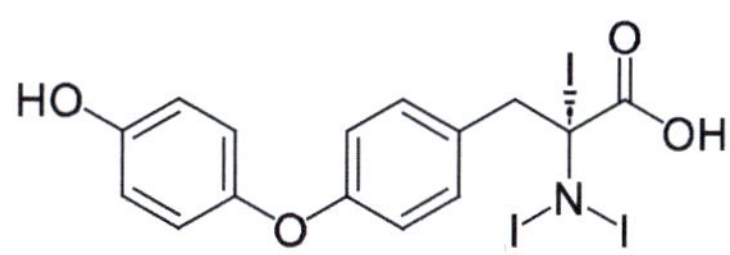

Triiodothyronine (T3)

In the late 1800s thyroid extracts were used to treat obesity [93]. It would do this by increasing metabolic rate and energy expenditure [94]. Thyroxine (T4)

Table 5.2 Obesity oral drugs.

Drug class	Drug name(s)	Date introduced	Mechanism of action
Nicotine	*Tobacco* (extract)	Late 1400s	Reduces appetite, food intake, and body weight
Thyroxine (thyroid hormone, T4)	• Levothyroxine	1893	Increases metabolic rate that can in turn induced body weight loss, via increased energy expenditure
Dinitrophenol	• Dinitrophenol	1933	Uncouples oxidative phosphorylation in mitochondria to increase metabolic rate and energy expenditure resulting in weight loss.
Amphetamines and CNS acting stimulants	• Benzedrine • Dextroamphetamine • Etilamfetamine • Lisdexamfetamine • Aminorex • Fenfluramine • Phentermine • Amfepramone • Sibutramine • Tesofensine • Mazindol • Mefenorex	1945	Act on certain hypothalamic neurons to release norepinephrine, dopamine, and/or serotonin, many via inhibiting monoamine transporters (norepinephrine (NETs); dopamine (DATs) or serotonin (SERTs) transporters) to prevent reuptake of these monoamine neurotransmitters. This results in increasing energy expenditure, decreasing appetite, and/or food intake, leading to body weight loss.
Amphetamines combinations	• "Fen-Phen" Fenfluramine + Phentermine	1984 proposed, and in much use in early 1990s. Combo never FDA approved; individually 1959 – Phentermine 1973 – Fenfluramine	Fenfluramine acts as a serotonin releasing agent. Causes the release of serotonin by disrupting vesicular storage, and reversing serotonin transporter function Phentermine, primarily a norepinephrine releasing agent, but also induces the release of serotonin and dopamine, to a far lesser extent. Causes the release of monoamines reverses transporter reuptake.
	• "Qsymia" Phentermine + Topiramate	2012 (USA)	Phentermine – (amphetamine) increases CNS hypothalamic neurons to release norepinephrine and, to a lesser extent, dopamine, and serotonin. Topiramate – a sulfamate modified sugar used to treat epilepsy and migraines. Mechanism unclear.

	• "Contrave" Bupropion + Naltrexone	2014 (USA & EU)	Bupropion – an atypical antidepressant primarily used to treat major depressive disorder and to support smoking cessation. Thought to be a norepinephrine–dopamine reuptake inhibitor (NDRI) and antagonist of several nicotinic acetylcholine receptors. Naltrexone – primarily used to manage alcohol/opioid use disorder by reducing cravings/feelings of euphoria linked with substance use disorder. An opioid receptor antagonist m-opioid receptor (MOR) > κ-opioid receptor (KOR) > > δ-opioid receptor. Augments Bupropion's increase of proopiomelanocortin (POMC) production (Melanocyte Stimulating Hormone, MSH).
Lipase inhibitors	• Orlistat	1999 (USA) 2007 (USA), OTC version 2009 (EU), OTC version	Reduces Free Fatty Acid (FFA) absorbance from the gut. Inhibits gastric and pancreatic lipases leading to excretion of lipids.
Cannabinoid receptor CB1 antagonists (inverse agonists)	• Rimonabant • Taranabant • Otenabant • Rosonabant	2006 (EU)	Antagonizes CB1Rs in the CNS, principally the hypothalamus, to reduce appetite and food intake resulting in weight loss. Rimonabant also found to antagonize of the μ-opioid receptor.
Serotonin receptor agonist	• Lorcaserin	2012	Increases proopiomelanocortin (POMC) production (Melanocyte Stimulating Hormone, MSH) and consequently promotes weight loss through increased satiety.
β(3)-adrenoceptor (ADRB3) agonists	• Mirbegron	2012 (USA & EU) for overactive bladder syndrome (OAB)	For obesity – Agonism of the β(3)-adrenoceptor leads to increased fatty acid oxidation, increased energy expenditure and subsequent weight loss.
Melanocortin 4 receptor (MC4R) agonist	• Setmelanotide	2020 (USA) 2021 (EU)	Activates MC4 receptors in the hypothalamus to reduce appetite, food intake, and consequently induce weight loss.

was approved for hypothyroidism, but never officially for weight loss in obesity. It can cause hyperthyroidism, cardiac palpitations and several other side effects. When triiodothyronine (T3) was discovered in 1952, it was also used to promote weight loss in obesity, but with limited effect [93, 95]. More recently, thyroid hormone receptor-β (THR-β) specific agonists have been generated that avoid cardiac effects which are mediated via THR-α [96]. While THR-β agonists may only have modest effects on weight loss [97], they show promise to treat other metabolic disease, such as metabolic-dysfunction associated steatohepatitis (MASH) [98].

Dinitrophenol

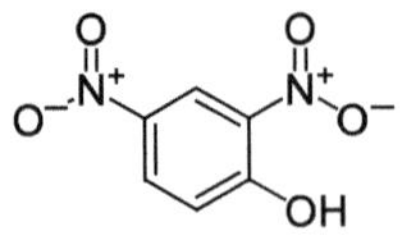

2,4-dinitrophenol

The use of 2,4-dinitrophenol (DNP) for body weight loss in obesity was introduced in the early 1930s [99–101]. Its mechanism of action is to uncouple oxidative phosphorylation in mitochondria that dissipates the proton gradient across the mitochondrial-membrane, linked to ATP production, and because of the loss of this proton-motive force, heat is generated instead of ATP. As such, energy expenditure is increased resulting in "burning off" internally stored fuels, like fat, and body weight loss is observed [94, 99, 100]. However, there are numerous serious adverse effects of taking DNP, including multiple organ failure and death [100, 102]. In 1938, the then recently passed Food, Drug and Cosmetic Act (FDCA) in the USA [103] labeled DNP as being "extremely dangerous and not fit for human consumption" [100]. The FDCA enabled the FDA to oversee and regulate production and use of foods, drugs, medical devices and cosmetics, which is still very active and essential for human health today [100]. Soon after 1938, prescriptions of DNP use for obesity halted and reports of poisonings due to taking it for weight loss dropped off [99, 100]. In the USA, DNP is legal to sell for chemical use, but not for human consumption. In the past DNP has been used as an antiseptic, herbicide and pesticide, but no longer in the USA or Europe today. As a precursor in the synthesis of 2,4,6-trinitrotoluene (TNT), DNP is a registered explosive in the USA and UK. Since 2023, DNP is classified as a regulated poison in the UK [104]. Although, the World Anti-Doping association has banned use of DNP since 2015, because of its "fat burning" effects, and despite the dangers of using it, DNP has continued use particularly among the body building and extreme dieting communities [105, 106]. There are some other chemical mitochondrial uncouplers in consideration to treat obesity [107], but this approach remains a strong safety concern [94].

Amphetamines

We have grouped this class of "anorexigens" together, since they are either amphetamines, or other stimulants which increase CNS monoamine neurotransmitter levels. Some of these (e.g., Amferpremone, Mefenorex) are "prodrugs" that are metabolically activated to an active amphetamine *in-vivo*. This amphetamine class act on certain hypothalamic neurons to release norepinephrine, dopamine and/or serotonin, mainly via inhibiting monoamine transporters (norepinephrin (NETs); dopamine (DATs) or serotonin (SERTs) transporters) to prevent reuptake of these monoamine neurotransmitters. This results in increasing energy expenditure, decreasing appetite and/or food intake, leading to body weight loss [108]. Amphetamines (notably Benzedrine, originally an inhaler for nasal congestion) were first used in the 1930s for weight loss, and several amphetamine-based small molecules were approved for treatment of obesity along with a reduce calorie diet and exercise regime to help lose weight in the mid 1940s [1].

However, concerns over adverse effects of using this amphetamine class for weight loss, including various cardiac problems, systemic and pulmonary hypertension, flushing and temperature increase, muscle cramping, mood and emotional problems, as well as addiction [109]. These adverse effects led to limiting approved amphetamine-based weight loss drugs to only short-term use (a few weeks) with label warnings of addiction in 1977 [1]. As a consequence, use of most molecules in this class to treat obesity declined, but with some notable exceptions in combinations (e.g., low dose phentermine plus fenfluramine, so-called "Phen-Fen") – see below (Figure 5.11).

It is worth noting that amphetamines have been a component of several combinations, including so-called "Rainbow Diet Pills" [110]. This was introduced in the 1940s as varying cocktail of amphetamines, thyroid hormone, diuretics, laxatives, phenolphthalein, herbal and other pharmacological ingredients, but caused many deaths and in the late 1960s were withdrawn in the USA by the FDA [110]. Despite this, they have continued use elsewhere in the world, and re-emerged as underground dietary supplements [110].

Centrally-Acting Combinations

Phentermine + Fenfluramine ("Phen-Fen") – was a popular combination used to treat obesity in the 1990s. Phentermine is an amphetamine that is primarily a norepinephrine releasing agent (but can also increase dopamine and serotonin) [1] that suppresses appetite. It is approved as a monotherapy for short-term weight loss treatment for obesity together with diet and exercise regimes [111]. It has fewer side effects, relative to other amphetamines, but only for limited use ($\geq$12 weeks) to deter from potential addiction [1, 112]. Fenfluramine is an amphetamine derivative that increases serotonin release and causes appetite suppression [113]. It was approved for treatment of obesity, along with diet and exercise in 1973, yet didn't

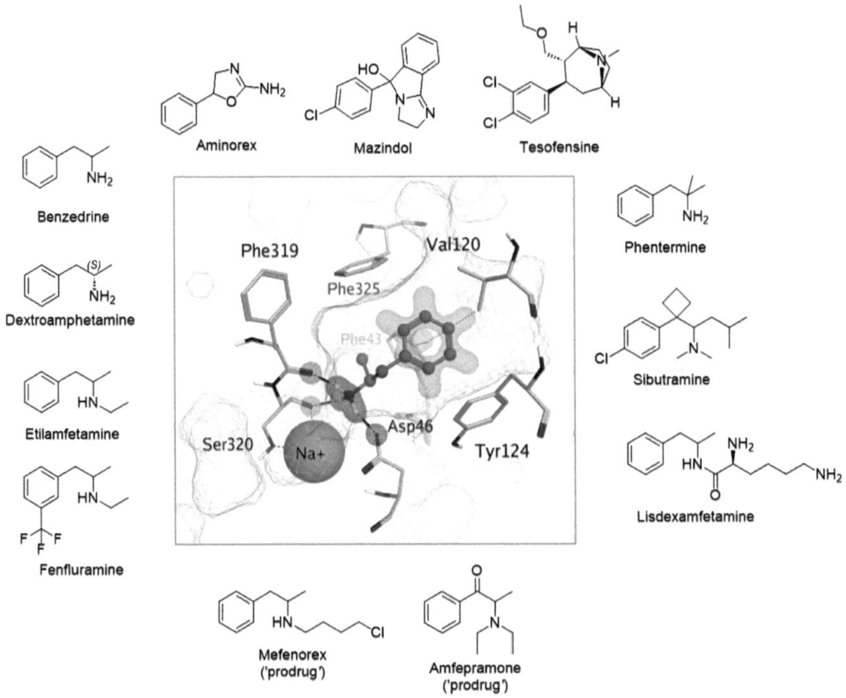

Figure 5.11 Overview of chemical structures of amphetamines and an example of Dextroamphetamine binding mode in complex with drosophila dopamine transporter (PDB ID: 4XP9).

gather traction as a monotherapy, mostly due to nausea and anxiety-inducing side effects [113]. In 1984, it was reported that a combination of Phentermine + Fenfluramine ('Phen-Fen') gave modest weight loss with less frequent adverse effects [114], and subsequently gained popular use although never had FDA approval as a combination [113]. In the early 1990s it emerged that Fenfluramine was associated with pulmonary hypertension, dyspnea, heart valve problems and cardiac fibrosis [115–117]. Consequently, in 1997 the FDA requested Fenfluramine be withdrawn [118], followed by many other countries around the world and the Phen-Fen combination stopped. However, phentermine monotherapy remains one of the few amphetamines still prescribed for short-term weight loss.

Phentermine + Topiramate ("Qsymia") – the action of phentermine is described above.

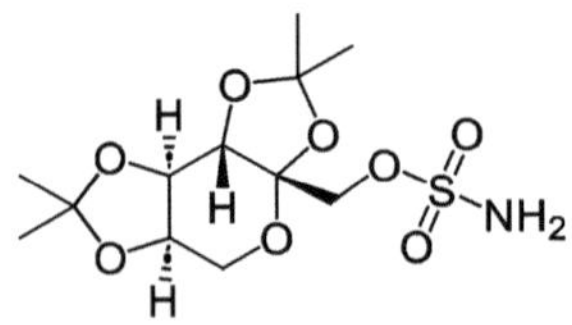

Topiramate

Topiramate is an anticonvulsant used to treat epilepsy [119]. Its mechanism of action is not well understood but thought to be a GABAnergic neuron agonist, that has some effect on suppressing appetite causing modest weight loss [111, 119, 120]. The combination ("Qsymia") has modest weight loss effects and was FDA approved for treatment of obesity in 2012, with the proviso that if ≤3% body weight loss is seen after three months the treatment be stopped [121]. It is not approved in Europe mostly due to safety concerns surrounding increased heart rate.

Bupropion + Naltrexone ("Contrave") – Bupropion is an atypical antidepressant primarily used to treat major depressive disorder.

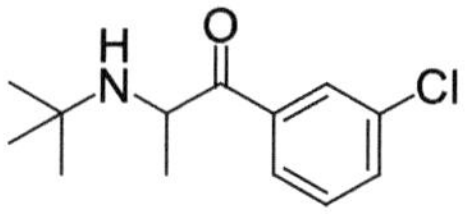

Bupropion

It is a norepinephrine–dopamine reuptake inhibitor (NDRI) and antagonist of several nicotinic acetylcholine receptors [122]. It can activate Proopiomelanocortin (POMC) neurons in the hypothalamus to increase α-Melanocyte Stimulating Hormone (α-MSH) levels to then suppress appetite [123]. Naltrexone is an μ-opioid receptor antagonist that prevents β-endorphin action to dampen autoinhibition of POMC-neurons to also increases hypothalamic α-MSH levels and suppress appetite [123]. These distinct, but complementary, mechanisms come together to promote some body weight loss in obesity. The bupropion/naltrexone combination (Contrave) was approved in USA and Europe in 2014 for management of obesity (BMI >30 kg/m^2) or overweight (BMI = 27–30 kg/m^2) with one obesity related comorbidity [123, 124]. The body weight loss is relatively modest and Contrave is not widely used, especially in Europe where it is not marketed despite EMA approval. Adverse side effects are mostly modest and manageable, including gastrointestinal, slight increases in pulse rate/blood pressure and some psychiatric symptoms like anxiety and depression [123].

Lorcaserin

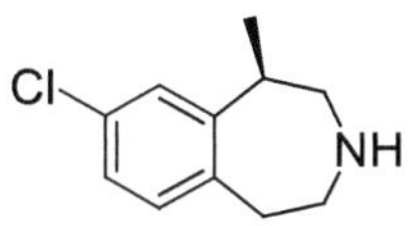

Lorcaserin

Lorcaserin is a small molecule selective serotonin (5-HTC2) receptor agonist, that also increases POMC production in the hypothalamus and consequently increases local α-MSH levels to suppress appetite [125]. It was approved in the USA, in 2012, a 10 mg dose twice a day for obesity (BMI >30 kg/m^2) or overweight (BMI = 27–30 kg/m^2) with one obesity related comorbidity along with a diet and exercise regime [126]. Because of its better serotonin receptor selectivity, lorcaserin had weight loss effects without triggering pulmonary hypertension or heart valve problems, like other less selective serotonin receptor agonists such as fenfluramine [126]. However, in clinical trials designed to monitor potential cardiac issues of lorcaserin, an increased risk of cancer was found [127]. In 2020, the FDA withdrew approval of lorcaserin for weight loss therapy [125, 126].

Orlistat

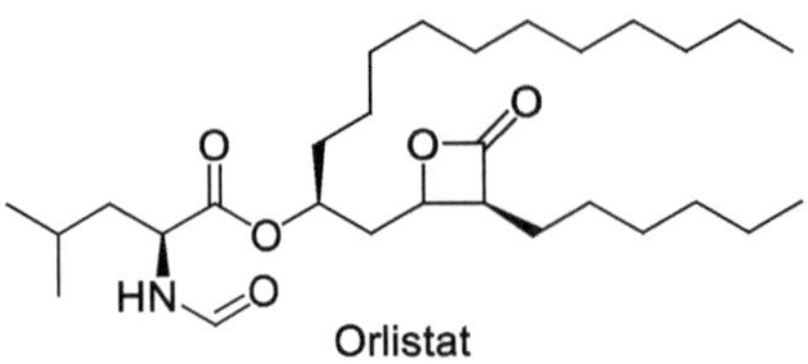

Orlistat

Orlistat is a synthetic derivative of a natural pancreatic lipase inhibitor, lipstatin, from *Streptomyces toxytricini* soil bacteria [128, 129]. As an oral medication inhibiting pancreatic lipase, it is taken three times a day with each meal. It works by inhibiting dietary triglycerides hydrolysis, which are then retained in the gut lumen and excreted [130]. With less fatty acids being absorbed from diet, less calories are taken on board and there is a consequential modest body weight loss [131]. Longer term use can also mildly alleviate some obesity associated symptoms such as T2D [132] and hypertension [133]. It was originally approved for obesity along with a hypocaloric/low fat diet in the USA in 1999, and since 2007 in the USA and 2009 in Europe orlistat has had "over-the-counter" (OTC) use, and as such is one of the most economic obesity treatments [134, 135]. However, it has problematic and uncomfortable gastrointestinal side effects, including steatorrhea, excessive flatulence and fecal incontinence [131], making it not in popular use.

Cannabinoid Receptor Antagonists

Cannabis plant extracts have been used for ancient medicinal and recreational purposes for centuries [136]. The active ingredient D^9- tetrahydrocannabinol (THC) was isolated and synthesized in the 1940s [136], that eventually led to the identification of the cannabinoid receptors CB1R [137] and CB2R [138] in the early 1990s. CB2R expression is restricted to the immune system, and it is CB1R that is predominately expressed in the CNS which was targeted for appetite suppression [139, 140]. A common effect of agonizing CB1R is an orexigenic effect [136, 141], so CBR1 antagonist approaches were pursued to suppress appetite [142, 143].

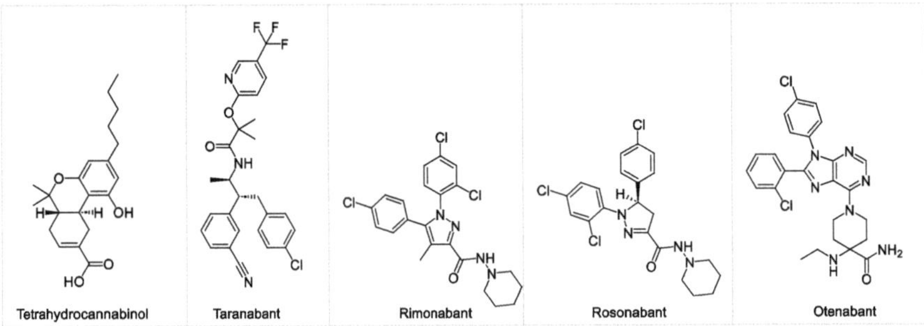

Rimonabant is a selective inverse agonist of the CBR1, that preferentially binds and holds CBR1 in an inactive state [139, 143]. It was approved for the treatment of obesity (and nicotine dependence) in Europe in 2006, but never in the USA [144]. Rimonabant did render significant weight loss [144, 145], and improved some obesity comorbidities [146]. However, there were serious adverse psychiatric effects of severe depression, anxiety and suicidal tendencies causing discontinuation of rimonabant use [147, 148]. In 2008, the EMA suspended use of rimonabant, and its approval was withdrawn in 2009 causing a suspension of rimonabant sales and use worldwide [144]. The pursuit of central CB1R antagonism as an obesity target has declined since.

β3-Adrenoreceptor Agonists

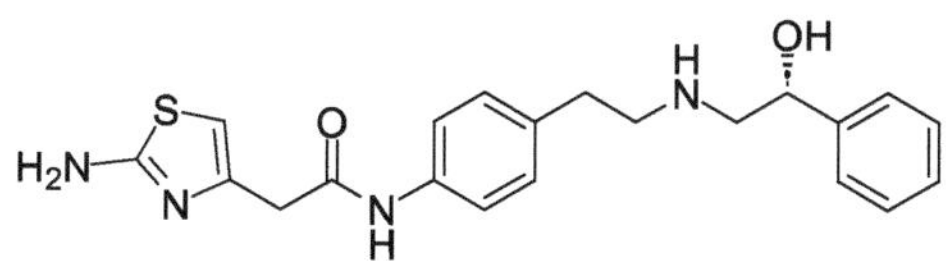

Mirabegron

Mirabegron, is β3-adrenoreceptor agonist, approved to treat overactive bladder syndrome in both the USA and Europe in 2012 [149]. Because β3-adrenoreceptor agonism can lead to increased lipolysis, fatty acid oxidation and mitochondrial respiration/uncoupling to increase energy expenditure this approach was also considered, off label, for body weight loss [150–152]. Side effects such as tachycardia, atrial fibrillation, hypertension, infections of the upper respiratory and urinary tracts, various gastrointestinal issues and fatigue are considered manageable [153]. Mirbegron has also been examined for heart failure indication but was found to have no beneficial effect, with adverse effects not significant [154].

Melanocortin 4 Receptor (MC4R) Agonist

Setmelanotide, is a small molecule peptide agonist of the MC4R (Figure 5.12) that is approved for rare disease obesity, including proopiomelanocortin (POMC), proprotein convertase subtilisin/kexin-1 (PCSK1) or leptin deficiencies [155]. It binds to MC4Rs in the hypothalamus associated with feeding behavior to reduce appetite, and perhaps increases energy expenditure, resulting in body weight loss in such patients [156]. The natural ligand of MC4R is α-melanocyte stimulating hormone (α-MSH) which is derived from proteolytic cleavage, by PCSK1, of the POMC proprotein substrate in the hypothalamus, skin, and intermediate lobe of the pituitary [157]. Hence, a synthetic MC4R agonist can bypass the need for α-MSH in certain POMC and PCSK1 deficiencies [155]. The α-MSH is also downstream of leptin neuronal signaling in the hypothalamus [158], so can also compensate for some forms of obesity associated with leptin deficiency [159]. Thus, setmelanotide is not effective for general obesity, only for rare genetic indications of obesity yet has relatively few adverse side effects [155].

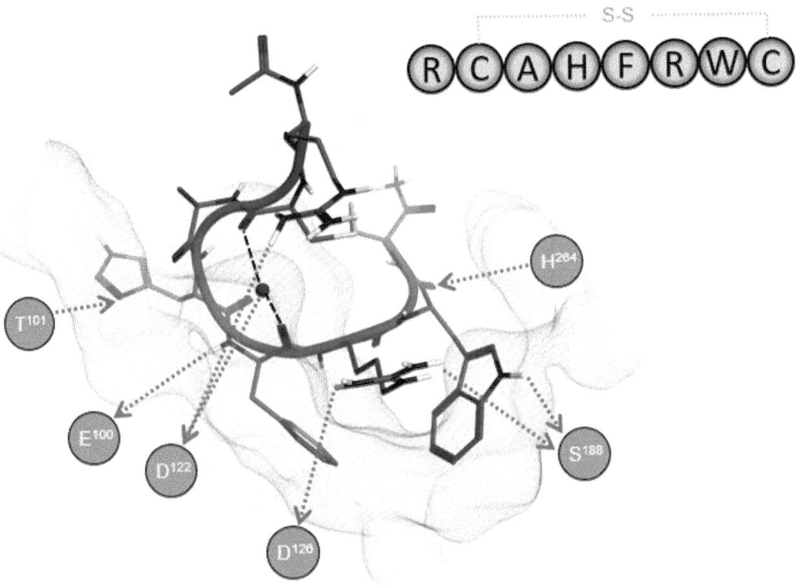

Figure 5.12 Setmelanotide is a stapled peptide, where two cysteines are connected via disulfide bridge. Complex between setmelanotide human Melanocortin receptor 4 (cryo-EM structure, PDB ID: 7AUE).

A Current Perspective for Oral Diabetes and Obesity Small Molecules

It is well appreciated that the obesity and T2D pandemics run hand-in-hand and that obesity-linked T2D is by far the most common form of T2D [160, 161]. As stated above, there are many small molecule oral therapeutics to treat T2D _or_ obesity, but there is currently not one that effectively treats T2D _and_ obesity [162, 163]. At least not as effective as the class of *injectable* GLP-1 analogs [162, 163]. GLP-1 analogs have the ability to potentiate glucose-induced insulin secretion to improve glycemia _and_ suppress appetite to induce quite impressive body weight loss as well as relieve some obesity related comorbidities [162–164]. However, incretin-based therapies are not for everyone with obesity-linked T2D [165–167], especially those with trypanophobia, and oral medications are preferred with better patient compliance [56]. As such, there has been a recent push for oral small molecule GLP-1 receptor (GLP-1R) agonists [168], which we will explore in the next section.

Small Molecule Glucagon-Like Peptide 1 Receptor (GLP-1R) Agonists

Introduction

The first peptide GLP-1R agonist, exenatide, was approved by the FDA in 2005, to improve glycemic control in patients with T2D as an adjunct to diet and exercise [169]. Multiple peptide GLP-1R agonists have since been approved for T2D, including exenatide extended-release (ER) once-weekly, dulaglutide once-weekly and semaglutide once-weekly, lixisenatide once-daily and liraglutide once-daily, all requiring subcutaneous administration. The subsequent approval by the FDA of semaglutide and liraglutide for weight management significantly expanded the market opportunity for the GLP-1R agonist class. Designed to overcome the need for subcutaneous administration, oral semaglutide (Rybelsus) was approved by the FDA for T2D in 2019, as a tablet containing the absorption enhancer sodium N-(8-[2-hydroxybenzoyl] amino) caprylate (SNAC) [170, 171]. By following the stringent dosing regimen which specifies administration with less than 120 ml of water after overnight fasting and with 30 minutes post-dose fasting, bioavailability of less than 1% is achieved [172]. Since the peptide agonists have extremely high GLP-1R potency, in the picomolar concentration range, such low oral exposure is sufficient to deliver an efficacious concentration. However, the oral formulation does still not deliver the higher systemic concentrations achieved with subcutaneous administration, which are required to deliver equivalent glucose lowering and body weight loss [173]. To address this and to offer a less restrictive dosing regimen, the pharmaceutical industry has been pursuing orally bioavailable small molecule GLP-1R agonists for the treatment of T2D and obesity for many years. Such therapies would also introduce opportunities for fixed dose combinations with other orally bioavailable small-molecule therapies for cardiometabolic diseases. However, unlike the discovery of small molecule class A GPCR agonists, the discovery of small molecule class B GPCR agonists with physicochemical properties amenable for oral dosing has been extremely challenging.

Peptide ligand binding to the extracellular domain (ECD) to initiate signaling of class B1 GPCRs is mechanistically different compared to class A receptors whose ligands primarily bind to residues located within the membrane spanning α-helical regions. Receptors of the class B1 incretin family contain a large and flexible ECD at their N-terminal that together with the transmembrane (TM) region is involved in binding of peptide ligands (Figure 5.13). For class B1 receptors, a complex two-step binding mechanism is required for receptor activation. Peptide ligands firstly bind to the ECD inducing changes in receptor dynamics allowing access and binding into the TM region. Engagement in the core of the TM bundle initiates an activation mechanism leading to outward movement of the intracellular side of TM helix 6, resulting in the receptor complexing with various intracellular binding partners (e.g. heterotrimeric G-proteins) and downstream signaling [174, 175].

The First Reported Small Molecule GLP-1R Agonists

One of the first reported small molecule GLP-1R agonists came from a group at the National Center for Drug Screening in Shanghai [176] from screening approximately 50 K synthetic and natural compounds in a rat GLP-1R luciferase reporter assay in HEK293 cells. A series of cyclobutane hits were discovered but only two hits were confirmed to elevate cyclic adenosine monophosphate (cAMP) levels. Interestingly, the agonist activity was driven by a cyclobutane product formed in the DMSO

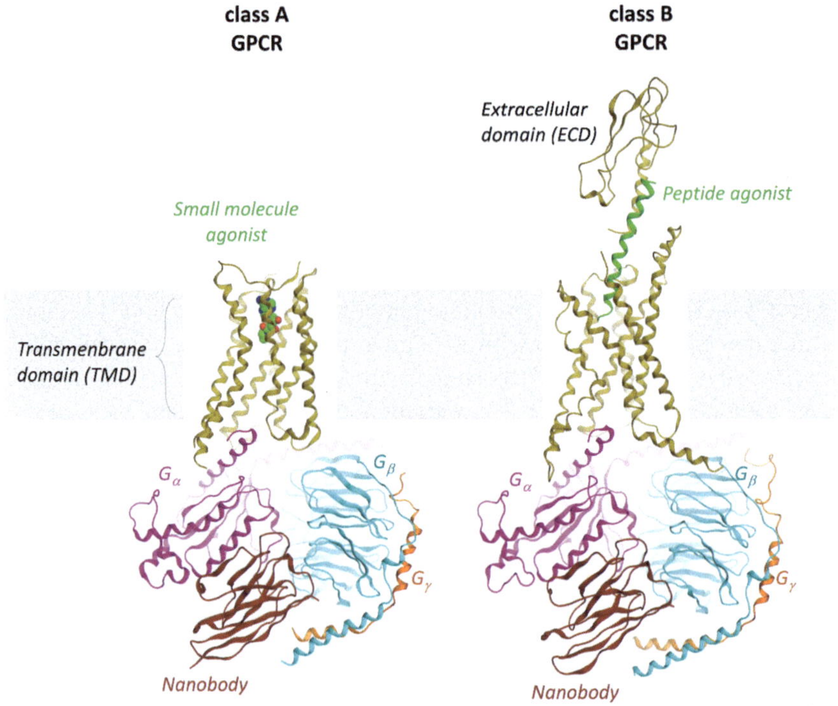

Figure 5.13 Comparison of class A and class B GPCRs in complex with G-proteins (PDB IDs: 6GDG and 8JIP, correspondently) to illustrate the challenges in corresponding small molecule agonist drug discovery: binding pocket of class A receptors located in transmembrane domain (TMD) and is relatively small, while orthosteric pocket (peptides' binding pocket) of class B receptors is much larger and is located at the interface of TMD and large and flexible extracellular domain (ECD).

solution from a dimerization of the initial alkene selected for screening. The lead compound Boc5 **1** is a full agonist in the cAMP/luciferase assay (estimated EC_{50} 2.7 μM), and equally active at both the human and rat GLP-1R. Boc5 showed no measurable activity at the GLP-2R or glucagon receptors. Displacement of [^{125}I]GLP-1 in receptor binding studies indicated that the agonist occupied the orthosteric GLP-1R binding site and this was confirmed several years later by cryo-electron microscopy (cryo-EM) structure of Boc5 in complex with the human GLP-1R and Gs protein (Figure 5.14) [177].

Boc5 induced glucose-stimulated insulin secretion in isolated rat pancreatic islets in a concentration dependent manner. Boc5 (3 μM) increased insulin secretion by approximately 2.5-fold following a glucose concentration increase from 3.3 to 25 mM, activity which is comparable to GLP-1 (100 nM). Boc5 also demonstrated GLP-1R mediated in-vivo efficacy in reducing HbA1c in db/db mice and food intake in wild-type mice. Daily injected doses (1 and 2 mg i.p.) reduced HbA1c in db/db mice to wild-type levels after four to six weeks. I.p. administration of Boc5 dose-dependently suppressed food intake up to 12 hours in wild type mice and up to 53% with the top dose (2 mg). The suppression was lost by pre-treatment with the

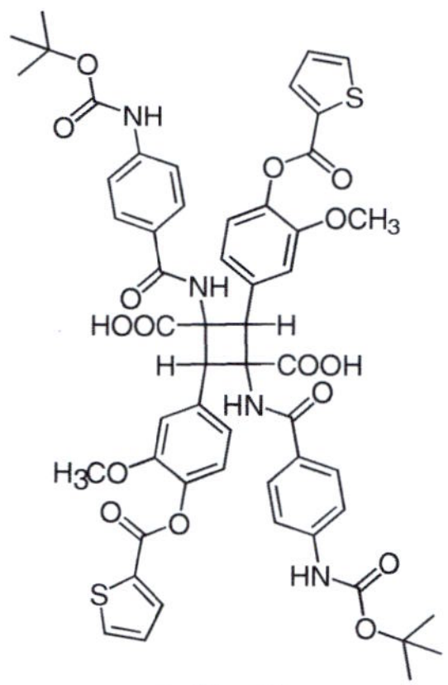

1 (Boc5)

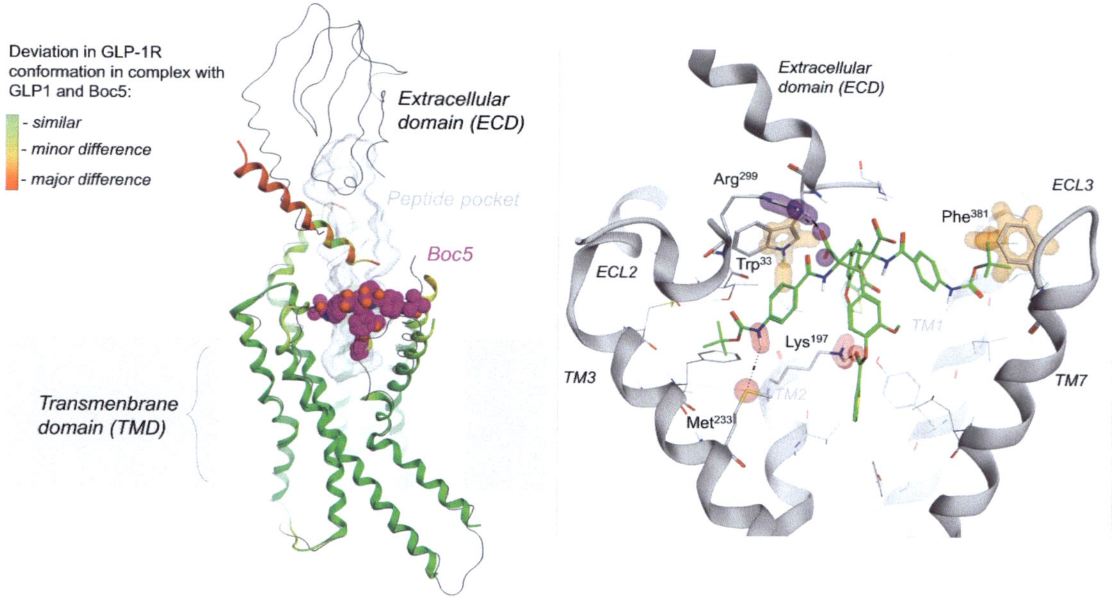

Figure 5.14 Boc5 in complex with the human GLP-1R (cryo-EM structure, PDB ID = 7X8R). Comparison of receptor conformations in complex with GLP-1 peptide and Boc5 (middle picture) indicated no significant changes in transmembrane domain (TMD) but rearrangement of the extracellular domain (ECD) interacting with Boc5 via Trp33. Peptide binding pocket is shown as grey mesh surface. One of thiophene-arms of Boc5 penetrated deep into the orthosteric ligand pocket (overlapping with GLP-1 peptide's N-terminal binding position), while tert-butyl carbamate arms occupied allosteric pockets between TM1-TM7 and TM2-TM3.

selective GLP-1R antagonist Exendin(9–39) demonstrating a GLP-1R driven in-vivo effect.

Further optimization of the series was able to deliver more potent analogues, with EC_{50} of approximately 100 nM in the reporter gene assay [178]. However, this modest potency coupled with unfavorable physicochemical properties, high molecular weight and high lipophilicity, would require significant optimization to deliver orally bioavailable clinical candidates. Nonetheless, this was the first report of a non-peptidic GLP-1R agonist demonstrating in-vivo efficacy in a preclinical model.

GLP-1R Agonists and Positive Allosteric Modulators

More recently, a number of small molecule GLP-1R positive allosteric modulators (PAMs) have been reported. PAMs are compounds that enhance the agonist efficacy of the endogenous ligand when bound to the receptor but have no effect alone. Since GLP-1 has a very short human half-life [179], such PAMs would lead to transient activation and only after meals when endogenous concentrations of GLP-1 are increased. A PAM that potentiates the activity of the GLP-1 metabolite GLP-1(9–36) would offer an attractive therapeutic approach since this metabolite accounts for the majority of postprandial GLP-1 in humans and has a significantly longer half-life compared to parental GLP-1, therefore potentially delivering prolonged receptor activation. However, GLP-1(9–36) is approximately 10 000-fold less potent than GLP-1, and hence a significant potentiation would be required for this to be a viable therapeutic approach [180].

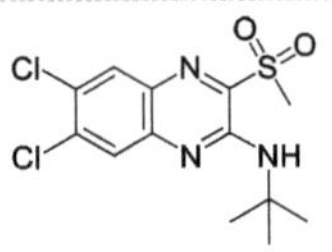	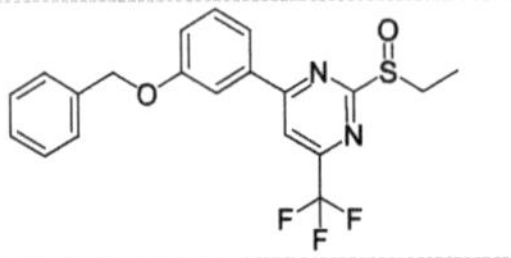
2	**3**
(Compound 2)	(BETP)

In 2007 Novo Nordisk reported a series of quinoxaline GLP-1R agonists [181]. An initial high throughput screen (HTS) of 500 K compounds via a radioligand binding assay ([^{125}I]GLP-1 displacement) failed to discover any agonists and hence Novo turned towards a functional cell assay measuring cAMP in membranes from baby hamster kidney cells expressing GLP-1R. A screen of 250 K compound diversity set led to the discovery of substituted quinoxalines, a series of potent non-competitive GLP-1R agonists. The sulfone **2** (compound 2) was the most potent analogue (EC_{50} approximately 100 nM) and a full agonist, albeit with a bell-shaped dose response curve. In HEK293 cells overexpressing human GLP-1R, **2** increased cAMP (EC_{50} 0.59 μM, Emax 88%) and caused less GLP-1R internalization compared to GLP-1 [182]. **2** was shown to stimulate insulin secretion from wild-type mouse islets, but not islets isolated from GLP-1R knockout mice confirming that the effect was GLP-1R dependent. **2** (1 μM) potentiated glucose (10 mM) induced insulin release threefold compared to glucose alone, an effect size comparable to that of 100 nM GLP-1.

In addition to being an agonist, **2** increased the binding affinity of GLP-1 to GLP-1R in a concentration dependent manner and was therefore characterized as an ago-allosteric modulator. The binding mode of **2** was confirmed by cryo-EM which showed that the compound binds covalently to Cys347 in TM6 of GLP-1R and introduces considerable steric bulk (Figure 5.15a) [183]. The mechanism of activation is possibly due to disruption of a hydrophobic lock between TM5 and TM6 (observed in glucagon receptor (GCGR)) [184]. The lock favors inactive receptor conformations, and its disruption therefore leads to a lowering of the energy barrier for receptor activation [184]. Although **2** increased the binding affinity of GLP-1, a corresponding increase in GLP-1 efficacy was not detected which the authors suggest may be due to a large receptor reserve in the over-expressing cell-line. Nonetheless this was an important milestone in the field, providing evidence that a small molecule agonist binding site exists on GLP-1R and is remote from the peptide ligand binding region. Several groups subsequently reported variations on the quinoxaline scaffold but their modest GLP-1R potency coupled with poor metabolic stability likely precluded clinical development [185–187].

A subsequent discovery in the GLP-1R agonist field was the work from Eli-Lilly in 2010 disclosing the small molecule agonist and PAM, 4-[3-(benzyloxy)phenyl]-2-ethylsulfinyl-6-(trifluoromethyl)-pyrimidine **3** (BETP), [188]. Lilly screened a small compound library, (~ 2000 compounds) derived from a 3D pharmacophore model built on previously reported GLP-1R agonists, against human GLP-1R in stably transfected HEK293 cells. Optimization of the initial partial agonist hit led to full agonist **3**, BETP, with improved potency (cAMP EC_{50} 0.66 μM). BETP has no activity at GLP-2R, gastric inhibitory polypeptide receptor (GIPR), or GCGR. Coincubation of BETP with GLP-1 induced both cAMP production in GLP-1R expressing HEK293 cells and insulin secretion in cultured pancreatic islets isolated from Sprague Dawley rats at 10 and 3 μM respectively. Consistent with these characteristics of an ago-allosteric modulator, BETP was unable to displace [^{125}I]GLP-1 binding to cell membranes expressing the human GLP-1R. Pfizer subsequently showed that BETP exerts its action by binding covalently to Cys347 in GLP-1R. This was shown by its inability to function as a PAM at the C347A – GLP-1R mutant [189]. Pfizer exploited BETP in their HTS which led to the discovery of danuglipron and will be discussed later. BETP is structurally similar to the earlier reported quinoxalines which share the same mode of action (Figure 5.15a).

BETP (10 mg/kg iv dose) increases insulin secretion in both the Sprague–Dawley rat intravenous glucose tolerance test (IVGTT) model and hyperglycemic clamp model, consistent with GLP-1R pharmacology.

A subsequent publication reports that BETP strongly potentiates the cAMP response of the weak GLP-1 metabolite GLP-1(9–36) with both an increase in potency, (pEC_{50} shift from 6.4 to 7.5) and efficacy (Emax shift from 15 to 99%) in a dose dependent manner (up to 30 mM BETP) [190]. This potentiation was also illustrated in-vivo in Wistar rats undergoing IVGTT. Coadministration of BETP

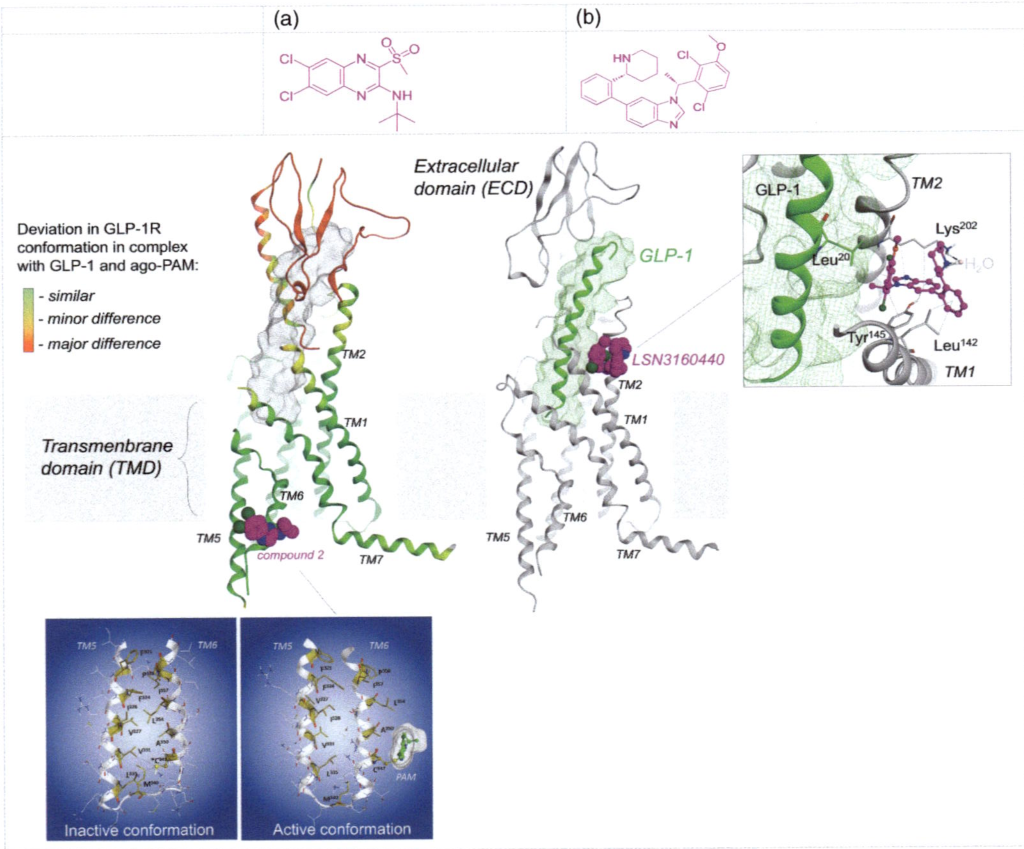

Figure 5.15 Positive allosteric modulators (PAMs) bound to GLP-1R. (a) Ago-allosteric modulator (compound 2) covalently bound to C^{347} (cryo-EM structure, PDB ID = 7DUR). It's mode of action is based on destabilization of a hydrophobic lock between TM5 and TM6 (subfigure in bottom-left). Comparison of receptor conformations in complex with GLP-1 peptide and compound 2 indicated no significant changes in transmembrane domain (TMD) but rearrangement of extracellular domain (ECD) with C-terminal α-helix overlapping with peptide's binding pocket (grey mesh surface). (b) Lilly's PAM (LSN3160440) bound in allosteric pocket between TM1 and TM2 (cryo-EM structure, PDB ID = 6VCB), the structure was obtained in the presence of GLP-1 and indicated peptide-PAM interactions (subfigure in top-right).

(5 mg/kg) with metabolite GLP-1(9–36) (150 nmol/kg) increased insulin secretion comparable to that achieved by parental GLP-1 (3 nmol/kg) whereas BETP alone had no impact on plasma insulin levels.

Since the discovery of BETP, several non-covalent chemotypes have been reported as GLP-1R PAMs. Vanderbilt University reported the tricyclic compound **4** (VU0453379) as a GLP-1R PAM discovered from a HTS [191]. The series had no calcium response in the absence of GLP-1 but potentiated an EC_{20} concentration of GLP-1 (EC_{50} = 1.3 μM, Emax 59%). The lead compound potentiated low dose exenatide to augment insulin secretion in primary mouse pancreatic islets.

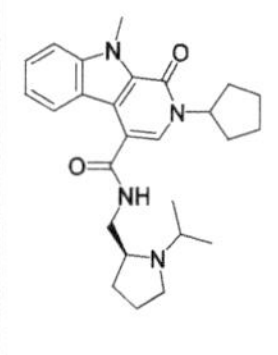	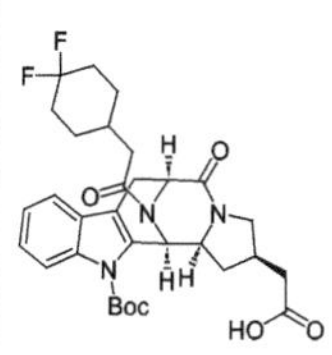	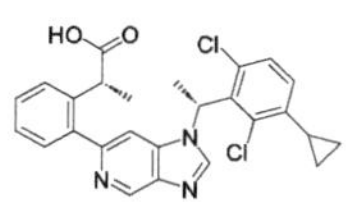	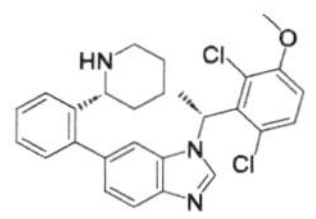	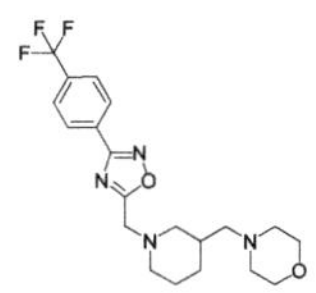
4 (VU0453379)	**5**	**6** (LSN3318839)	**7** (LSN3160440)	**8** (V-0219)

Sanofi disclosed a series of indole PAMs claimed to bind to a region overlapping with the orthosteric pocket [180]. The lead compound **5** had no effect on cAMP levels when tested alone in HEK293 cells overexpressing GLP-1R but did potentiate an EC_{20} concentration of GLP-1(9–36) metabolite (EC_{50} 5 nM; Emax 100%) and shifted the EC_{50} by 2215-fold (at 3 μM). **5** proved to be a selective potentiator of GLP-1(9–36) and it had no effect on the biological response of GLP-1. The compound suffers from transporter-mediated poor oral bioavailability in rodents and hence required coadministration of rifampicin, an OATP/MRP2 inhibitor, to achieve sufficient oral exposure in an ob/ob mouse oral glucose-tolerance test (OGTT). **5** alone had no effect on blood glucose concentration in the absence of rifampicin and/or GLP-1(9–36). Intraperitoneal administration of GLP-1(9–36) to the combination of rifampicin and **5** produced a significant reduction in blood glucose concentration. In contrast, the peptide GLP-1(9–36) alone had no effect with or without addition of rifampicin on blood glucose concentration.

Lilly disclosed a series of benzimidazole PAMs showing biased pharmacology [192]. In INS-1832-3 cells, compound **6** (LSN3318839), produced only a marginal improvement of the cAMP accumulation produced by GLP-1 (2 to 2.7-fold, 0.1 μM **6**) but had a significant effect on the GLP-1(9–36) response. GLP-1(9–36) had no measurable cAMP activity in INS-1832-3 cells whereas **6** (3 μM) increased the potency (EC_{50} 7 nM) and efficacy (Emax 87%) of the peptide. The potentiation of **6** is predominantly biased toward G-protein signaling. In HEK293 cells, **6** (6 μM) produced a potent effect (EC_{50} 12 nM) on β-arrestin recruitment by GLP-1(9–36) but with low efficacy (Emax 10%). In cultures of INS-1832-3 cells, the combination of **6** (3 μM) and GLP-1(9–36) in the presence of high glucose profoundly increased insulin levels in the media with an effect comparable to that produced by GLP-1.

The structure of GLP-1R bound to a close analogue **7** (LSN3160440) in complex with full-length GLP-1, heterotrimeric Gs and the Camelid antibody Nb35 was determined using cryo-EM (Figure 5.15b) [193]. **7** binds at the extracellular side of the helical bundle in a pocket formed by residues in the interface between TM1 and TM2. Interestingly, **7** forms several interactions with GLP-1, explaining the molecular basis for the probe dependence of **7** for GLP-1(9-36) versus oxyntomodulin which is driven by a single residue on the peptide.

6 was profiled in an OGTT in GIP-R KO mice to determine the GLP-1R-mediated control of a glucose excursion. A 30 mg/kg oral dose of **6** delivered a significant reduction in glucose. An additive glucose lowering effect (65% AUC) was observed when **6** (30 mg/kg) was co-administered with 10 mg/kg sitagliptin, a DPP4 inhibitor that prevents the degradation of GLP-1 to GLP-1(9–36). Given that the circulating levels of GLP-1(9–36) are negligible in animals treated with sitagliptin, the authors suggest that the efficacy was likely due to activation of GLP-1R by the combined effect of **6** and GLP-1 only. Importantly this was the first reported PAM to produce GLP-1R-dependent glucose lowering by potentiating endogenous concentrations of GLP-1. However, **6** (30 mg/kg) had no effect on body weight when administered alone, or in combination with 10 mg/kg sitagliptin, to DIO mice for 14 days.

More recently in 2022, a group from Madrid published a highly potent series of GLP-1R PAMs identified from a focused screen measuring potentiation of the effect of GLP-1 (EC_{25}) on calcium mobilization in HEK293 cells stably expressing human GLP-1R [194]. The lead compound **8** (V-0219) achieved a maximal effect on GLP-1 cAMP production at 0.1 nM, 42% higher than that of GLP-1 alone, however changes in the GLP-1 EC_{50} were not significant. 0.1 nM of **8** also delivered the maximal effect in potentiating insulin secretion in rat INS-1 B-cells, 1.8-fold potentiation of efficacy of GLP-1 mediated insulin secretion (EC_{50} 0.25 nM) was observed. **8** also showed excellent selectivity across a panel of 54 GPCRs, showing less than 50% binding at 10 mM. **8** also had moderate oral bioavailability in rat (39%). The compound (0.1 mg/kg i.p.) reduced blood glucose in wild-type C57BL/6 N mice following a glucose load but had no effect in GLP-1R KO mice. In addition, an intracerebroventricular dose (1 μg/kg) of **8** potentiated the feeding inhibition induced by the GLP-1R agonist exendin-4 in male Wistar rats, reducing its ID_{50} from 394 to 89 ng.

Although several different GLP-1R PAMs have been reported, none have entered clinical development to date. This is possibly due to two reasons. Firstly, transient receptor activation driven by endogenous GLP-1 may be insufficient to deliver the required efficacy. Lilly highlighted that constant activation of GLP-1R is predicted to be more efficacious than PAM potentiators in T2D and obesity. Their studies in DIO mice also suggest that transient activation of the receptor is likely insufficient for GLP-1R related body weight reduction [192]. They also argued that clinical data generated with long-acting peptides such as semaglutide, versus short-acting analogues such as exenatide, suggest that constant activation of the GLP-1R produces higher efficacy. Secondly, a significant potentiation (estimated to be approximately 2500-fold by Sanofi) of the longer acting, but much weaker, metabolite GLP-1(9-36) would be required to deliver efficacy, [180]. Furthermore, with the exception on **8**, the reported GLP-1R PAMs are relatively weakly potent, requiring concentrations in the micromolar range to illicit a functional modulation of receptor activity.

Small Molecule GLP-1R Agonists in Clinical Development

TTP273 from vTv Therapeutics

The first small molecule GLP-1R agonist to enter clinical development was the investigational drug TTP273 from vTv Therapeutics. This series of molecules was first disclosed in the patent literature in 2009 [195]. The exact chemical structure of the clinical candidate is unknown but is assumed to be an analogue from the series exemplified by compound **9**, TT-OAD2 (Figure 5.16). Very little preclinical data is available for TTP273 although the patents claim potency up to EC_{50} 2 nM for the series in a cAMP HEK293 cell assay. A 12-week phase 2 clinical study in subjects with T2D on a stable dose of metformin met its primary endpoint of change in HbA1c from baseline at 12 weeks. A once daily oral dose (150 mg) achieved up to 0.87% reduction in HbA1c and a body weight loss of up to 2.47 kg in subjects weighing greater than 100 kg with negligible GI side effects being reported [196]. However, a subsequent publication in 2020 showed that **9** was a relatively weak partial GLP-1R agonist (approx. EC_{50} 100 nM cAMP, Emax 50%) (Zhao et al. 2020). There was no detectable recruitment of β-arrestin and very weak activity in an intracellular calcium mobilization assay suggesting biased agonism. The authors also solved the ligand-bound structure by cryo-EM confirming that TT-OAD2 occupied an allosteric binding site between TM2 andTM3 with minimal overlap with the GLP-1 binding site (Figure 5.16). No further clinical reports have emerged for TTP273 since the phase 2 study completed in 2016.

Danuglipron and Lotiglipron

In October 2017, Pfizer initiated phase 1 clinical trials with danuglipron (PF-06882961), which is a member of a new class of highly potent small molecule GLP-1R agonists. The group from Pfizer indicated that numerous screening approaches had previously proven unsuccessful in finding GLP-1R agonists. The hit from which danuglipron was derived, was discovered via an innovative screening approach exploiting a sensitized functional assay [168]. In this assay BETP (**3**) was used to lower the activation barrier of the receptor in order to enable the detection of weakly potent agonists that would otherwise go undiscovered [189]. The BETP-sensitized cAMP HTS identified the fluoropyrimidine compound **10** (hit-2) (Figure 5.17) which produced a 70% response at 20 μM and which was inactive in the absence of BETP. Subsequent optimization of this very weak series of agonists, using less sensitive functional cell assays with a GLP-1R density comparable to endogenous tissue levels, led to the discovery of danuglipron (**11**). Danuglipron is a potent full agonist on the cAMP pathway (EC_{50} 13 nM) but a weak partial agonist in recruiting β-arrestin (EC_{50} 490 nM; Emax 36%). Radiolabel binding studies confirm a high affinity for the GLP-1R (Ki 80 nM) consistent with the cAMP potency. Danuglipron was equipotent at the cynomolgus monkey GLP-1R but inactive at rodent receptors due to a Trp33Ser mutation in the binding pocket (Figure 5.17).

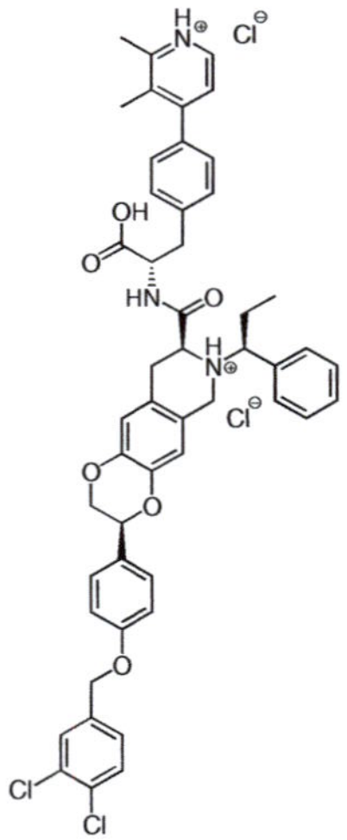

9 (TT-OAD2)

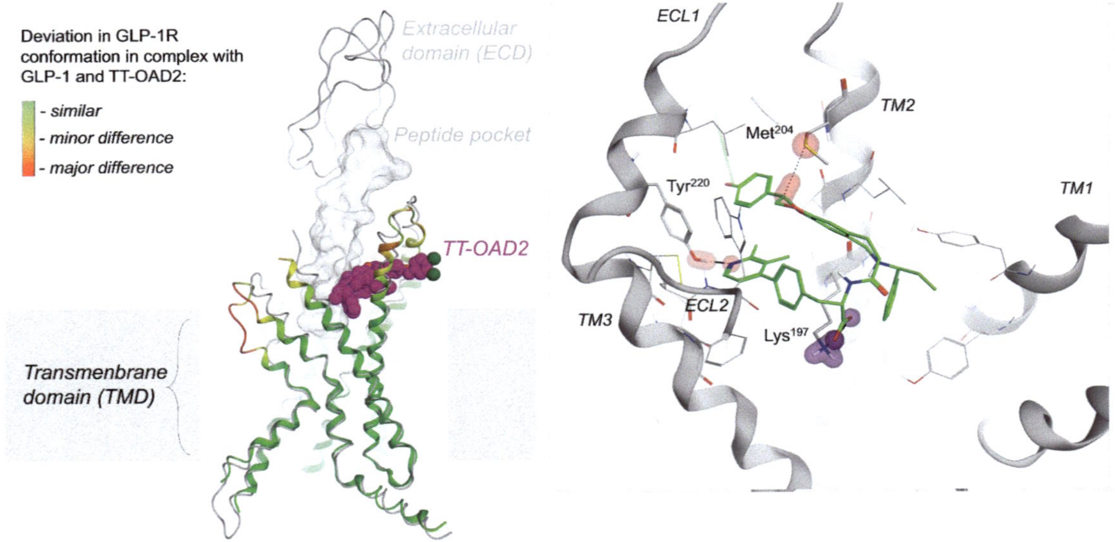

Figure 5.16 TT-OAD2 in complex with the GLP-1R (cryo-EM structure, PDB ID = 6ORV). Comparison of receptor conformations in complex with GLP-1 peptide (grey mesh surface) and TT-OAD2 indicated no significant changes in transmembrane domain (TMD). TT-OAD2 occupied an allosteric binding site between TM2-TM3 with minimal overlap with the peptide's binding pocket (mesh grey surface). Extracellular domain (ECD) was not resolved in the cryo-EM indicating remaining high conformational flexibility of the domain despite the complex formation.

The danuglipron-bound GLP-1R cryoEM structure revealed several changes in the GLP-1R conformation (Figure 5.17). Upon ligand binding, extracellular loops 1 and 3 (ECL-1 and ECL-3) together with the extracellular domain (ECD) move closer to each other, changing the size of the orthosteric pocket and inducing a binding site suitable for a small molecule. One of the key structural changes from HTS hit to danuglipron was introduction of a carboxylic group on the benzimidazole that forms a strong salt bridge interaction with Arg380 (ECL-3) and induces pocket closing. Moreover, the structure revealed a well-resolved water-network below the danuglipron binding position that extends deep into the orthosteric pocket. The waters facilitated interactions with the central polar network of the receptor which play critical roles for GLP-1R activation [197].

Importantly Pfizer were able to deliver such potency with significantly improved physicochemical properties (MW 555.6 g/mol, logD 1.8) compared to the previously reported TT-OAD2 series. The lower lipophilicity led to excellent selectivity against the human ether-à-go-go-related gene (hERG) ion channel (>100 μM) and relatively low intrinsic metabolic clearance in human liver microsomes and hepatocytes. However, relatively short half-lives and low to moderate dose-dependent oral bioavailability was observed in rat ($t_{1\backslash 2}$ 1.1 hours, 11–39% F) and monkey ($t_{1\backslash 2}$ 1.9 hours, 5–9% F). In a humanized GLP-1R mouse model, danuglipron stimulated glucose-dependent insulin release and suppressed food intake with efficacy comparable to injectable peptidic GLP-1R agonists. In an IPGTT in humanized GLP-1R mice, danuglipron (30 mg/kg s.c.) displayed improved glucose tolerance, reduced blood glucose and increased plasma insulin. In a separate study, food intake was significantly reduced in humanized GLP-1R mice at 2.5, 5.5 and 15.5 hours after dosing (30 mg/kg s.c.) [198]. Oral doses of danuglipron (100 mg/kg) in monkey afforded systemic concentrations achieving receptor occupancy comparable to that achieved by clinically efficacious doses of liraglutide and enhanced glucose-stimulated insulin secretion. Furthermore, once-daily subcutaneous administration of danuglipron (2.9 mg/kg) for two days significantly reduced food intake compared to vehicle-treated monkeys.

Phase 1 clinical trial pharmacokinetic data indicated that danuglipron required twice daily oral dosing to achieve sufficient receptor occupancy over 24 hours, with a mean human half-life ranging from 4.3 to 6.1 hours [168, 198]. However, unlike oral semaglutide, danuglipron can be dosed without regard to food. In 2020 a phase 2b study was initiated in adults with T2D inadequately controlled by diet and exercise, with or without metformin treatment [199]. Participants received placebo or oral danuglipron, 2.5, 10, 40, 80, or 120 mg twice daily with food for 16 weeks. All doses significantly reduced HbA1c and fasting plasma glucose (FPG) at week 16. The top dose of 120 mg twice daily reduced HbA1c and FPG by 1.16% and 33.24 mg/dl respectively compared to placebo. Body weight was significantly reduced at week 16 in the 80-mg twice daily (2.04 kg) and 120 mg twice daily (4.17 kg) groups only. The most commonly reported adverse events were typical of GLP-1R agonist therapeutics, such as nausea, diarrhea, and vomiting.

After completing a Phase 2b study in non-diabetic obese participants that demonstrated placebo-adjusted weight reductions up to 13% at 32 weeks, Pfizer announced that the twice-daily formulation of danuglipron would not be progressed due to high discontinuation rates of greater than 50% across all doses compared to 40% with placebo. The company was developing a slow-release formulation to reduce side effects.

To address the short human half-life of danuglipron and the requirement for twice daily oral dosing, Pfizer subsequently developed lotiglipron (PF-07081532) (**12** Figure 5.17) in collaboration with Sosei Heptares. Lotiglipron is from the same chemical series as danuglipron and was shown to have a human half-life supportive of once-daily dosing in participants with T2D (180 mg dose, $t_{1/2}$ 23.1 hours) and obesity (180 mg dose, $t_{1/2}$ 20.7 hours) [200]. 180 mg once daily dosing of lotiglipron for four to six weeks reduced HbA1c by 1.61% in participants with T2D. Body weight reductions of up to approximately 5.5% were observed in participants with T2D and approximately 5.2% in participants with obesity.

In June 2023 Pfizer announced the decision to terminate the clinical development of lotiglipron based on pharmacokinetic data from Phase 1 drug–drug-interaction studies and laboratory measurements of elevated transaminases in these Phase 1 and Phase 2 studies [201].

Orforglipron

Eli-Lilly's orforglipron **13** (LY3502970/OWL833) became the first FDA approved oral, non-peptide GLP-1R agonist for weight management in April 2026 [201b]. Eli-Lilly licensed the compound from Chugai Pharmaceuticals in 2018 [202]. Chugai discovered the hit series via a cell-based screening method employing LLC-PK1 cells expressing human GLP-1R and using urokinase-type plasminogen activator expression as a readout [203]. Orforglipron is a highly potent and selective GLP-1R partial agonist (cAMP EC_{50} 3.1 nM; Emax 24.5%) demonstrating biased pharmacology towards G-protein activation in HEK293 cells expressing various densities of human GLP-1R with no measurable activity in the β-arrestin assay [173]. Orforglipron shows no measurable activity at other class B GPCRs.

A cryo-EM structure revealed that orforglipron has a much larger binding pocket with a different binding pose (more parallel to the membrane) to danuglipron (Figure 5.18) [173]. Several structural waters were detected deep in the binding pocket; however, they did not form a continuous network extending to the ligand. The fluoromethyl indazole and dimethyl tetrahydropyran moieties of orforglipron extend beyond the orthosteric pocket and occupy pockets in-between TM helixes: (1) TM1 – TM2 similar to Lilly's PAM, LSN3318839 (Figure 5.15b); (2) TM2 – TM3 similar to TT-OAD2 (Figure 5.17) and Boc5 (Figure 5.14).

Although orforglipron has relatively high molecular weight (MW 883 g/mol) and lipophilicity, outside the typical range for good oral exposure, it has moderate oral bioavailability in both rat and cynomolgus monkeys of 33–43% and 21–28% respectively, and a half-life following oral administration of 10.4–12.4 hours in rats and 3.4–4.6 hours in cynomolgus monkeys [173]. Like danuglipron, orforglipron is inactive at mouse GLP-1R and therefore a humanized mouse model was developed to

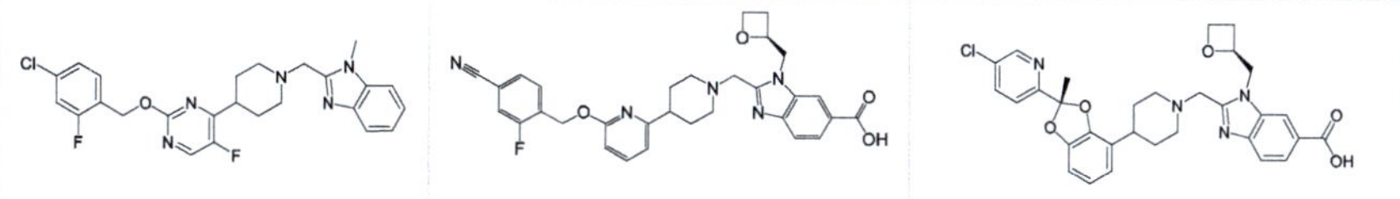

10	11	12
(hit-2)	Danuglipron (PF-06882961)	Lotiglipron (PF-07081532)

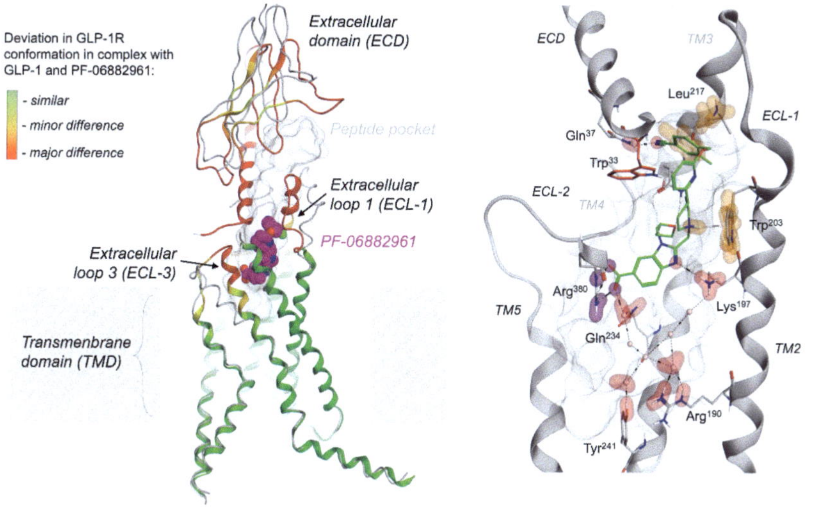

Figure 5.17 Danuglipron (PF-06882961) in complex with GLP-1R (cryoEM structure, PDB ID = 6X1A). Peptide binding pocket is shown with grey mesh surface. Comparison of receptor conformations in complex with GLP-1 peptide and danuglipron indicated significant shift in extracellular loops 1 and 3 (ECL-1 and ECL-3). Together with rearrangement of extracellular domain (ECD) these conformational changes in the receptor led to a reduction in the pocket size, which is more favourable for a small molecule binding. One of ECD's residues interacting with danuglipron (Trp33, highlighted in red) is mutated to Ser in mouse and rat, which may explain lack of danuglipron activity at the rodent receptors.

assess in-vivo efficacy. Orforglipron shows robust glucose lowering at doses from 0.1 to 10 mg/kg in hGLP-1R knock-in mice challenged with intraperitoneally injected glucose. Interestingly, the 0.1 mg/kg dose achieves the same glucose lowering as both the 10 mg/kg highest dose and the approved peptide exenatide, indicating that maximal efficacy is achieved from a low blood concentration (0.1 mg/kg achieves 8 nM blood concentration). In cynomolgus monkeys, orforglipron enhances glucose-stimulated insulin secretion (steady-state concentration: 9.1 ± 0.8 nM) comparable to that stimulated by high-dose exenatide (43.0 ± 4.1 pmol/l). Furthermore, oral doses of orforglipron achieved a dose-dependent reduction of food intake in monkeys similar to that of exenatide. Importantly, these studies demonstrate that a small molecule partial agonist for cAMP activation delivers comparable in-vivo efficacy to the full agonist exenatide in preclinical models. Lilly proposed that the GLP-1 system has substantial receptor reserve in-vivo, enabling a full biological response to be achieved from a partial agonist.

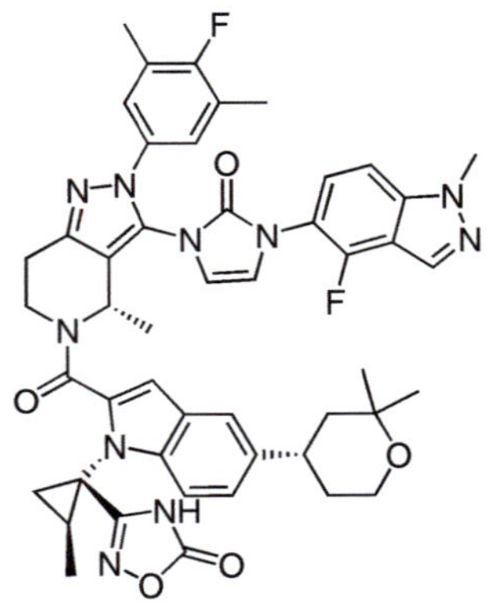

13
(Orforglipron)
(LY3502970 / OWL833)

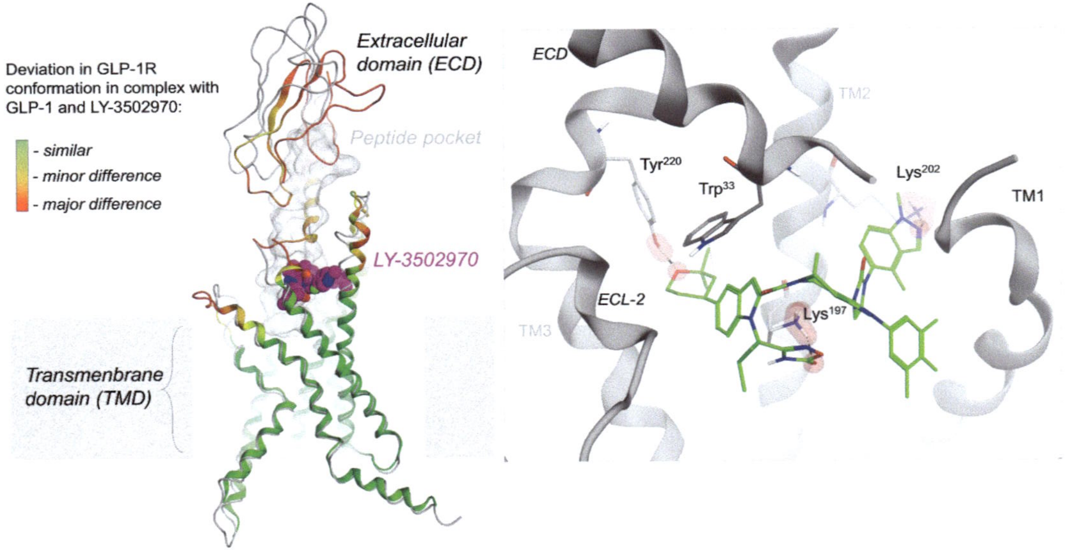

Figure 5.18 Orforglipron (LY3502970/OWL833) in complex with the GLP-1R (cryoEM structure, PDB ID = 6XOX). Comparison of receptor conformations in complex with GLP-1 peptide and orforglipron indicated no significant changes in transmembrane domain (TMD) but rearrangement of extracellular domain (ECD) interacting with orforglipron via Trp^{33}. Peptide binding pocket is shown with grey mesh surface. Two orforglipron's substituents (fluoromethyl indazole and dimethyl tetrahydropyran) extend beyond the orthosteric pocket and occupy allosteric pockets between TM1-TM2 and TM2-TM3.

A phase 1a single and multiple-ascending-dose study in healthy participants confirmed a pharmacokinetic profile supportive of once daily oral dosing [204]. The mean half-life was 24.6 to 35.3 hours following a single dose (0.3–6 mg) which extended to 48.1 to 67.5 hours on day 28 across the dose range (2–24 mg). Dose-dependent reductions in OGTT glucose values were observed after 2 hours on Day 1, ranging from 27.0 to 79.3 mg/dl, statistically significant for all doses, and maintained on Day 28 in the higher dose groups, ranging from 51.0 to 63.6 mg/dl. Substantial reductions in body weight of up to 5.4 kg were observed after four weeks in orforglipron-treated healthy subjects (BMI 20–40 kg/m^2), compared to a reduction of 2.4 kg with placebo. The most common adverse events were gastrointestinal tract-related typical of the GLP-1R agonist class.

In September 2021 Lilly initiated a 26-week phase 2 trial enrolling participants with type 2 diabetes treated with diet and exercise, with or without metformin, and with a HbA1c of 7.0–10.5% and stable BMI of 23 kg/m^2 or more [205]. Participants were randomly assigned dulaglutide 1.5 mg once per week, or orforglipron 3, 12, 24, 36 or 45 mg oral daily dose. At week 26, mean reduction in HbA1c with orforglipron was up to 2.10% versus 1.10% with dulaglutide and statistically significant versus placebo (0.43%). Mean bodyweight reduction up to 10.1 kg was achieved with orforglipron versus 2.2 kg for placebo and 3.9 kg for dulaglutide. The majority of adverse events were again gastrointestinal related.

Orforglipron led to improvement in all prespecified weight-related and cardiometabolic measures in a phase 2 trial in adults with obesity, or overweight adults with at least one weight-related coexisting condition, but without diabetes. Participants were randomly assigned to receive orforglipron (12, 24, 36, or 45 mg) or placebo once daily for 36 weeks [206]. At week 36, the mean body weight change ranged from −9.4% to −14.7% with orforglipron treatment compared to −2.3% with placebo. The most common adverse events reported were gastrointestinal events, which were mild to moderate, occurred primarily during dose escalation, and led to discontinuation of orforglipron in 10 to 17% of participants across dose cohorts.

Summary of the GLP-1R Small Molecule Agonist Landscape

Orforglipron is currently the only approved oral small molecule GLP-1R agonist [214]. Pfizer's leading asset, danuglipron, was terminated in 2023. Both compounds have high affinity for the GLP-1R and comparable potency at stimulating cAMP accumulation. However, their signaling profiles differ significantly. Relative to GLP-1, danuglipron is a full agonist for cAMP production whereas Lilly report that orforglipron demonstrated partial agonist behaviour [173]. Danuglipron is a partial agonist in recruiting β-arrestin and has been shown to induce receptor internalization [168]. In contrast, orforglipron displayed no measurable recruitment of β-arrestin, a feature that Lilly suggest may enhance clinical efficacy. It remains to be proven whether this biased signaling profile offers any clinical advantage in treating T2D or obesity.

Although both compounds are considerably less potent than GLP-1 and the approved peptide agonists [197] they are able to achieve sufficient plasma concentrations from an oral dose to elicit a pharmacological response and deliver clinical efficacy in T2D and obesity.

Since the disclosure of the danuglipron and orforglipron chemical structures, there has been a wave of activity across the biotechnology and pharma industry with multiple small molecule agonists entering clinical development. AstraZeneca and Eccogene entered into an exclusive license agreement for ECC5004/AZD5004 (elecoglipron), an oral once daily GLP-1R agonist currently in phase 3 [207]. Roche acquired Carmot Therapeutics giving the pharma company access to a portfolio of incretins including CT-996, a once-daily oral GLP-1R receptor agonist currently in Phase-2 [208]. In addition, Structure Therapeutics (GSBR-1290 / aleniglipron) [209], Sciwind Biosciences (XW014) [210], Regor Therapeutics (RGT-075) [211], are all in clinical development with oral small molecule GLP-1R agonists. Tern Therapeutics discontinued the development of their small molecule GLP-1R agonist (TERN-601) in 2025 [212].

Outlook for GLP-1R Small Molecule Agonists and Beyond

An oral therapeutic has advantages over injectables for obesity-linked T2D [56], particularly in terms of patient compliance, convenience and potentially cost. Another advantage is better feasibility for fixed dose combinations on top of a small molecule GLP-1R agonist foundation, like addition of a SGLT2 inhibitor. Considering the promise of small molecule GLP-1R agonists there will undoubtedly be attempts to investigate other related hormone receptor targets, such as the glucose-insulinotropic polypeptide (GIP) receptor (GIPR), for small molecule agonism. Given the good effectiveness of injectable GLP-1R/GIPR dual agonist in Tirzepatide [213] we would not be surprised if a combination of small molecules for GLP-1R *and* GIPR agonism emerges in the not too distant future. For patients dealing with obesity and/or T2D better treatment options of those conditions should be soon coming.

References

1 Haslam, D. (2016). Weight management in obesity – past and present. *Int. J. Clin. Pract.* 70 (3): 206–217. https://doi.org/10.1111/ijcp.12771.

2 Wibisono, A., Lestari, A.N., Sorensen, L., and Hill, P. (2017). Fear of injections among people with type 2 diabetes: overview of the problem. *J. Diabetes Nurs.* 21 (3): 91–95.

3 Cordiner, R. and Pearson, E. (2019). Reflections on the sulphonylurea story: a drug class at risk of extinction or a drug class worth reviving? *Diabetes Obes. Metab.* 21 (4): 761–771. https://doi.org/10.1111/dom.13596.

4 Prendergast, B. (1984). Glyburide and glipizide, second-generation oral sulfonylurea hypoglycemic agents. *Clin. Pharm.* 3 (5): 473–485.

5 Apovian, C., Okemah, J., and O'Neil, P.M. (2019). Body weight considerations in the management of type 2 diabetes. *Adv. Ther.* 36 (1): 44–58. https://doi.org/10.1007/s12325-018-0824-8.

6 Proks, P., Reimann, F., Green, N. et al. (2002). Sulfonylurea stimulation of insulin secretion. *Diabetes* 51 (suppl_3): S368–S376. https://doi.org/10.2337/diabetes.51.2007.S368.

7 Del Prato, S. and Pulizzi, N. (2006). The place of sulfonylureas in the therapy for type 2 diabetes mellitus. *Metabolism* 55: S20–S27. https://doi.org/10.1016/j.metabol.2006.02.003.

8 Lamos, E., Stein, S., and Davis, S. (2013). Sulfonylureas and meglitinides: historical and contemporary issues. *Panminerva Med.* 55 (3): 239–251.

9 Alarcon, C., Wicksteed, B., and Rhodes, C. (2006). Exendin 4 controls insulin production in rat islet beta cells predominantly by potentiation of glucose-stimulated proinsulin biosynthesis at the translational level. *Diabetologia* 49 (12): 2920–2929. https://doi.org/10.1007/s00125-006-0433-y.

10 Kahn, S., Haffner, S., Heise, M. et al. (2006). Glycemic durability of rosiglitazone, metformin, or glyburide monotherapy. *N. Engl. J. Med.* 355 (23): 2427–2443. https://doi.org/10.1056/NEJMoa066224.

11 Kahn, S., Lachin, J., Zinman, B. et al. (2011). Effects of rosiglitazone, glyburide, and metformin on β-cell function and insulin sensitivity in ADOPT. *Diabetes* 60 (5): 1552–1560. https://doi.org/10.2337/db10-1392.

12 Kampouraki, M., Mavridou, K., Bakola, M. et al. (2023). Can sulfonylureas for agricultural use cause diabetes? A report of three cases. *Cureus* 15 (3): e35938. https://doi.org/10.7759/cureus.35938.

13 Mohan, V., Saboo, B., Khader, J. et al. (2022). Position of sulfonylureas in the current ERA: review of national and international guidelines. *Clin. Med. Insights Endocrinol. Diabetes* 15: 1–8. https://doi.org/10.1177/11795514221074663.

14 Tomlinson, B., Patil, N., Fok, M. et al. (2022). The role of sulfonylureas in the treatment of type 2 diabetes. *Expert. Opin. Pharmacother.* 23 (3): 387–403. https://doi.org/10.1080/14656566.2021.1999413.

15 Broome, D., Pantalone, K., Kashyap, S. et al. (2021). Approach to the patient with MODY-monogenic diabetes. *J. Clin. Endocrinol. Metab.* 106 (1): 237–250. https://doi.org/10.1210/clinem/dgaa710.

16 Bowman, P., Flanagan, S., and Hattersley, A. (2018). Future roadmaps for precision medicine applied to diabetes: rising to the challenge of heterogeneity. *J. Diabetes Res.* 2018: e3061620. https://doi.org/10.1155/2018/3061620.

17 Witters, L. (2001). The blooming of the French lilac. *J. Clin. Invest.* 108 (8): 1105–1107. https://doi.org/10.1172/JCI14178.

18 Rathke, B. (1879). Ueber Biguanid. *Ber. Dtsch. Chem. Ges.* 12 (1): 776–784. https://doi.org/10.1002/cber.187901201219.

19 Bailey, C. (2017). Metformin: historical overview. *Diabetologia* 60 (9): 1566–1576. https://doi.org/10.1007/s00125-017-4318-z.

20 World Health Organization (2023). *WHO Model List of Essential Medicines – 23rd List*. WHO Tech doc. 26 July.

21 American Diabetes Association (2022). Standards of care in diabetes—2023 abridged for primary care providers. *Clin. Diabetes* 41 (1): 4–31. https://doi.org/10.2337/cd23-as01.

22 LaMoia, T. and Shulman, G. (2021). Cellular and molecular mechanisms of Metformin action. *Endocr. Rev.* 42 (1): 77–96. https://doi.org/10.1210/endrev/bnaa023.

23 UK Prospective Diabetes Study (UKPDS) Group (1998). Effect of intensive blood-glucose control with Metformin on complications in overweight patients with type 2 diabetes (UKPDS 34). *Lancet* 352 (9131): 854–865. https://doi.org/10.1016/S0140-6736(98)07037-8.

24 Holman, R., Paul, S., Bethel, M. et al. (2008). 10-year follow-up of intensive glucose control in type 2 diabetes. *N. Engl. J. Med.* 359 (15): 1577–1589. https://doi.org/10.1056/NEJMoa0806470.

25 Foretz, M., Guigas, B., and Viollet, B. (2023). Metformin: update on mechanisms of action and repurposing potential. *Nat. Rev. Endocrinol.* 19 (8): 460–476. https://doi.org/10.1038/s41574-023-00833-4.

26 Herzig, S. and Shaw, R. (2018). AMPK: guardian of metabolism and mitochondrial homeostasis. *Nat. Rev. Mol. Cell Biol.* 19 (2): 121–135. https://doi.org/10.1038/nrm.2017.95.

27 Foretz, M., Hébrard, S., Leclerc, J. et al. (2010). Metformin inhibits hepatic gluconeogenesis in mice independently of the LKB1/AMPK pathway via a decrease in hepatic energy state. *J. Clin. Invest.* 120 (7): 2355–2369. https://doi.org/10.1172/JCI40671.

28 Miller, R., Chu, Q., Xie, J. et al. (2013). Biguanides suppress hepatic glucagon signaling by decreasing production of cyclic AMP. *Nature* 494 (7436): 256–260. https://doi.org/10.1038/nature11808.

29 Barzilai, N., Crandall, J., Kritchevsky, S. et al. (2016). Metformin as a tool to target aging. *Cell Metab.* 23 (6): 1060–1065. https://doi.org/10.1016/j.cmet.2016.05.011.

30 Mohammed, I., Hollenberg, M., Ding, H. et al. (2021). A critical review of the evidence that Metformin is a putative anti-aging drug that enhances healthspan and extends lifespan. *Front. Endocrinol.* 12: 718942. https://doi.org/10.3389/fendo.2021.718942.

31 Derosa, G. and Maffioli, P. (2012). α-glucosidase inhibitors and their use in clinical practice. *Arch. Med. Sci.* 8 (5): 899–906. https://doi.org/10.5114/aoms.2012.31621.

32 Van de Laar, F., Lucassen, P., Akkermans, R. et al. (2005). Alpha-glucosidase inhibitors for type 2 diabetes mellitus. *Cochrane Database Syst. Rev.* 2005 (2): CD003639. https://doi.org/10.1002/14651858.CD003639.pub2.

33 Kumar, R. and Sinha, V. (2012). Newer insights into the drug delivery approaches of α-glucosidase inhibitors. *Expert Opin. Drug Deliv.* 9 (4): 403–416. https://doi.org/10.1517/17425247.2012.663080.

34 Black, C., Donnelly, P., McIntyre, L. et al. (2007). Meglitinide analogues for type 2 diabetes mellitus. *Cochrane Database Syst. Rev.* 2: CD004654. https://doi.org/10.1002/14651858.CD004654.pub2.

35 Dornhorst, A. (2001). Insulinotropic meglitinide analogues. *Lancet* 358 (9294): 1709–1716. https://doi.org/10.1016/S0140-6736(01)06715-0.

36 Derosa, G., Mugellini, A., Ciccarelli, L. et al. (2003). Comparison of glycaemic control and cardiovascular risk profile in patients with type 2 diabetes during treatment with either Repaglinide or Metformin. *Diabetes Res. Clin. Pract.* 60 (3): 161–169. https://doi.org/10.1016/S0168-8227(03)00057-3.

37 Grygiel-Górniak, B. (2014). Peroxisome proliferator-activated receptors and their ligands: nutritional and clinical implications – a review. *Nutr. J.* 13 (1): 17. https://doi.org/10.1186/1475-2891-13-17.

38 Davidson, M., Mattison, D., Azoulay, L. et al. (2018). Thiazolidinedione drugs in the treatment of type 2 diabetes mellitus: past, present and future. *Crit. Rev. Toxicol.* 48 (1): 52–108. https://doi.org/10.1080/10408444.2017.1351420.

39 Ferré, P. (2004). The biology of peroxisome proliferator-activated receptors: relationship with lipid metabolism and insulin sensitivity. *Diabetes* 53 (Suppl 1): S43–S50. https://doi.org/10.2337/diabetes.53.2007.s43.

40 Shulman, G. (2014). Ectopic fat in insulin resistance, dyslipidemia, and cardiometabolic disease. *N. Engl. J. Med.* 371 (12): 1131–1141. https://doi.org/10.1056/NEJMra1011035.

41 Colca, J. and Scherer, P. (2022). The metabolic syndrome, thiazolidinediones, and implications for intersection of chronic and inflammatory disease. *Mol. Metabol.* 55: 101409. https://doi.org/10.1016/j.molmet.2021.101409.

42 Straub, L. and Scherer, P. (2019). Metabolic messengers: adiponectin. *Nat. Metab.* 1 (3): 334–339. https://doi.org/10.1038/s42255-019-0041-z.

43 Jonas, D., Van Scoyoc, E., Gerrald, K. et al. (2011). *Newer Diabetes Medications, TZDs, and Combinations*. Portland, US: Drug Class Reviews.

44 Loke, Y., Singh, S., and Furberg, C. (2009). Long-term use of thiazolidinediones and fractures in type 2 diabetes: a meta-analysis. *Can. Med. Assoc. J.* 180 (1): 32–39. https://doi.org/10.1503/cmaj.080486.

45 Li, Y., Jin, D., Xie, W. et al. (2018). PPAR-γ and Wnt regulate the differentiation of MSCs into adipocytes and osteoblasts respectively. *Current Stem Cell Res. Ther.* 13 (3): 185–192.

46 Nissen, S. and Wolski, K. (2007). Effect of Rosiglitazone on the risk of myocardial infarction and death from cardiovascular causes. *N. Engl. J. Med.* 356 (24): 2457–2471. https://doi.org/10.1056/NEJMoa072761.

47 Home, P., Pocock, S., Beck-Nielsen, H. et al. (2009). Rosiglitazone evaluated for cardiovascular outcomes in oral agent combination therapy for type 2 diabetes (RECORD): a multicentre, randomised, open-label trial. *Lancet* 373 (9681): 2125–2135. https://doi.org/10.1016/S0140-6736(09)60953-3.

48 Stone, J., Furuya-Kanamori, L., Barendregt, J. et al. (2015). Was there really any evidence that Rosiglitazone increased the risk of myocardial infarction or death from cardiovascular causes? *Pharmacoepidemiol. Drug Saf.* 24 (3): 223–227. https://doi.org/10.1002/pds.3736.

49 DeFronzo, R., Inzucchi, S., Abdul-Ghani, M. et al. (2019). Pioglitazone: the forgotten, cost-effective cardioprotective drug for type 2 diabetes. *Diab. Vasc. Dis. Res.* 16 (2): 133–143. https://doi.org/10.1177/1479164118825376.

50 Rajan T., Ferro, E.G., and Elshazly M.B. (2021). *2020 FDA Guidance for Diabetes Drug Development: Cardiorenal Populations and Outcomes: Lessons Learned and Future Directions*. www.acc.org (accessed 28 February 2024).

51 Drucker, D. (2013). Incretin action in the pancreas: potential promise, possible perils, and pathological pitfalls. *Diabetes* 62 (10): 3316–3323. https://doi.org/10.2337/db13-0822.

52 Drucker, D. and Holst, J. (2023). The expanding incretin universe: from basic biology to clinical translation. *Diabetologia* 66 (10): 1765–1779. https://doi.org/10.1007/s00125-023-05906-7.

53 Deacon, C. (2004). Circulation and degradation of GIP and GLP-1. *Horm. Metab. Res.* 36 (11–12): 761–765. https://doi.org/10.1055/s-2004-826160.

54 Drucker, D. (2007). Dipeptidyl peptidase-4 inhibition and the treatment of type 2 diabetes: preclinical biology and mechanisms of action. *Diabetes Care* 30 (6): 1335–1343. https://doi.org/10.2337/dc07-0228.

55 Thornberry, N. and Weber, A. (2007). Discovery of JANUVIA (Sitagliptin), a selective dipeptidyl peptidase IV inhibitor for the treatment of type 2 diabetes. *Curr. Top. Med. Chem.* 7 (6): 557–568. https://doi.org/10.2174/156802607780091028.

56 Boye, K., Ross, M., Mody, R. et al. (2021). Patients' preferences for once-daily oral versus once-weekly injectable diabetes medications: the REVISE study. *Diabetes Obes. Metab.* 23 (2): 508–519. https://doi.org/10.1111/dom.14244.

57 Staels, B. (2009). A review of bile acid sequestrants: potential mechanism(s) for glucose-lowering effects in type 2 diabetes mellitus. *Postgrad. Med.* 121 (3 Suppl 1): 25–30. https://doi.org/10.3810/pgm.2009.05.suppl53.290.

58 Brighton, C., Rievaj, J., Kuhre, R. et al. (2015). Bile acids trigger GLP-1 release predominantly by accessing basolaterally located G Protein–Coupled bile acid receptors. *Endocrinology* 156 (11): 3961–3970. https://doi.org/10.1210/en.2015-1321.

59 González-Regueiro, J., Moreno-Castañeda, L., Uribe, M. et al. (2017). The role of bile acids in glucose metabolism and their relation with diabetes. *Ann. Hepatol.* 16 (Suppl. 1): S15–S20. https://doi.org/10.5604/01.3001.0010.5494.

60 Dereje, B. and Nardos, A. (2023). Dopamine 2 agonists for the management of type 2 diabetes: a systematic review and meta-analysis. *J. Diabetes Metab. Disord.* 22 (2): 931–943. https://doi.org/10.1007/s40200-023-01230-4.

61 García-Tornadú, I., Ornstein, A., Chamson-Reig, A. et al. (2010). Disruption of the dopamine D2 receptor impairs insulin secretion and causes glucose intolerance. *Endocrinology* 151 (4): 1441–1450. https://doi.org/10.1210/en.2009-0996.

62 Lamos, E., Levitt, D., and Munir, K. (2016). A review of dopamine agonist therapy in type 2 diabetes and effects on cardio-metabolic parameters. *Prim. Care Diabetes* 10 (1): 60–65. https://doi.org/10.1016/j.pcd.2015.10.008.

63 Cincotta, A. (2023). Brain dopamine-clock interactions regulate cardiometabolic physiology: mechanisms of the observed cardioprotective effects of circadian-timed bromocriptine-QR therapy in type 2 diabetes subjects. *Int. J. Mol. Sci.* 24 (17): 13255. https://doi.org/10.3390/ijms241713255.

64 Von Mering, J. (1886). Über künstlichen diabetes. *Centralbl MedWiss* 22: 531.

65 Rossetti, L., Smith, D., Shulman, G. et al. (1987). Correction of hyperglycemia with phlorizin normalizes tissue sensitivity to insulin in diabetic rats. *J. Clin. Invest.* 79 (5): 1510–1515. https://doi.org/10.1172/JCI112981.

66 Chao, E. and Henry, R. (2010). SGLT2 inhibition — a novel strategy for diabetes treatment. *Nat. Rev. Drug Discov.* 9 (7): 551–559. https://doi.org/10.1038/nrd3180.

67 Ferrannini, E. (2017). Sodium-glucose co-transporters and their inhibition: clinical physiology. *Cell Metab.* 26 (1): 27–38. https://doi.org/10.1016/j.cmet.2017.04.011.

68 Haas, B., Eckstein, N., Pfeifer, V. et al. (2014). Efficacy, safety and regulatory status of SGLT2 inhibitors: focus on canagliflozin. *Nutr. Diabetes* 4 (11): e143. https://doi.org/10.1038/nutd.2014.40.

69 Boland, B., Brown, C., Boland, M. et al. (2019). Pancreatic β-cell rest replenishes insulin secretory capacity and attenuates diabetes in an extreme model of obese type 2 diabetes. *Diabetes* 68 (1): 131–140. https://doi.org/10.2337/db18-0304.

70 Zheng, H., Liu, M., Li, S. et al. (2021). Sodium-glucose co-transporter-2 inhibitors in non-diabetic adults with overweight or obesity: a systematic review and meta-analysis. *Front. Endocrinol.* 12: 706914. https://doi.org/10.3389/fendo.2021.706914.

71 Jhund, P., Kondo, T., Butt, J. et al. (2022). Dapagliflozin across the range of ejection fraction in patients with heart failure: a patient-level, pooled meta-analysis of DAPA-HF and DELIVER. *Nat. Med.* 28 (9): 1956–1964. https://doi.org/10.1038/s41591-022-01971-4.

72 Rosano, G., Quek, D., and Martínez, F. (2020). Sodium-glucose co-transporter 2 inhibitors in heart failure: recent data and implications for practice. *Card. Fail. Rev.* 6: e31. https://doi.org/10.15420/cfr.2020.23.

73 Zannad, F., Ferreira, J., Pocock, S. et al. (2020). SGLT2 inhibitors in patients with heart failure with reduced ejection fraction: a meta-analysis of the EMPEROR-reduced and DAPA-HF trials. *Lancet* 396 (10254): 819–829. https://doi.org/10.1016/S0140-6736(20)31824-9.

74 Heerspink, H., Stefánsson, B., Correa-Rotter, R. et al. (2020). Dapagliflozin in patients with chronic kidney disease. *N. Engl. J. Med.* 383 (15): 1436–1446. https://doi.org/10.1056/NEJMoa2024816.

75 Maxson, R., Starr, J., Sewell, J. et al. (2024). SGLT2 inhibitors to slow chronic kidney disease progression: a review. *Clin. Ther.* 46 (1): e23–e28. https://doi.org/10.1016/j.clinthera.2023.10.014.

76 American Diabetes Association Professional Practice Committee (2021). 9. Pharmacologic approaches to glycemic treatment: standards of medical care in diabetes—2022. *Diabetes Care* 45 (Suppl_1): S125–S143. https://doi.org/10.2337/dc22-S009.

77 Konkwo, C. and Perry, R. (2021). Imeglimin – current development and future potential in type 2 diabetes. *Drugs* 81 (2): 185–190. https://doi.org/10.1007/s40265-020-01434-5.

78 Yanai, H., Adachi, H., Hakoshima, M. et al. (2023). Glucose-lowering effects of imeglimin and its possible beneficial effects on diabetic complications. *Biology* 12 (5): 726. https://doi.org/10.3390/biology12050726.

79 Dubourg, J., Fouqueray, P., Quinslot, D. et al. (2022). Long-term safety and efficacy of imeglimin as monotherapy or in combination with existing antidiabetic agents in Japanese patients with type 2 diabetes (TIMES 2): a 52-week, open-label, multicentre phase 3 trial. *Diabetes Obes. Metab.* 24 (4): 609–619. https://doi.org/10.1111/dom.14613.

80 Cheng, C., Jabri, S., Taoka, B. et al. (2020). Small molecule glucagon receptor antagonists: an updated patent review (2015-2019). *Expert Opin. Ther. Pat.* 30 (7): 509–526. https://doi.org/10.1080/13543776.2020.1769600.

81 Manchem, V., Goldfine, I., Kohanski, R. et al. (2001). A novel small molecule that directly sensitizes the insulin receptor in vitro and in vivo. *Diabetes* 50 (4): 824–830. https://doi.org/10.2337/diabetes.50.4.824.

82 Rani, L., Grewal, A., Sharma, N. et al. (2021). Recent updates on free fatty acid receptor 1 (GPR-40) agonists for the treatment of type 2 diabetes mellitus. *Mini Rev. Med. Chem.* 21 (4): 426–470. https://doi.org/10.2174/1389557520666201023141326.

83 Nema, P., Asati, V., Kendya, P. et al. (2023). Structural insight on GPR119 agonist as potential therapy for type II diabetes: a comprehensive review. *Mini Rev. Med. Chem.* 23 (21): 2008–2040. https://doi.org/10.2174/1389557523666230302140658.

84 Liu, R., Mathieu, C., Berthelet, J. et al. (2022). Human protein tyrosine phosphatase 1B (PTP1B): from structure to clinical inhibitor perspectives. *Int. J. Mol. Sci.* 23 (13): 7027. https://doi.org/10.3390/ijms23137027.

85 Boyle, D. (2008). Recent advances in the discovery of 11beta-HSD1 inhibitors. *Curr. Opin. Drug Discov. Devel.* 11 (4): 495–511.

86 Toulis, K., Nirantharakumar, K., Pourzitaki, C. et al. (2020). Glucokinase activators for type 2 diabetes: challenges and future developments. *Drugs* 80 (5): 467–475. https://doi.org/10.1007/s40265-020-01278-z.

87 Syed, Y. (2022). Dorzagliatin: first approval. *Drugs* 82 (18): 1745–1750. https://doi.org/10.1007/s40265-022-01813-0.

88 Charlton, A. (2004). Medicinal uses of tobacco in history. *J. R. Soc. Med.* 97 (6): 292–296. https://doi.org/10.1258/jrsm.97.6.292.

89 Jun, H., Yu, H., Gong, J. et al. (2018). An immune-beige adipocyte communication via nicotinic acetylcholine receptor signaling. *Nat. Med.* 24 (6): 814–822. https://doi.org/10.1038/s41591-018-0032-8.

90 Jarvik, M. (1991, 2023). Beneficial effects of nicotine. *Br. J. Addict.* 86 (5): 571–575. https://doi.org/10.1111/j.1360-0443.1991.tb01810.x. American Society of Health-System Pharmacists. Nicotine (Monograph). https://www.drugs.com/monograph/nicotine.html (accessed 27 February 2024).

91 American Society of Health-System Pharmacists (2023). Nicotine (Monograph). https://www.drugs.com/monograph/nicotine.html (accessed 27 February 2024).

92 Sanner, T. and Grimsrud, T. (2015). Nicotine: carcinogenicity and effects on response to cancer treatment – a review. *Front. Oncol.* 5: 196. https://doi.org/10.3389/fonc.2015.00196.

93 Bray, G. and Purnell, J. (2000). *An Historical Review of Steps and Missteps in the Discovery of Anti-Obesity Drugs*. In: Feingold KR, Adler RA, Ahmed SF, et al., editors. *Endotext [Internet]*. South Dartmouth (MA): MDText.com, Inc.; Available from: https://www.ncbi.nlm.nih.gov/books/NBK581942/.

94 Harper, J., Dickinson, K., and Brand, M. (2001). Mitochondrial uncoupling as a target for drug development for the treatment of obesity. *Obes. Rev.* 2 (4): 255–265. https://doi.org/10.1046/j.1467-789X.2001.00043.x.

95 Goodman, N.G. (1969). Triiodothyronine and placebo in the treatment of obesity. A study of fifty-five patients. *Med. Ann. Dist. Columbia* 38 (12): 658–662. passim.

96 Li, L., Song, Y., Shi, Y. et al. (2023). Thyroid hormone receptor-β Agonists in NAFLD therapy: possibilities and challenges. *J. Clin. Endocrinol. Metab.* 108 (7): 1602–1613. https://doi.org/10.1210/clinem/dgad072.

97 Lin, S., Huang, S., Deng, Z. et al. (2023). Discovery of a novel, liver-targeted thyroid hormone receptor-β agonist, CS271011, in the treatment of lipid metabolism disorders. *Front. Endocrinol.* 14: 1109615. https://doi.org/10.3389/fendo.2023.1109615.

98 Younossi, Z., Stepanova, M., Taub, R. et al. (2022). Hepatic fat reduction due to resmetirom in patients with nonalcoholic steatohepatitis is associated with improvement of quality of life. *Clin. Gastroenterol. Hepatol.* 20 (6): 1354–1361.e7. https://doi.org/10.1016/j.cgh.2021.07.039.

99 Bleasdale, E., Thrower, S., and Petróczi, A. (2018). Would you use it with a seal of approval? Important attributes of 2,4-Dinitrophenol (2,4-DNP) as a hypothetical pharmaceutical product. *Front. Psych.* 9: 124. https://doi.org/10.3389/fpsyt.2018.00124.

100 Grundlingh, J., Dargan, P., and El-Zanfaly, M. (2011). 2,4-Dinitrophenol (DNP): a weight loss agent with significant acute toxicity and risk of death. *J. Med. Toxicol.* 7 (3): 205–212. https://doi.org/10.1007/s13181-011-0162-6.

101 Tainter, M., Stockton, A., and Cutting, W. (1933). Use of dinitrophenol in obesity and related conditions: a progress report. *JAMA J. Am. Med. Assoc.* 101 (19): 1472–1475. https://doi.org/10.1001/jama.1933.02740440032009.

102 Sousa, D., Carmo, H., Bravo, R. et al. (2020). Diet aid or aid to die: an update on 2,4-dinitrophenol (2,4-DNP) use as a weight-loss product. *Arch. Toxicol.* 94 (4): 1071–1083. https://doi.org/10.1007/s00204-020-02675-9.

103 Lam, C. and Patel, P. (2024). *Food, Drug, and Cosmetic Act*. Treasure Island (FL), US: StatPearls.

104 Wickware, C. (2023). Government to change law to reclassify so-called "diet drug" as a poison. *Pharm. J.* 310 (7969): https://doi.org/10.1211/PJ.2023.1.173336.

105 McVeigh, J., Germain, J., and Van Hout, M. (2017). 2,4-Dinitrophenol, the inferno drug: a netnographic study of user experiences in the quest for leanness. *J. Subst. Abus.* 22 (2): 131–138. https://doi.org/10.3109/14659891.2016.1149238.

106 Petróczi, A., Ocampo, J., Shah, I. et al. (2015). Russian roulette with unlicensed fat-burner drug 2,4-dinitrophenol (DNP): evidence from a multidisciplinary study of the internet, bodybuilding supplements and DNP users. *Subst. Abuse Treat. Prev. Policy* 10: 39. https://doi.org/10.1186/s13011-015-0034-1.

107 Alexopoulos, S., Chen, S.-Y., Brandon, A. et al. (2020). Mitochondrial uncoupler BAM15 reverses diet-induced obesity and insulin resistance in mice. *Nat. Commun.* 11 (1): 2397. https://doi.org/10.1038/s41467-020-16298-2.

108 Heal, D., Smith, S., Gosden, J. et al. (2013). Amphetamine, past and present – a pharmacological and clinical perspective. *J. Psychopharmacol.* 27 (6): 479–496. https://doi.org/10.1177/0269881113482532.

109 Greene, S., Kerr, F., and Braitberg, G. (2008). Review article: amphetamines and related drugs of abuse. *Emerg. Med. Australas.* 20 (5): 391–402. https://doi.org/10.1111/j.1742-6723.2008.01114.x.

110 Cohen, P., Goday, A., and Swann, J. (2012). The return of rainbow diet pills. *Am. J. Public Health* 102 (9): 1676–1686. https://doi.org/10.2105/AJPH.2012.300655.

111 Narayanaswami, V. and Dwoskin, L. (2017). Obesity: current and potential pharmacotherapeutics and targets. *Pharmacol. Ther.* 170: 116–147. https://doi.org/10.1016/j.pharmthera.2016.10.015.

112 Glazer, G. (2001). Long-term pharmacotherapy of obesity 2000: a review of efficacy and safety. *Arch. Intern. Med.* 161 (15): 1814–1824. https://doi.org/10.1001/archinte.161.15.1814.

113 Samanta, D. (2022). Fenfluramine: a review of pharmacology, clinical efficacy, and safety in epilepsy. *Children* 9 (8): 1159. https://doi.org/10.3390/children9081159.

114 Weintraub, M., Hasday, J., Mushlin, A. et al. (1984). A double-blind clinical trial in weight control. Use of fenfluramine and phentermine alone and in combination. *Arch. Intern. Med.* 144 (6): 1143–1148.

115 Connolly, H., Crary, J., McGoon, M. et al. (1997). Valvular heart disease associated with fenfluramine–phentermine. *N. Engl. J. Med.* 337 (9): 581–588. https://doi.org/10.1056/NEJM199708283370901.

116 Douglas, J., Munro, J., Kitchin, A. et al. (1981). Pulmonary hypertension and fenfluramine. *Br. Med. J.* 283 (6296): 881–883. https://doi.org/10.1136/bmj.283.6296.881.

117 Steffee, C., Singh, H., and Chitwood, W. (1999). Histologic changes in three explanted native cardiac valves following use of fenfluramines. *Cardiovasc. Pathol.* 8 (5): 245–253. https://doi.org/10.1016/S1054-8807(99)00019-8.

118 Centers for Disease Control and Prevention (1997). Cardiac valvulopathy associated with exposure to fenfluramine or dexfenfluramine: U.S. Department of Health and Human Services interim public health recommendations. *MMWR Morb. Mortal Wkly. Rep.* 46: 1061–1066.

119 Wajid, I., Vega, A., Thornhill, K. et al. (2023). Topiramate (Topamax): evolving role in weight reduction management: a narrative review. *Life (Basel).* 13 (9): 1845. https://doi.org/10.3390/life13091845.

120 Lee, S., Sziklas, V., Andermann, F. et al. (2003). The effects of adjunctive topiramate on cognitive function in patients with epilepsy. *Epilepsia* 44 (3): 339–347. https://doi.org/10.1046/j.1528-1157.2003.27402.x.

121 Cosentino, G., Conrad, A., and Uwaifo, G. (2011). Phentermine and topiramate for the management of obesity: a review. *Drug Des. Devel. Ther.* 7: 267–278. https://doi.org/10.2147/DDDT.S31443.
122 Stahl, S., Pradko, J., Haight, B. et al. (2004). A review of the neuropharmacology of bupropion, a dual norepinephrine and dopamine reuptake inhibitor. *Primary Care Companion to The Journal of Clinical Psychiatry.* 6 (4): 159–166. https://doi.org/10.4088/pcc.v06n0403.
123 Billes, S., Sinnayah, P., and Cowley, M. (2014). Naltrexone/bupropion for obesity: an investigational combination pharmacotherapy for weight loss. *Pharmacol. Res.* 84: 1–11. https://doi.org/10.1016/j.phrs.2014.04.004.
124 Dahlberg, S., Chang, E., Weiss, S. et al. (2022). Use of contrave, naltrexone with bupropion, bupropion, or naltrexone and major adverse cardiovascular events: a systematic literature review. *Diabetes Metabol. Syndr. Obesity Targets Therapy* 15: 3049–3067. https://doi.org/10.2147/DMSO.S381652.
125 Higgins, G., Fletcher, P., and Shanahan, W. (2020). Lorcaserin: a review of its preclinical and clinical pharmacology and therapeutic potential. *Pharmacol. Ther.* 205: 107417. https://doi.org/10.1016/j.pharmthera.2019.107417.
126 Tak, Y. and Lee, S. (2021). Long-term efficacy and safety of anti-obesity treatment: where do we stand? *Curr. Obes. Rep.* 10 (1): 14–30. https://doi.org/10.1007/s13679-020-00422-w.
127 Sharretts, J., Galescu, O., Gomatam, S. et al. (2020). Cancer risk associated with Lorcaserin – the FDA's review of the CAMELLIA-TIMI 61 trial. *N. Engl. J. Med.* 383 (11): 1000–1002. https://doi.org/10.1056/NEJMp2003873.
128 Bialecka-Florjanczyk, E., Fabiszewska, A., Krzyczkowska, J. et al. (2018). Synthetic and natural lipase inhibitors. *Mini Rev. Med. Chem.* 18 (8): 672–683. https://doi.org/10.2174/1389557516666160630123356.
129 Weibel, E., Hadvary, P., Hochuli, E. et al. (1987). Lipstatin, an inhibitor of pancreatic lipase, produced by Streptomyces toxytricini. I. Producing organism, fermentation, isolation and biological activity. *J. Antibiot.* 40 (8): 1081–1085. https://doi.org/10.7164/antibiotics.40.1081.
130 Heck, A., Yanovski, J., and Calis, K. (2000). Orlistat, a new lipase inhibitor for the management of obesity. *Pharmacotherapy* 20 (3): 270–279. https://doi.org/10.1592/phco.20.4.270.34882.
131 Hvizdos, K. and Markham, A. (1999). Orlistat: a review of its use in the management of obesity. *Drugs* 58 (4): 743–760. https://doi.org/10.2165/00003495-199958040-00015.
132 Gillies, C., Abrams, K., Lambert, P. et al. (2007). Pharmacological and lifestyle interventions to prevent or delay type 2 diabetes in people with impaired glucose tolerance: systematic review and meta-analysis. *BMJ* 334 (7588): 299. https://doi.org/10.1136/bmj.39063.689375.55.
133 Siebenhofer, A., Winterholer, S., Jeitler, K. et al. (2021). Long-term effects of weight-reducing drugs in people with hypertension. *Cochrane Database Syst. Rev.* 17 (1): CD007654. https://doi.org/10.1002/14651858.CD007654.pub5.
134 Finkelstein, E., Chodavadia, P., and Strombotne, K. (2023). A systematic review of the economic value proposition for commercially available nonsurgical

weight-loss interventions. *Obesity* 31 (7): 1725–1733. https://doi.org/10.1002/oby.23760.

135 Xue, Y., Zou, H., Ruan, Z. et al. (2023). Pharmacoeconomic evaluation of anti-obesity drugs for chronic weight management: a systematic review of literature. *Front. Endocrinol.* 14: 1254398. https://doi.org/10.3389/fendo.2023.1254398.

136 Pertwee, R. (2006). Cannabinoid pharmacology: the first 66 years. *Br. J. Pharmacol.* 147 (Suppl 1): S163–S171. https://doi.org/10.1038/sj.bjp.0706406.

137 Matsuda, L., Lolait, S., Brownstein, M. et al. (1990). Structure of a cannabinoid receptor and functional expression of the cloned cDNA. *Nature* 346 (6284): 561–564. https://doi.org/10.1038/346561a0.

138 Munro, S., Thomas, K., and Abu-Shaar, M. (1993). Molecular characterization of a peripheral receptor for cannabinoids. *Nature* 365 (6441): 61–65. https://doi.org/10.1038/365061a0.

139 Lange, J. and Kruse, C. (2005). Keynote review: medicinal chemistry strategies to CB1 cannabinoid receptor antagonists. *Drug Discov. Today* 10 (10): 693–702. https://doi.org/10.1016/S1359-6446(05)03427-6.

140 Zou, S. and Kumar, U. (2018). Cannabinoid receptors and the endocannabinoid system: signaling and function in the central nervous system. *Int. J. Mol. Sci.* 19 (3): 833. https://doi.org/10.3390/ijms19030833.

141 Koch, M. (2017). Cannabinoid receptor signaling in central regulation of feeding behavior: a mini-review. *Front. Neurosci.* 11: 293. https://doi.org/10.3389/fnins.2017.00293.

142 Antel, J., Gregory, P., and Nordheim, U. (2006). CB1 cannabinoid receptor antagonists for treatment of obesity and prevention of comorbid metabolic disorders. *J. Med. Chem.* 49 (14): 4008–4016. https://doi.org/10.1021/jm058238r.

143 Carai, M., Colombo, G., and Gessa, G. (2005). Rimonabant: the first therapeutically relevant cannabinoid antagonist. *Life Sci.* 77 (19): 2339–2350. https://doi.org/10.1016/j.lfs.2005.04.017.

144 Sam, A., Salem, V., and Ghatei, M. (2011). Rimonabant: from RIO to Ban. *J. Obes.* 2011: 432607. https://doi.org/10.1155/2011/432607.

145 Van Gaal, L., Rissanen, A., Scheen, A. et al. (2005). Effects of the cannabinoid-1 receptor blocker rimonabant on weight reduction and cardiovascular risk factors in overweight patients: 1-year experience from the RIO-Europe study. *Lancet* 365 (9468): 1389–1397. https://doi.org/10.1016/S0140-6736(05)66374-X.

146 Rosenstock, J., Hollander, P., Chevalier, S. et al. (2008). SERENADE: the study evaluating rimonabant efficacy in drug-naive diabetic patients: effects of monotherapy with rimonabant, the first selective CB1 receptor antagonist, on glycemic control, body weight, and lipid profile in drug-naive type 2 diabetes. *Diabetes Care* 31 (11): 2169–2176. https://doi.org/10.2337/dc08-0386.

147 Christensen, R., Kristensen, P., Bartels, E. et al. (2007). Efficacy and safety of the weight-loss drug rimonabant: a meta-analysis of randomised trials. *Lancet* 370 (9600): 1706–1713. https://doi.org/10.1016/S0140-6736(07)61721-8.

148 King, A. (2010). Neuropsychiatric adverse effects signal the end of the line for rimonabant. *Nat. Rev. Cardiol.* 7 (11): 602–602. https://doi.org/10.1038/nrcardio.2010.148.

149 Sacco, E., Bientinesi, R., Tienforti, D. et al. (2014). Discovery history and clinical development of mirabegron for the treatment of overactive bladder and urinary incontinence. *Expert Opin. Drug Discov.* 9 (4): 433–448. https://doi.org/10.1517/17460441.2014.892923.

150 Bel, J., Tai, T., Khaper, N. et al. (2021). Mirabegron: the most promising adipose tissue beiging agent. *Physiol. Rep.* 9 (5): e14779. https://doi.org/10.14814/phy2.14779.

151 Liu, Y., Toubro, S., Astrup, A. et al. (1995). Contribution of beta 3-adrenoceptor activation to ephedrine-induced thermogenesis in humans. *Int. J. Obes. Relat. Metab. Disord.* 19 (9): 678–685.

152 Zhao, X., Liu, Y., Zhang, X. et al. (2023). The combined effect of metformin and mirabegron on diet-induced obesity. *Media Commun.* 4 (2): e207. https://doi.org/10.1002/mco2.207.

153 Bragg, R., Hebel, D., Vouri, S. et al. (2014). Mirabegron: a beta-3 agonist for overactive bladder. *Consult. Pharm.* 29 (12): 823–837. https://doi.org/10.4140/TCP.n.2014.823.

154 Balligand, J.-L., Brito, D., Brosteanu, O. et al. (2023). Repurposing the β3-adrenergic receptor agonist mirabegron in patients with structural cardiac disease: the beta3-LVH phase 2b randomized clinical trial. *JAMA Cardiol.* 8 (11): 1031–1040. https://doi.org/10.1001/jamacardio.2023.3003.

155 Clément, K., van den Akker, E., Argente, J. et al. (2020). Efficacy and safety of setmelanotide, an MC4R agonist, in individuals with severe obesity due to LEPR or POMC deficiency: single-arm, open-label, multicentre, phase 3 trials. *Lancet Diabetes Endocrinol.* 8 (12): 960–970. https://doi.org/10.1016/S2213-8587(20)30364-8.

156 Hainer, V., Hainerová, I., Kunešová, M. et al. (2020). Melanocortin pathways: suppressed and stimulated melanocortin-4 receptor (MC4R). *Physiol. Res.* 69 (Suppl 2): S245–S254. https://doi.org/10.33549/physiolres.934512.

157 Harno, E., Gali Ramamoorthy, T., Coll, A.P. et al. (2018). POMC: the physiological power of hormone processing. *Physiol. Rev.* 98 (4): 2381–2430. https://doi.org/10.1152/physrev.00024.2017.

158 Farooqi, I. and O'Rahilly, S. (2008). Mutations in ligands and receptors of the leptin–melanocortin pathway that lead to obesity. *Nat. Clin. Pract. Endocrinol. Metab.* 4 (10): 569–577. https://doi.org/10.1038/ncpendmet0966.

159 Clément, K., Biebermann, H., Farooqi, I. et al. (2018). MC4R agonism promotes durable weight loss in patients with leptin receptor deficiency. *Nat. Med.* 24 (5): 551–555. https://doi.org/10.1038/s41591-018-0015-9.

160 Magliano, D.J. and Boyko, E.J. (2025). Diabetes Atlas 11th edition scientific committee. Diabetes Atlas [Internet]. In: *3. The global picture of diabetes*, 11the. Brussels: International Diabetes Federation Available from: https://www.ncbi.nlm.nih.gov/books/NBK618744/.

161 Collaborators GBDD (2023). Global, regional, and national burden of diabetes from 1990 to 2021, with projections of prevalence to 2050: a systematic analysis for the global burden of disease study 2021. *Lancet* 402 (10397): 203–234. https://doi.org/10.1016/S0140-6736(23)01301-6.

162 Chetty, A., Rafi, E., Bellini, N. et al. (2023). A review of incretin therapies approved and in late-stage development for overweight and obesity management. *Endocr. Pract.* S1530-891X(23)00790-5 30 (3): 292–303. https://doi.org/10.1016/j.eprac.2023.12.010.

163 Mariam, Z. and Niazi, S. (2024). Glucagon-like peptide agonists: a prospective review. *Endocrinol. Diabetes Metabol.* 7 (1): e462. https://doi.org/10.1002/edm2.462.

164 Ussher, J. and Drucker, D. (2023). Glucagon-like peptide 1 receptor agonists: cardiovascular benefits and mechanisms of action. *Nat. Rev. Cardiol.* 20 (7): 463–474. https://doi.org/10.1038/s41569-023-00849-3.

165 Liu, S., Liu, J., Si, L. et al. (2023). Patient preferences for anti-hyperglycaemic medication for type 2 diabetes mellitus in China: findings from a national survey. *BMJ Glob. Health* 8 (4): e010942. https://doi.org/10.1136/bmjgh-2022-010942.

166 Marx, N., Husain, M., Lehrke, M. et al. (2022). GLP-1 receptor agonists for the reduction of atherosclerotic cardiovascular risk in patients with type 2 diabetes. *Circulation* 146 (24): 1882–1894. https://doi.org/10.1161/CIRCULATIONAHA.122.059595.

167 Sikirica, M., Martin, A., Wood, R. et al. (2017). Reasons for discontinuation of GLP1 receptor agonists: data from a real-world cross-sectional survey of physicians and their patients with type 2 diabetes. *Diabetes Metab. Syndr. Obes.* 10: 403–412. https://doi.org/10.2147/DMSO.S141235.

168 Griffith, D., Edmonds, D., Fortin, J.-P. et al. (2022). A small-molecule oral agonist of the human glucagon-like peptide-1 receptor. *J. Med. Chem.* 65 (12): 8208–8226. https://doi.org/10.1021/acs.jmedchem.1c01856.

169 Sheahan, K., Wahlberg, E., and Gilbert, M. (2020). An overview of GLP-1 agonists and recent cardiovascular outcomes trials. *Postgrad. Med. J.* 96 (1133): 156–161. https://doi.org/10.1136/postgradmedj-2019-137186.

170 Davies, M., Pieber, T., Hartoft-Nielsen, M.-L. et al. (2017). Effect of oral semaglutide compared with placebo and subcutaneous semaglutide on Glycemic Control in patients with type 2 diabetes: a randomized clinical trial. *JAMA* 318 (15): 1460–1470. https://doi.org/10.1001/jama.2017.14752.

171 Hedrington, M. and Davis, S. (2019). Oral semaglutide for the treatment of type 2 diabetes. *Expert. Opin. Pharmacother.* 20 (2): 133–141. https://doi.org/10.1080/14656566.2018.1552258.

172 Overgaard, R., Navarria, A., Ingwersen, S. et al. (2021). Clinical pharmacokinetics of oral semaglutide: analyses of data from clinical pharmacology trials. *Clin. Pharmacokinet.* 60 (10): 1335–1348. https://doi.org/10.1007/s40262-021-01025-x.

173 Kawai, T., Sun, B., Yoshino, H. et al. (2020). Structural basis for GLP-1 receptor activation by LY3502970, an orally active nonpeptide agonist. *Proc. Natl. Acad. Sci.* 117 (47): 29959–29967. https://doi.org/10.1073/pnas.2014879117.

174 Cary, B., Zhang, X., Cao, J. et al. (2023). New insights into the structure and function of class B1 GPCRs. *Endocr. Rev.* 44 (3): 492–517. https://doi.org/10.1210/endrev/bnac033.

175 Wootten, D., Christopoulos, A., Marti-Solano, M. et al. (2018). Mechanisms of signalling and biased agonism in G protein-coupled receptors. *Nat. Rev. Mol. Cell Biol.* 19 (10): 638–653. https://doi.org/10.1038/s41580-018-0049-3.

176 Chen, D., Liao, J., Li, N. et al. (2007). A nonpeptidic agonist of glucagon-like peptide 1 receptors with efficacy in diabetic db/db mice. *Proc. Natl. Acad. Sci. USA* 104 (3): 943–948. https://doi.org/10.1073/pnas.0610173104.

177 Cong, Z., Zhou, Q., Li, Y. et al. (2022). Structural basis of peptidomimetic agonism revealed by small-molecule GLP-1R agonists Boc5 and WB4–24. *Proc. Natl. Acad. Sci.* 119 (20): e2200155119. https://doi.org/10.1073/pnas.2200155119.

178 Liu, Q., Li, N., Yuan, Y. et al. (2012). Cyclobutane derivatives as novel nonpeptidic small molecule agonists of glucagon-Like peptide-1 receptor. *J. Med. Chem.* 55 (1): 250–267. https://doi.org/10.1021/jm201150j.

179 Lee, S. and Lee, D.Y. (2017). Glucagon-like peptide-1 and glucagon-like peptide-1 receptor agonists in the treatment of type 2 diabetes. *Annals Pediatr. Endocrinol. Metabol.* 22 (1): 15. https://doi.org/10.6065/apem.2017.22.1.15.

180 Méndez, M., Matter, H., Defossa, E. et al. (2020). Design, synthesis, and pharmacological evaluation of potent positive allosteric modulators of the glucagon-like peptide-1 receptor (GLP-1R). *J. Med. Chem.* 63 (5): 2292–2307. https://doi.org/10.1021/acs.jmedchem.9b01071.

181 Knudsen, L., Kiel, D., Teng, M. et al. (2007). Small-molecule agonists for the glucagon-like peptide 1 receptor. *Proc. Natl. Acad. Sci.* 104 (3): 937–942. https://doi.org/10.1073/pnas.0605701104.

182 Coopman, K., Huang, Y., Johnston, N. et al. (2010). Comparative effects of the endogenous agonist glucagon-like peptide-1 (GLP-1)-(7-36) amide and the small-molecule ago-allosteric agent “compound 2” at the GLP-1 receptor. *J. Pharmacol. Exp. Ther.* 334 (3): 795–808. https://doi.org/10.1124/jpet.110.166009.

183 Cong, Z., Chen, L.-N., Ma, H. et al. (2021). Molecular insights into ago-allosteric modulation of the human glucagon-like peptide-1 receptor. *Nat. Commun.* 12 (1): 3763. https://doi.org/10.1038/s41467-021-24058-z.

184 Yin, Y., de Waal, P.W., He, Y. et al. (2017). Rearrangement of a polar core provides a conserved mechanism for constitutive activation of class B G protein-coupled receptors. *J. Biol. Chem.* 292 (24): 9865–9881. https://doi.org/10.1074/jbc.M117.782987.

185 Teng, M., Johnson, M.D., Thomas, C. et al. (2007). Small molecule ago-allosteric modulators of the human glucagon-like peptide-1 (hGLP-1) receptor. *Bioorg. Med. Chem. Lett.* 17 (19): 5472–5478. https://doi.org/10.1016/j.bmcl.2007.06.086.

186 Kopin, A.S. and Beinborn, M. (2004). Methods and Compositions for the Treatment of Metabolic Disorders. WO Patent 2, 004, 103, 310, filed 20 May 2004 and issued 02 December 2004.

187 Moon, H.-S., Yang, J. S., Kim, M. K. et al. (2011). Novel Quinoxaline Derivatives. WO Patent 2, 011,122, 815, filed 28 March 2011 and issued 6 October 2011.

188 Sloop, K., Willard, F., Brenner, M. et al. (2010). Novel small molecule glucagon-like peptide-1 receptor agonist stimulates insulin secretion in rodents and from human islets. *Diabetes* 59 (12): 3099–3107. https://doi.org/10.2337/db10-0689.

189 Nolte, W., Fortin, J.-P., and Stevens, B. (2014). A potentiator of orthosteric ligand activity at GLP-1R acts via covalent modification. *Nat. Chem. Biol.* 10 (8): 629–631. https://doi.org/10.1038/nchembio.1581.

190 Wootten, D., Savage, E., Valant, C. et al. (2012). Allosteric modulation of endogenous metabolites as an avenue for drug discovery. *Mol. Pharmacol.* 82 (2): 281–290. https://doi.org/10.1124/mol.112.079319.

191 Morris, L., Nance, K., Gentry, P. et al. (2014). Discovery of (S)-2-Cyclopentyl-N-((1-isopropylpyrrolidin2-yl)-9-methyl-1-oxo-2,9-dihydro-1H-pyrrido[3,4-b]indole-4-carboxamide (VU0453379): a novel, CNS penetrant glucagon-like peptide 1 receptor (GLP-1R) positive allosteric modulator (PAM). *J. Med. Chem.* 57 (23): 10192–10197. https://doi.org/10.1021/jm501375c.

192 Willard, F., Wainscott, D., Showalter, A. et al. (2021). Discovery of an orally efficacious positive allosteric modulator of the glucagon-like peptide-1 receptor. *J. Med. Chem.* 64 (6): 3439–3448. https://doi.org/10.1021/acs.jmedchem.1c00029.

193 Bueno, A., Sun, B., Willard, F. et al. (2020). Structural insights into probe-dependent positive allosterism of the GLP-1 receptor. *Nat. Chem. Biol.* 16 (10): 1105–1110. https://doi.org/10.1038/s41589-020-0589-7.

194 Decara, J., Vázquez-Villa, H., Brea, J. et al. (2022). Discovery of V-0219: a small-molecule positive allosteric modulator of the glucagon-like peptide-1 receptor toward oral treatment for "Diabesity.". *J. Med. Chem.* 65 (7): 5449–5461. https://doi.org/10.1021/acs.jmedchem.1c01842.

195 Mjalli, A., Polisetti, D. R., Yokum, T. S. et al. (2009). Oxadiazoanthracene compounds for the treatment of diabetes. WO Patent 2, 009, 111, 700, filed 06 March 2009 and issued 11 September 2009.

196 Freeman, J., Dvergsten, C., Dunn, I. et al. (2017). TTP273, Investigational Oral (Non-Peptide) GLP-1R Agonist: Improved Glycemic Control without Nausea and Vomiting in Phase 2. Poster presented at the American Diabetes Association 77th Scientific Sessions, San Diego (9–13 June 2017).

197 Zhang, X., Belousoff, M., Zhao, P. et al. (2020). Differential GLP-1R binding and activation by peptide and non-peptide agonists. *Mol. Cell* 80 (3): 485–500.e7. https://doi.org/10.1016/j.molcel.2020.09.020.

198 Saxena, A., Gorman, D., Esquejo, R. et al. (2021). Danuglipron (PF-06882961) in type 2 diabetes: a randomized, placebo-controlled, multiple ascending-dose phase 1 trial. *Nat. Med.* 27 (6): 1079–1087. https://doi.org/10.1038/s41591-021-01391-w.

199 Saxena, A., Frias, J., Brown, L. et al. (2023). Efficacy and safety of oral small molecule glucagon-like peptide 1 receptor agonist Danuglipron for glycemic control among patients with type 2 diabetes: a randomized clinical trial. *JAMA Netw. Open* 6 (5): e2314493. https://doi.org/10.1001/jamanetworkopen.2023.14493.

200 Sessa, B., Saxena, A., Schmeltz, A. et al. (2022). Analyst and Investor Call to Review Oral GLP-1 Data. Data presented at European Association for the Study of Diabetes (EASD) Annual Meeting in Stockholm, Sweden (21 September 2022).

201 Pfizer (2023). Pfizer provides update on GLP-1-RA clinical development program for adults with obesity and type 2 diabetes mellitus. Press release (26 June).

202 Sato, T. et al. (2018). Pyrazolopyridine derivative having glp-1 receptor agonist effect. WO Patent 2, 018, 056, 453, filed 26 September 2017 and issued 29 March 2018.

203 Tamura, T., Noda, H., Joyashiki, E. et al. (2016). Identification of an orally active small-molecule PTHR1 agonist for the treatment of hypoparathyroidism. *Nat. Commun.* 7 (1): 13384. https://doi.org/10.1038/ncomms13384.

204 Pratt, E., Ma, X., Liu, R. et al. (2023). Orforglipron (LY3502970), a novel, oral non-peptide glucagon-like peptide-1 receptor agonist: a Phase 1a, blinded, placebo-controlled, randomized, single- and multiple-ascending-dose study in healthy participants. *Diabetes Obes. Metab.* 25 (9): 2634–2641. https://doi.org/10.1111/dom.15184.

205 Frias, J., Hsia, S., Eyde, S. et al. (2023). Efficacy and safety of oral orforglipron in patients with type 2 diabetes: a multicentre, randomised, dose-response, phase 2 study. *Lancet* 402 (10400): 472–483. https://doi.org/10.1016/S0140-6736(23)01302-8.

206 Wharton, S., Blevins, T., Connery, L. et al. (2023). Daily oral GLP-1 receptor agonist Orforglipron for adults with obesity. *N. Engl. J. Med.* 389 (10): 877–888. https://doi.org/10.1056/NEJMoa2302392.

207 AstraZeneca (2023). AstraZeneca licenses novel agent for the treatment of cardiometabolic conditions and obesity. Press release (9 November).

208 Carmot Therapeutics (2023). Carmot therapeutics enters into definitive merger agreement with Roche. Press release (3 December).

209 Structure Therapeutics (2023). Structure therapeutics announces positive results from phase 1b clinical study of oral GLP-1 receptor agonist GSBR-1290 and provides program update. Press release (29 September).

210 Sciwind Biosciences (2022). Sciwind biosciences announces initiation of dosing in phase 1 clinical trial evaluating XW014, an oral small molecule GLP-1 receptor agonist for the treatment of obesity and type 2 diabetes. Press release (09 October).

211 Regor Therapeutics (2022). Regor announces the first patient dosed in the U.S. in the Phase II clinical trial for RGT-075, a novel small molecule GLP-1R agonist. Press release (12 April).

212 Terns Pharmaceuticals (2023). Terns pharmaceuticals to highlight new preclinical data for tern-601 program in obesity at the American diabetes association's 83rd annual scientific sessions. Press release (22 May).

213 Jastreboff, A.M., Aronne, L.J., and Ahmad, N.N. (2022). Tirzepatide once weekly for the treatment of obesity. *N. Engl. J. Med.* 387 (3): 205–216. https://doi.org/10.1056/NEJMoa2206038.

214 U.S. Food and Drug Administration. (April 2026). FDA Approves First New Molecular Entity Under National Priority Voucher Program. FDA press announcement. https://www.fda.gov/news-events/press-announcements/fda-approves-first-new-molecular-entity-under-national-priority-voucher-program.

6

Trends in the Field of Insulin Drug Design

Thomas Hoeg-Jensen

Eli Lilly and Company, Protomer Technologies, Inc., 26 N. Euclid Ave., Pasadena, CA 91101, USA

Introduction

Insulin was discovered in 1921 [1], and this lifesaving two-chain 6 kDa disulfide crosslinked hormone is the most powerful drug for control of blood glucose [2]. Native insulin is however not ideal for pharmaceutical application due to problems of timing of exposure to food intake as well as risk of hypoglycemia (life-threatening low blood glucose) [3]. Furthermore, insulin drugs must be administered by injection since oral dosing leads to insulin degradation and poor absorption. An assortment of insulin variants with optimized time-action profiles are now available to people with diabetes for control of glucose spikes after meals (fast-acting insulin, bolus insulin) as well as basal insulin drugs for glucose control around the clock (long-acting insulin). Notably, insulin dosing is a challenge, since both mealtime and basal insulin must be titrated to fit individual insulin sensitivity (with fasting blood glucose as readout), and meal insulin doses must be matched to the size and character of each meal. In order to lower the risk of long-term complications from diabetes, insulin dosing should aim to match the native insulin secretion patterns stylized in Figure 6.1 [4]. However, intense insulin dosing comes with increased risk of hypoglycemia [5]. People with type 1 diabetes have no insulin secretion due to auto-immune destruction of the insulin producing beta cells, so they must use both basal and meal insulin multiple times daily. People with type 2 diabetes have low insulin sensitivity and an assortment of treatments are available for management of type 2 diabetes. Type 2 is however a progressive disorder, and most type 2 diabetes patients progress to insulin drugs at some stage. Type 2 patients typically use only basal insulin initially, while relying on their internal insulin secretion to cover meals. However, many people with type 2 diabetes progress to basal/bolus insulin treatment at some point.

The current review will discuss the design of insulin analogues with optimized pharmacokinetics, along with developments towards engineering of tissue-selective

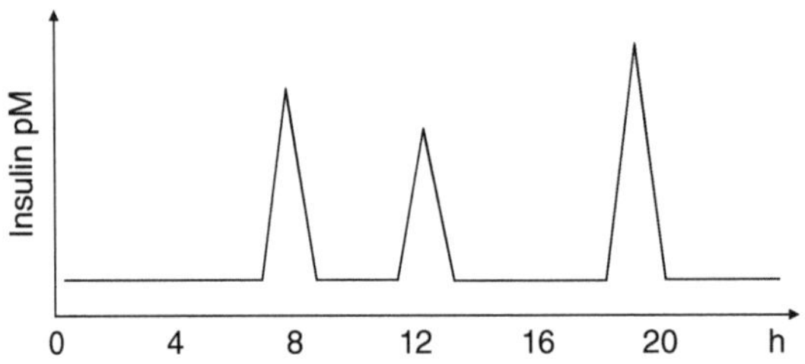

Figure 6.1 Stylized native insulin secretion pattern, showing basal insulin level around the clock and peaks after each meal. Modern insulin analogues help simulate this pattern by providing long-acting and fast-acting insulin types. However, getting multiple daily doses right to match prevailing glucose is always difficult. Dosing too much or too little insulin can be harmful long-term or acutely dangerous due to hyperglycemia or hypoglycemia.

insulin, oral insulin and glucose-sensitive insulin for lowering the risk of hypoglycemia. Contrary to the many academic reviews of insulin science that were published in connection with the centurial celebration of insulin discovery [6], the given chapter will focus on insulin structural drug design including patent references, which have been largely ignored in prior texts. Instead of providing a long introduction to insulin chemistry and biology, these basics of insulin science will be brought up as needed to follow the drug engineering story.

Native Insulin

From the 1920s to the 1990s insulin for pharmaceutical use was isolated from animal pancreas, mainly from pigs. Insulin sequences from a plethora of animals have been characterized [7], and bovine insulin also found some pharmaceutical use. However, bovine insulin has three mutations relative to human insulin, and bovine insulin is considered more immunogenic than pig insulin [8], which has only one residue different (B30A/T, see Figure 6.2). Reverse proteolysis using trypsin or ALP alias Lys-C enzyme for amino acid exchange at B29Lys can transform pig insulin to human insulin [9, 10], which came to the market in the early 1990s. The native insulin types are however not ideal with regard to pharmacokinetics neither for meal nor basal use since administered by subcutaneous injection (SC). Insulin is generally formulated with Zn(II) to get insulin hexamer, which is more stable long-term both chemically and physically, and also the native storage form of insulin in beta cells. Insulin drugs must generally have two years stability in solution with high purity standards. Slow dissociation of insulin hexamers during absorption from the SC injection site leads to mismatch of insulin action relative to glucose spikes after meals. This is contrary to the quick dissociation of insulin hexamer that happens upon insulin secretion from beta cells to blood in people who do not have diabetes. Native insulin drug should therefore best be injected approximately 30 minutes before each meal, where the user does not necessarily know the meal character or size, nor the exact time of meal serving. Faster-acting insulin types were therefore a clinical wish for many years.

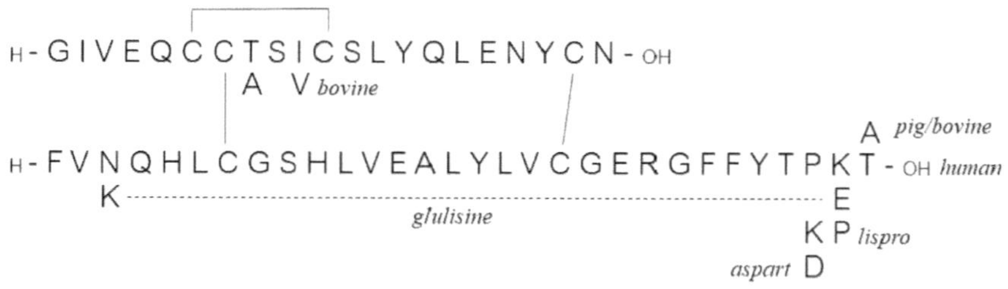

Figure 6.2 Structures of fast-acting insulin drugs, insulin lispro (B28K B29P), insulin aspart (B28D), insulin glulisine (B3K B29E) along with pig and bovine insulin (B30A and A8A A10V B30A) versus human insulin (B30T).

Meal Insulin Designs and Formulations

The advent of recombinant expression of proteins around 1990 enabled engineering of proteins with altered sequences [11]. 3D structures of insulin hexamers were known from x-ray crystallographic work in the 1960s [12] and gave the basis for rational design of insulin analogues that could form weaker complexing insulin hexamers, thus leading to faster hexamer dissociation after injection and thus faster insulin absorption [13]. Meal insulin lispro (B28K B28P) [14, 15], insulin aspart (B28D) [16–18] and insulin glulisine (B3K B29E) [19, 20] have been on the market since the early 2000s and have largely replaced human insulin for meal use, see Figure 6.2. T_{max} for the meal insulin drugs are around 60 minutes versus 120 minutes for human insulin. The given insulin drugs can thus be injected with the meal instead of 30 minutes before. The meal variants are also the preferred insulin types for pump use, where fast response to meal doses or fast adjustments to basal insulin patterns are desired.

Optimized formulations of insulin lispro and aspart with even faster onset of action (T_{max} near 30 minutes) came to the market around 2015, based on reformulations with vasodilators and other excipients, among other increasing blood flow at the injection site, treprostinil for lispro and niacinamide for insulin aspart [21–24]. These reformulated meal insulin drugs can be taken during or after the meal, when precise meal size is known, and more precise dosing of meal insulin is thereby possible.

Once-Daily Basal Insulin Designs

Insulin has isoelectric point of approximately 5, and co-crystallization of insulin with the basic protein protamine (originally isolated from fish sperm) can provide solids that dissolve slowly after injection of their suspensions [25]. The main type is called NPH for neutral protamine Hagedorn, and the NPH protraction principle can give insulin profiles with half-life of approximately six hours. NPH insulin must thus be used twice daily in order to get 24 hours basal coverage, but NPH has the advantage that it can be co-formulated with meal insulin [26]. Such co-formulations

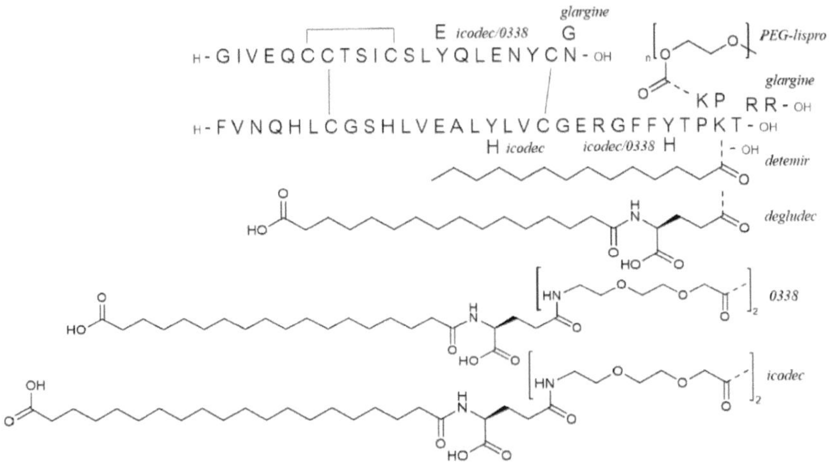

Figure 6.3 Structures of basal insulin drugs. Insulin detemir, degludec, 0338 and icodec are all desB30 analogues, as illustrated with -OH from B29K. PEG-Lispro uses 20 kDa PEG.

retain the individual timing profiles of the components (basal and meal), thus saving the patient a few injections per day. The injection of suspended solids like NPH has however the limitation that dosing is not very precise, and injection of too much insulin can happen, leading to dangerous hypoglycemia. There was thus for many years a clinical wish for soluble long-acting insulin drug, which would allow more precise dosing.

Addition of basic residues like arginine to the insulin sequence can change its isoelectric point from 5 to 7, and thereby lower insulin solubility at neutral pH, while securing good solubility at slightly acidic conditions, pH 4–5. Insulin glargine is A21G B31R B32R insulin (Figure 6.3), and it is soluble at acidic pH, while precipitating upon injection by neutralization of pH to form a SC depot [27–29]. A21N can slowly deamidate at acidic pH, so A21G is used in glargine to circumvent such degradation during storage. The half-life of glargine is around 12 hours, thus covering almost 24 hours when used once daily. Glargine has been available since around year 2000, and a more concentrated form of glargine was introduced around 2015, providing full 24 hours coverage (300 insulin units/ml ~ 10 mg/ml instead of 100 units/ml ~ 3.5 mg/ml) [30]. The bioavailability of U300 glargine is lower than for U100, so users that change from glargine U100 to U300 must be aware that they will likely need to titrate to higher molar dose of U300 than U100 to get the same glycemic control.

Insulin detemir is chemically modified desB30 human insulin, made by acylation of B29Lys N-epsilon with myristic acid (C14 fatty acid, see Figure 6.3) [31–33]. This modification changes the oligomer properties of insulin detemir towards dihexamer and enables binding to the native transport protein albumin (human serum albumin, HSA), which helps protract both the SC absorption and the circulation time of insulin detemir [34]. In humans, insulin detemir has half-life of approximately seven hours, so it must typically be used twice daily for basal coverage, although some patients use it once daily. The fatty acid acylation technology has become a general platform for peptide and protein drug protraction, now used with other drugs than insulin [35]. Insulin detemir has the special property that it is weight neutral [36], meaning that patients that start insulin therapy with insulin detemir do not gain weight contrary to other insulin types where small weight gains typically are observed after insulin initiation. The reason for the weight neutral property of insulin detemir is not clear, but weak liver preferential action has been suggested [37]. Noteworthy, insulin detemir has low potency in humans, around 25% relative to human insulin, probably due to unspecific clearance of this very hydrophobic conjugate by non-insulin-receptor mediated routes [38]. The commercial concentration of insulin detemir is 2.4 mmol/l in order to compensate for the lower glycodynamic potency, whereas other insulin products are used at 600 umol/l (defined as 100 U/ml). Insulin detemir has been available since around 2005. Neither insulin detemir nor insulin glargine tolerate co-formulation with meal insulin since the higher concentration of insulin detemir and the acidic pH of insulin glargine formulation alters the absorption profiles of co-formulated meal insulin.

Insulin degludec has C16 fatty diacid attached to B29Lys *N*-epsilon of desB30 human insulin via a gamma-L-glutamyl linker (Figure 6.3) [39, 40]. The use of a fatty diacid (contrary to the mono-fatty acid of detemir) and γ-Glu linker makes insulin degludec as polar as human insulin itself. The fatty diacid also gives stronger albumin binding than for the corresponding mono-fatty acid conjugation. Insulin degludec further has the special property that it forms soluble multihexamers after SC injection, which leads to very slow absorption and thus very long pharmacokinetics. The multihexamer formation happens when the conservation excipients phenol and meta-cresol defuse away from insulin degludec upon SC injection. All insulin products must contain bacteriostatic excipients like phenol/cresol because insulin pens and vials are multi-use. An opened insulin vial or pen can be used around one month. Phenol and cresol defuse quickly away from the SC injection site because these compounds are small and amphipolar. Insulin degludec shows half-life in humans around 25 hours, so it can be dosed "flexibly," [41] which means that the user does not need to dose this basal insulin at the same time every day (contrary to other basal insulins), and this can be convenient when travelling or sleeping late. The polarity of insulin degludec ensures that it has glycodynamic potency like normal insulin (contrary to insulin detemir), and it is available in co-formulation with insulin aspart for simultaneous basal and meal coverage [42]. The individual pharmacokinetic kinetic profiles or insulin degludec and insulin aspart are retained when dosing their co-formulation.

Once-Weekly Insulin Designs

Use of a once-weekly insulin will reduce the number of injections by 313 per year compared to a once-daily insulin [43]. For people with type 2 diabetes, there are many treatment options, from oral anti-diabetic medications like metformin and sodium-linked glucose transporter-2 inhibitors (SGLT-2i) to glucagon-like peptide-1 agonists (GLP-1) [44, 45]. The latter not only helps control blood glucose but can also give weight loss and cardiovascular benefits. However, type 2 diabetes is a progressive disorder, and many type 2 patients move to basal insulin in later stages of their treatment. As mentioned in the introduction, people with type 1 diabetes need both basal insulin and multiple daily injections of fast-acting insulin with every meal.

Insulin icodec is a derivative of desB30 human insulin, which uses γ-Glu and short PEG-like linkers to conjugate a strongly albumin binding fatty diacid, eicosane dioic acid (C20 diacid) to B29Lys (Figure 6.3) [46, 47]. Insulin icodec furthermore has three mutations relative to human insulin, A14E B16H B25H, which stabilize against insulin disulfide degradation during the week-long circulation [48], as well as decreased insulin receptor affinity. The receptor affinity of insulin icodec in the presence of albumin is 30.000 times lower than that of human insulin [46]. Since both the glucose-lowering effect and clearance of insulin happens via binding to insulin receptor followed by cellular internalization, it was discovered that very low receptor affinity can help prolong the circulation time of insulin analogues like insulin icodec. This "low receptor affinity" drug design principle can appear counter-intuitive since high receptor affinity is typically an aim in drug design in pursuit of high drug potency. However, insulin icodec has the same molar glycodynamic potency as normal insulin because insignificant amounts of insulin icodec are lost to unspecific clearance despite week-long circulation. Insulin icodec has completed phase 3 clinical trials and is now approved in many countries. The half-life of insulin icodec in humans is around eight days. In type 2 patients, the glycemic control from once-weekly dosing of insulin icodec was found to be at least on par with the once-daily insulin comparators (insulin glargine and degludec) [49].

Insulin efsitora alfa (basal insulin Fc) consists of two single-chain insulin analog sequences fused to a dimeric Fc domain (fragment crystallizable) of an immunoglobulin G2 antibody (IgG2), see Figure 6.4 [50, 51]. Antibodies are generally recirculated by the neonatal receptor system (FcRn), so fusions of peptides to Fc will generally prolong their circulation time. Native proinsulin as expressed in the beta cells is a single-chain insulin precursor having a long C-peptide connecting the B-chain C-terminal of insulin with the A-chain N-terminal [52]. Proinsulin is considered inactive, and it only becomes active after processing in the beta cells to two-chain insulin by enzymatic removal of the 30-residue C-peptide. Insulin efsitora alfa on the other hand uses a short linker between its B- and A-chain insulin segments and retains insulin bioactivity in its single-chain form. The B27-B30 segment of human insulin is replaced with GGGG in the insulin B-chain of efsitora, and the short peptide linker of efsitora, GGSGGGG, is placed between B30G and A1. In addition to this, insulin efsitora alfa has insulin backbone mutations A10T A14D A21G B16E B25H that improve chemical and physical stability as well as lower the insulin receptor affinity. The half-life of insulin efsitora alfa in humans was found to be approximately 17 days [53], so efsitora provides a very flat basal insulin profile with a low peak-to-trough ratio [54]. Insulin efsitora alfa has completed phase 3 clinical trials [55], and is currently awaiting regulatory reviews (May 2026).

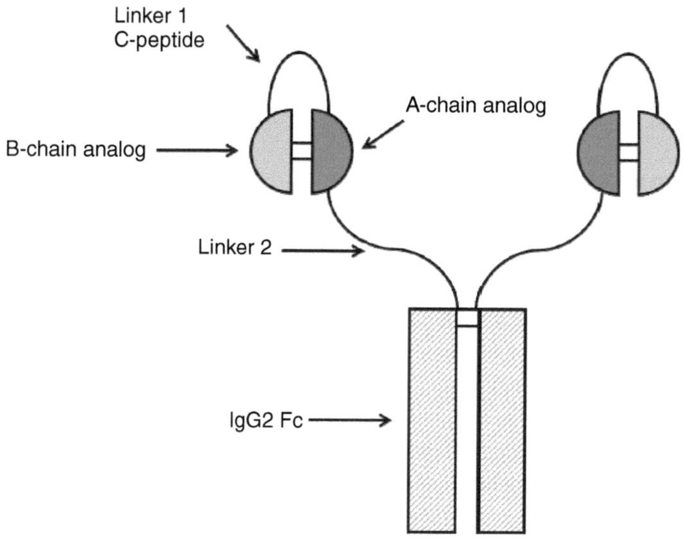

Figure 6.4 Structure of once-weekly candidate insulin efsitora alfa. The single-chain insulin has the mutations A10T A14D A21G B16E B25H B27G B28G B29G B30G and peptide linker G2SG4 between B30 and A1 (linker 1). Linker 2 from A21 to Fc domain is (G4Q)3G5. Diabetes Obes. Metab. credits: Adapted from Donnelly, 2023.

Tissue Selective and Functionally Selective Insulin

Native, pancreatic insulin secretion delivers the hormone directly to the liver, where approximately half of the insulin action takes place (glucose absorption, formation of glycogen, and down-regulation of gluconeogenesis). The insulin that passes through the liver takes effects on the rest of the body, mainly promoting glucose uptake in fat and muscle cells. However, when insulin drug is injected SC, there is relatively less effect on the liver and more effect on the periphery. It has therefore been a clinical wish to get a liver preferential insulin drug, and several approaches have been tried. 20 kDa PEGylation of insulin lispro gave an insulin with large hydrodynamic volume, namely apparent molecular weight around 60 kDa (BIL, basal insulin lispro, Figure 6.3) [56, 57]. The slow diffusion of BIL from SC to the circulation and high retention in the central compartment due to slow diffusion to peripheral tissue, was shown to give liver preferential effects. This led to lower risk of hypoglycemia and less weight-gain than seen with comparator insulin. Unfortunately, longer term, BIL gave increased liver enzyme blood values and triglyceride levels, so BIL was abandoned in late-stage development [58]. Strongly albumin binding insulin by fatty acid acylation at A22K has also been pursued with liver preferential aim, but these efforts were stopped at early clinical trials [59, 60]. Formulation of insulin with hepatic directed vehicles are currently pursued in clinical trials [61].

Insulin signaling happens via several biological pathways, mainly the metabolic AKT and mitogenic ERK routes, and it has been speculated that functionally selective insulin or partial insulin receptor agonists could improve diabetes outcome or hypoglycemia risk. However, both the AKT-selective basal insulin NN-1965 as well as the partial receptor agonist insulin dimer MK-1092 were stopped in early phase clinical trials due to unconvincing results [62–64].

Oral and Pulmonary Insulin

Insulin injections are not as bad as most people think [65]. Handy pens and very small injection volumes (few microliters) with very thin needles make insulin injections not painful, contrary to for example vaccine injections, which require large volumes (up to milliliters) and large needles. Nevertheless, if insulin could be dosed by oral route, it would be convenient. Oral dosing could help compliance and could theoretically give liver preferential action, since the portal vein leads from the gut to the liver. Being a protein, insulin is easily degraded by the proteolytic environment in the gut, and since insulin is relatively large, it is not well absorbed through the gut wall. Also, dose-to-dose variations of insulin absorption from the gut are significant. Oral dosing of native insulin has been attempted many times with different types of formulations [66], but native insulin is not what the patients need. Oral insulin would make most sense for people with type 2 diabetes, who typically use only long-acting insulin. The most successful trial for oral insulin used a basal, fatty diacid-conjugated insulin similar to insulin degludec and icodec. The lead molecule 0338 is identical to insulin icodec except having C18 fatty diacid and native B16Y, Figure 6.3 [67]. The clinical studies showed that once-daily dosing of 0338 caprate tablets could provide glucose control on par with injected basal insulin. The long profile of 0338 in the circulation helped smooth the variations from gut absorption. However, the oral bioavailability of 0338 was not surprisingly low, ~5% [68], and the 0338 program was stopped after phase 2 clinic for financial reasons.

Pulmonary insulin (lung dosed insulin) would similarly have benefited from use of long-acting insulin because type 2 diabetes patients would be the most likely users. However, the pulmonary insulin products that have reached the market are based on human insulin, thus for meal use, and these products have not been commercially successful [69]. The first product was withdrawn from the market after short time, and the second product, which is still available, has gained little market share.

Glucose-Sensitive Insulin

The main adverse effect of insulin drugs is occasional hypoglycemia, low blood glucose, which can be dangerous [3]. The idea of engineering an insulin that will change its biological activity in response to fluctuating glucose levels has been pursued since the 1970s [70], but with little success in terms of drug development. Hundreds of academic papers have described glucose-sensitive sustained release by formulating insulin with polymers that can encapsulate insulin in a SC depot and release the hormone in response to increasing glucose levels, Figure 6.5a [71]. However, the response from such systems will always be slow due to the need for glucose

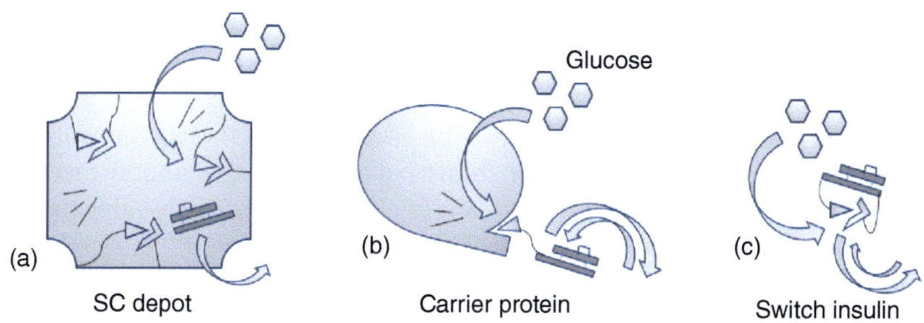

Figure 6.5 Glucose-sensitive insulin concepts: (a). Subcutaneous depot with insulin encapsulation in glucose-sensitive polymer. At increasing glucose levels, the polymer becomes more open and releases more insulin. However, the process is slow and irreversible. (b). Glucose-sensitive binding to a native protein or receptor (often multivalent but here illustrated as monovalent). At higher glucose, more insulin is released from the carrier protein (reversibly). (c). Insulin with a switch composed of a glucose binder and a binding partner (the switch can be multivalent). At low glucose, the switch is mainly in the closed form, which blocks the receptor binding surfaces of insulin or pulls insulin to a less bioactive conformation. At higher glucose, the switch opens and equilibrates insulin to a more bioactive form (reversibly). Notably, concepts (b) and (c) are both equilibria, which seems important for the compounds to respond reversibly to fluctuations in blood glucose levels (both up and down).

diffusion from the blood to the SC compartment and into the polymer, in addition to insulin diffusing the other way. Furthermore, once insulin is released from such systems, it is no longer glucose sensitive. Insulin derivatives that can respond reversibly to glucose fluctuations in the circulation seem a better idea. Two main concepts have been pursued, either glucose responsive binding to a carrier protein present in the circulation or switch-based alteration of insulin bioactivity, Figure 6.5b,c. A switch consists of a glucose binding motif in combination with a binding partner such as a glucoside, both conjugated to insulin at suitable positions (Figure 6.5c). At low blood glucose, the switch should be in a closed form, leading to low insulin bioactivity due to the switch either blocking the receptor binding surfaces of insulin, and/or due to the closed switch pulling insulin to conformations of low bioactivity. At higher blood glucose values, the switch should bind glucose and open, thus equilibrating insulin to a higher bioactive state. Switch systems require access to a small glucose binding motif that has affinity for glucose matching the narrow physiological range for blood glucose, which is roughly 2 to 20 mM in diabetes patients. There are few options in this regard. Boronic acids are known to bind glucose with displacement constant (Kd) in the low millimolar range (Kd $\sim$ 20 mM), whereas they bind stronger to fructose (Kd $\sim$ 1 mM). Insulin with a monoboronic acid + polyol-based switch at positions A1/B29 was shown to be responsive to fructose, but not to glucose [72]. Diboronic acids can bind glucose stronger, as vastly studied in research towards optic glucose monitors [73], but incorporation of diboronates into switch-based systems with insulin has so far not worked well enough for progression to drug development.

A macrocycle designed to bind glucose [74] has been used for engineering the switch-based insulin NNC2215 [75], which was shown to give attenuation of hypoglycemia as well as partial meal coverage in animal models when compared to non-glucose sensitive insulin.

Oligofucosyl/mannosyl insulin derivatives were found to bind to native mannose receptor [76, 77] and to be released by increasing blood glucose, thereby providing glucose-sensitive delivery in the circulation from a balance between mannose receptor and insulin receptor binding [78]. However, in clinical trials the glycodynamic potency of the lead compound (MK-2640) was found to be very low, 25 times lower than comparator, probably due to high background clearance via the mannose receptor [79], and the program was stopped after phase 1 clinic.

Diboronate insulin conjugates have been discovered to bind albumin in glucose dependent fashion with good response over the physiological glucose range [80, 81], and a few such compounds are now in early-stage development as glucose-sensitive insulin drugs (Figure 6.5b).

Insulin Pumps and Cell-Based Therapy

Insulin pumps are well established and still undergo improvements. The dream is to develop closed-looped systems that via continuous SC glucose monitoring can autonomously deliver insulin as needed [82]. However, timing of insulin meal delivery is a fundamental problem for closed-loop systems since the pump does not know when and what the person eats. Therefore, meal announcements seem required. Also, the lag of glucose transport from blood to the SC space (where the glucose monitor is inserted) as well as the lag of insulin transport to the circulation gives delay of insulin delivery of roughly one hour, which is a problem for autonomous pump meal-time doses. Still, pumps that can autonomously stop insulin delivery in response to measured dropping blood glucose is a big step forward for lowering hypoglycemic risk [83]. There can be occasional mechanical failures with pumps and sensors as well as the hassle of wearing such devices (pump + glucose monitor with two different catheters). Besides, the sterile catheters must be changed every three to four days since local irritation can happen if the inserts are left at the SC insertion site for longer time. Not least, pumps and their sterile accessories are rather expensive. The paraphernalia cost more than the insulin drug itself, so pumps are not a solution for all patients.

Cell-based therapy like beta cells replacement could be the ultimate solution for diabetes (the cure), but despite progress, this solution seems years off commercial approval [84]. Immune reactions to donated cells are a problem, so immunosuppressive drugs must generally be used, and several clinical setbacks have recently occurred. Cell therapy also appears to become an expensive solution, so it will hardly reach all patients.

Conclusions

Insulin engineering has pioneered several technologies in general protein science and has provided people with diabetes improved options for glucose control both in terms of basal and meal needs. Once-weekly insulin drugs seem likely to impact the basal insulin market at least for type 2 diabetes. If glucose sensitive insulin development succeeds, it should lower the risk of hypoglycemia, and thus allow the patients to treat their glucose fluctuations more aggressively, thereby hopefully resulting in better outcomes for people with insulin-treated diabetes.

Abbreviations

ALP	achromobacter lyticus protease
Fc	fragment crystallizable domain of antibody
HSA	human serum albumin
IgG2	immunoglobulin G2 antibody
kDa	kilo Dalton
NPH	Neutral protamine Hagedorn
SC	subcutaneous

Biography

Thomas Hoeg-Jensen studied organic chemistry at University of Copenhagen with a one-year visit to University of Louisville, Kentucky, and received his Ph.D. in 1995. After being hired by Novo Nordisk, Thomas worked with insulin drug design, and he is co-inventor of insulin degludec (once-daily insulin marketed as Tresiba) and insulin icodec (once-weekly insulin Awiqli now approved in many countries, but USA for type 2 diabetes only). Thomas is also a long-time pioneer in glucose-sensitive insulin science. In 2012, Thomas was appointed adjunct professor at University of Copenhagen, and he has supervised multiple students and postdocs from Denmark, United Kingdom, Holland, Greece, and United States. In 2023, Thomas was hired by Protomer Technologies and E. Lilly in Pasadena, Los Angeles, California.

References

1 Banting, F.G., Best, C.H., Collip, J.B. et al. (1922). Pancreatic extracts in the treatment of diabetes mellitus. *Can. Med. Assoc. J.* 12 (3): 141–146.

2 Kurtzhals, P., Nishimura, E., Haahr, H. et al. (2021). Commemorating insulin's centennial: engineering insulin pharmacology towards physiology. *Trends Pharmacol. Sci.* 42 (8): 620–639. https://doi.org/10.1016/j.tips.2021.05.005.

3 Hoeg-Jensen, T. (2021). Review: glucose-sensitive insulin. *Mol Metab.* 46: 101107. https://doi.org/10.1016/j.molmet.2020.101107.

4 Polonsky, K.S., Given, B.D., and Van Cauter, E. (1988). Twenty-four-hour profiles and pulsatile patterns of insulin secretion in normal and obese subjects. *J. Clin. Invest.* 81 (2): 442–448. https://doi.org/10.1172/jci113339.

5 Zaykov, A.N., Mayer, J.P., and DiMarchi, R.D. (2016). Pursuit of a perfect insulin. *Nat. Rev. Drug Discov.* 15 (6): 425–439. https://doi.org/10.1038/nrd.2015.36.
6 Sims, E.K., Carr, A.L.J., Oram, R.A. et al. (2021). 100 years of insulin: celebrating the past, present and future of diabetes therapy. *Nat. Med.* 27 (7): 1154–1164. https://doi.org/10.1038/s41591-021-01418-2.
7 Irwin, D.M. (2021). Evolution of the insulin gene: changes in gene number, sequence, and processing. *Front. Endocrinol. (Lausanne)* 12: 649255. https://doi.org/10.3389/fendo.2021.649255.
8 Reeves, W.G. and Kelly, U. (1982). Insulin antibodies induced by bovine insulin therapy. *Clin. Exp. Immunol.* 50 (1): 163–170.
9 Morihara, K., Oka, T., and Tsuzuki, H. (1979). Semi-synthesis of human insulin by trypsin-catalysed replacement of Ala-B30 by Thr in porcine insulin. *Nature* 280 (5721): 412–413. https://doi.org/10.1038/280412a0.
10 Markussen, J., Damgaard, U., Pingel, M. et al. (1983). Human insulin (Novo): chemistry and characteristics. *Diabetes Care* 6 (Suppl 1): 4–8.
11 Goeddel, D.V., Kleid, D.G., Bolivar, F. et al. (1979). Expression in Escherichia coli of chemically synthesized genes for human insulin. *Proc. Natl. Acad. Sci. USA* 76 (1): 106–110. https://doi.org/10.1073/pnas.76.1.106.
12 Adams, M.J., Blundell, T.L., Dodson, E.J. et al. (1969). Structure of rhombohedral 2 zinc insulin crystals. *Nature* 224 (5218): 491–495. https://doi.org/10.1038/224491a0.
13 Brange, J., Ribel, U., Hansen, J.F. et al. (1988). Monomeric insulins obtained by protein engineering and their medical implications. *Nature* 333 (6174): 679–682. https://doi.org/10.1038/333679a0.
14 DiMarchi, R.D., Chance, R.E., Long, H.B. et al. (1994). Preparation of an insulin with improved pharmacokinetics relative to human insulin through consideration of structural homology with insulin-like growth factor I. *Horm. Res.* 41 (Suppl 2): 93–96. https://doi.org/10.1159/000183967.
15 Chance, R.E., Dimarchi, R.D., Frank, B.H.et al. (1993). Insulin analogs modified at position 29 of the B chain. Patent Application US5618913.
16 Lindholm, A. and Jacobsen, L.V. (2001). Clinical pharmacokinetics and pharmacodynamics of insulin aspart. *Clin. Pharmacokinet.* 40 (9): 641–659. https://doi.org/10.2165/00003088-200140090-00002.
17 Brange, J., Norris, K., Hansen, M.T., Novo, A.S.1986). Insulin analogues. Patent Application US5618913.
18 Norup, E., Langkjaer, L., Havelund, S., Novo Nordisk, A.S.1997). Insulin preperations containing NaCl. Patent Application WO1997048414.
19 Becker, R.H. (2007). Insulin glulisine complementing basal insulins: a review of structure and activity. *Diabetes Technol. Ther.* 9 (1): 109–121. https://doi.org/10.1089/dia.2006.0035.
20 Ertl, J., Habermann, P., Geisen, K.et al. (1998). Insulin derivatives having a rapid onset of action. Patent Application US6221633.
21 Heise, T., Linnebjerg, H., Coutant, D. et al. (2020). Ultra rapid lispro lowers postprandial glucose and more closely matches normal physiological glucose response compared to other rapid insulin analogues: a phase 1 randomized,

crossover study. *Diabetes Obes. Metab.* 22 (10): 1789–1798. https://doi.org/10.1111/dom.14094.

22 Kildegaard, J., Buckley, S.T., Nielsen, R.H. et al. (2019). Elucidating the mechanism of absorption of fast-acting insulin aspart: the role of niacinamide. *Pharm. Res.* 36 (3): 49. https://doi.org/10.1007/s11095-019-2578-7.

23 Olsen, H.B., Havelund, S., Ribel, U.et al. (2010). Preparation comprising insulin, nicotinamide and an amino acid. Patent Application WO2010149772.

24 Christie, M.E., Hardy, T.A.; Eli, Lilly, and Company. (2015). Rapid-acting insulin composition. Patent Application WO2015171484.

25 Hagedorn, H.C. (1937). Protamine insulinate: (Section of therapeutics and pharmacology). *Proc. R. Soc. Med.* 30 (6): 805–814.

26 Roach, P. and Woodworth, J.R. (2002). Clinical pharmacokinetics and pharmacodynamics of insulin lispro mixtures. *Clin. Pharmacokinet.* 41 (13): 1043–2057. https://doi.org/10.2165/00003088-200241130-00003.

27 Pieber, T.R., Eugène-Jolchine, I., and Derobert, E. (2000). Efficacy and safety of HOE 901 versus NPH insulin in patients with type 1 diabetes. The European Study Group of HOE 901 in type 1 diabetes. *Diabetes Care* 23 (2): 157–162. https://doi.org/10.2337/diacare.23.2.157.

28 Dorchung M, Hoechst. (1988). A21 B30 modified insulin derivatives having an altered action profile. Patent Application DE3837825.

29 Langkjar, L., Norris, K., Markussen, J. et al. (1988). A21 insulin derivatives. Patent Application WO198806599.

30 Becker, R.H., Dahmen, R., Bergmann, K. et al. (2015). New insulin glargine 300 units mL-1 provides a more even activity profile and prolonged glycemic control at steady state compared with insulin glargine 100 units · mL-1. *Diabetes Care* 38 (4): 637–643. https://doi.org/10.2337/dc14-0006.

31 Kurtzhals, P., Havelund, S., Jonassen, I. et al. (1996). Albumin binding and time action of acylated insulins in various species. *J. Pharm. Sci.* 85 (3): 304–308. https://doi.org/10.1021/js950412j.

32 Markussen, J., Jonassen, I., Havelund, S.et al. (1996). Insulin derivatives. Patent Application WO1996029344.

33 Havelund, S., Halstrom, J., Jonassen, I.et al. (1995). Acylated insulin. Patent Application US5750497.

34 Havelund, S., Plum, A., Ribel, U. et al. (2004). The mechanism of protraction of insulin detemir, a long-acting, acylated analog of human insulin. *Pharm. Res.* 21 (8): 1498–1504. https://doi.org/10.1023/b:pham.0000036926.54824.37.

35 Kurtzhals, P., Oestergaard, S., Nishimura, E., and Kjeldsen, T. (2023). Derivatization with fatty acids in peptide and protein drug discovery. *Nat. Rev. Drug Discov.* 22 (1): 59–80. https://doi.org/10.1038/s41573-022-00529-w.

36 Russell-Jones, D., Danne, T., Hermansen, K. et al. (2015). Weight-sparing effect of insulin detemir: a consequence of central nervous system-mediated reduced energy intake? *Diabetes Obes. Metab.* 17 (10): 919–927. https://doi.org/10.1111/dom.12493.

37 Hermansen, K. and Davies, M. (2007). Does insulin detemir have a role in reducing risk of insulin-associated weight gain? *Diabetes Obes. Metab.* 9 (3): 209–217. https://doi.org/10.1111/j.1463-1326.2006.00665.x.

38 Brand, C.L. and Sturis, J. (2023). Probing the mechanism of reduced in vivo potency of insulin detemir. *Expert Opin. Drug Metab. Toxicol.* 19 (4): 225–228. https://doi.org/10.1080/17425255.2023.2219389.

39 Jonassen, I., Havelund, S., Hoeg-Jensen, T. et al. (2012). Design of the novel protraction mechanism of insulin degludec, an ultra-long-acting basal insulin. *Pharm. Res.* 29 (8): 2104–2114. https://doi.org/10.1007/s11095-012-0739-z.

40 Jonassen, I., Hoeg-Jensen, T., Havelund, S.et al. (2005). Novel insulin derivatives. Patent Application WO2005012347.

41 Josse, R.G. and Woo, V. (2013). Flexibly timed once-daily dosing with degludec: a new ultra-long-acting basal insulin. *Diabetes Obes. Metab.* 15 (12): 1077–1084. https://doi.org/10.1111/dom.12114.

42 Havelund, S., Ribel, U., Hubálek, F. et al. (2015). Investigation of the physico-chemical properties that Enable Co.-formulation of basal insulin degludec with fast-acting insulin aspart. *Pharm. Res.* 32 (7): 2250–2258. https://doi.org/10.1007/s11095-014-1614-x.

43 Rosenstock, J., Juneja, R., Beals, J.M. et al. (2024). The basis for weekly insulin therapy: evolving evidence with insulin Icodec and insulin Efsitora Alfa. *Endocr. Rev.* 1–35. https://doi.org/10.1210/endrev/bnad037.

44 Lau, J., Bloch, P., Schaffer, L. et al. (2015). Discovery of the once-weekly glucagon-like peptide-1 (GLP-1) analogue semaglutide. *J. Med. Chem.* 58 (18): 7370–7380. https://doi.org/10.1021/acs.jmedchem.5b00726.

45 Coskun, T., Sloop, K.W., Loghin, C. et al. (2018). LY3298176, a novel dual GIP and GLP-1 receptor agonist for the treatment of type 2 diabetes mellitus: from discovery to clinical proof of concept. *Mol Metab.* 18: 3–14. https://doi.org/10.1016/j.molmet.2018.09.009.

46 Kjeldsen, T.B., Hubálek, F., Hjoerringgaard, C.U. et al. (2021). Molecular engineering of insulin icodec, the first acylated insulin analog for once-weekly administration in humans. *J. Med. Chem.* 64 (13): 8942–8950. https://doi.org/10.1021/acs.jmedchem.1c00257.

47 Madsen, P., Kjeldsen, T.B., Hoeg-Jensen, T.et al. (2009). Protease stablized, acylated insulin analogues. Patent Application WO2009115469.

48 Hubálek, F., Cramer, C.N., Helleberg, H. et al. (2024). Enhanced disulphide bond stability contributes to the once-weekly profile of insulin icodec. *Nat. Commun.* 15 (1): 6124. https://doi.org/10.1038/s41467-024-50477-9.

49 Philis-Tsimikas, A., Bajaj, H.S., Begtrup, K. et al. (2023). Rationale and design of the phase 3a development programme (ONWARDS 1–6 trials) investigating once-weekly insulin icodec in diabetes. *Diabetes Obes. Metab.* 25 (2): 331–341. https://doi.org/10.1111/dom.14871.

50 Moyers, J.S., Hansen, R.J., Day, J.W. et al. (2022). Preclinical characterization of LY3209590, a novel weekly basal insulin Fc-fusion protein. *J. Pharmacol. Exp. Ther.* 382 (3): 346–355. https://doi.org/10.1124/jpet.122.001105.

51 Baldwin, D.B., Beals, J.M., Day, J.W.et al. (2016). Insulin fusions. Patent Application WO2016178905.

52 Steiner, D.F., Cunningham, D., Spigelman, L., and Aten, B. (1967). Insulin biosynthesis: evidence for a precursor. *Science* 157 (3789): 697–700. https://doi.org/10.1126/science.157.3789.697.

53 Heise, T., Chien, J., Beals, J.M. et al. (2023). Pharmacokinetic and pharmacodynamic properties of the novel basal insulin Fc (insulin efsitora alfa), an insulin fusion protein in development for once-weekly dosing for the treatment of patients with diabetes. *Diabetes Obes. Metab.* 25 (4): 1080–1090. https://doi.org/10.1111/dom.14956.

54 Kazda, C.M., Bue-Valleskey, J.M., Chien, J. et al. (2023). Novel once-weekly basal insulin Fc achieved similar glycemic control with a safety profile comparable to insulin degludec in patients with type 1 diabetes. *Diabetes Care* 46 (5): 1052–1059. https://doi.org/10.2337/dc22-2395.

55 Wysham, C., Bajaj Harpreet, S., Del Prato, S. et al. Insulin Efsitora versus Degludec in type 2 diabetes without previous insulin treatment. *N. Engl. J. Med.* https://doi.org/10.1056/NEJMoa2403953.

56 Moore, M.C., Smith, M.S., Sinha, V.P. et al. (2014). Novel PEGylated basal insulin LY2605541 has a preferential hepatic effect on glucose metabolism. *Diabetes* 63 (2): 494–504. https://doi.org/10.2337/db13-0826.

57 Beals, J.M., Cutler, G.B., Doyle, B.et al. (2009). Pegylated insulin lispro compounds. Patent Application WO2009152128.

58 Cusi, K., Sanyal, A.J., Zhang, S. et al. (2016). Different effects of basal insulin peglispro and insulin glargine on liver enzymes and liver fat content in patients with type 1 and type 2 diabetes. *Diabetes Obes. Metab.* 18 (Suppl 2): 50–58. https://doi.org/10.1111/dom.12751.

59 Gregory, J.M., Kraft, G., Scott, M.F. et al. (2019). Peripherally delivered hepatopreferential insulin analog insulin-406 mimics the hypoglycaemia-sparing effect of portal vein human insulin infusion in dogs. *Diabetes Obes. Metab.* 21 (10): 2294–2304. https://doi.org/10.1111/dom.13808.

60 Edgerton, D.S., Scott, M., Farmer, B. et al. (2019). Targeting insulin to the liver corrects defects in glucose metabolism caused by peripheral insulin delivery. *JCI Insight* 5 (7): https://doi.org/10.1172/jci.insight.126974.

61 Weinstock, R.S., Bode, B.W., Garg, S.K. et al. (2022). Reduced hypoglycaemia using liver-targeted insulin in individuals with type 1 diabetes. *Diabetes Obes. Metab.* 24 (9): 1762–1769. https://doi.org/10.1111/dom.14761.

62 Olsen, G.S., Hansen, B.F., Schaffer, L.et al. (2019). Functionally selective insulin. Patent Application WO2019034726.

63 Lin, S., Yan, L., Huo, P.et al. (2016). Insulin receptor partial agonists. Patent Application WO2016081670.

64 Pissarnitski, D.A., Kekec, A., Yan, L. et al. (2022). Discovery of insulin receptor partial agonists MK-5160 and MK-1092 as novel basal insulins with potential to improve therapeutic index. *J. Med. Chem.* 65 (7): 5593–5605. https://doi.org/10.1021/acs.jmedchem.1c02073.

65 Miyakoshi, M., Kamoi, K., Iwanaga, M. et al. (2007). Comparison of patient's preference, pain perception, and usability between Micro Fine Plus 31-gauge needle and Microtapered NanoPass 33-gauge needle for insulin therapy. *J. Diabetes Sci. Technol.* 1 (5): 718–724. https://doi.org/10.1177/193229680700100516.

66 Brayden, D.J. (2021). The centenary of the discovery of insulin: an update on the quest for oral delivery. Mini review. *Frontiers in Drug Delivery.* 1: https://doi.org/10.3389/fddev.2021.726675.

67 Kjeldsen, T.B., Hubálek, F., Tagmose, T.M. et al. (2021). Engineering of orally available, ultralong-acting insulin analogues: discovery of OI338 and OI320. *J. Med. Chem.* 64 (1): 616–628. https://doi.org/10.1021/acs.jmedchem.0c01576.

68 Hubálek, F., Refsgaard, H.H.F., Gram-Nielsen, S. et al. (2020). Molecular engineering of safe and efficacious oral basal insulin. *Nat. Commun.* 11 (1): 3746. https://doi.org/10.1038/s41467-020-17487-9.

69 Oleck, J., Kassam, S., and Goldman, J.D. (2016). Commentary: why was inhaled insulin a failure in the market? *Diabetes Spectr.* 29 (3): 180–184. https://doi.org/10.2337/diaspect.29.3.180.

70 Brownlee, M. and Cerami, A. (1979). A glucose-controlled insulin-delivery system: semisynthetic insulin bound to lectin. *Science* 206 (4423): 1190–1191. https://doi.org/10.1126/science.505005.

71 Zhang, Y. and Hung-Chieh, C.D. (2023). From natural insulin to designed analogs: a chemical biology exploration. *Chembiochem* 24 (24): e202300470. https://doi.org/10.1002/cbic.202300470.

72 Chen, Y.S., Gleaton, J., Yang, Y. et al. (2021). Insertion of a synthetic switch into insulin provides metabolite-dependent regulation of hormone-receptor activation. *Proc. Natl. Acad. Sci. USA* 118 (30): https://doi.org/10.1073/pnas.2103518118.

73 Sun, X. and James, T.D. (2015). Glucose sensing in supramolecular chemistry. *Chem. Rev.* 115 (15): 8001–8037. https://doi.org/10.1021/cr500562m.

74 Tromans, R.A., Carter, T.S., Chabanne, L. et al. (2019). A biomimetic receptor for glucose. *Nat. Chem.* 11 (1): 52–56. https://doi.org/10.1038/s41557-018-0155-z.

75 Hoeg-Jensen, T., Kruse, T., Brand, C.L. et al. (2024). Glucose-sensitive insulin with attenuation of hypoglycaemia. *Nature* 634 (8035): 944–951. https://doi.org/10.1038/s41586-024-08042-3.

76 Lin, S., Yan, L., Kekec, A.et al. (2015). Glucose-responsive insulin conjugates. Patent Application WO2015051052.

77 Murikipudi, S., Lancaster, T.M., Zion, T.C., Smartcells Inc.d. (2012). Uses of macrophage mannose receptor to screen compounds and uses of these compounds. Patent Application WO2012050822.

78 Kaarsholm, N.C., Lin, S., Yan, L. et al. (2018). Engineering glucose responsiveness into insulin. *Diabetes* 67 (2): 299–308. https://doi.org/10.2337/db17-0577.

79 Moore, M.C., Kelley, D.E., Camacho, R.C. et al. (2018). Superior glycemic control with a glucose-responsive insulin analog: hepatic and nonhepatic impacts. *Diabetes* 67 (6): 1173–1181. https://doi.org/10.2337/db18-0099.

80 Hoeg-Jensen, T., Behrens, C., Clo, E.et al. (2020). Glucose sensitive insulin derivatives. Patent Application WO2020201041.

81 Spencer, R.K., Chen, D., Mali, S.et al. (2022). Aromatic boron containing compounds and insulin analogs. Patent Application WO2022109078.
82 Freckmann, G., Waldenmaier, D., and Heinemann, L. (2024). Head-to-head evaluation of continuous glucose monitoring and automated insulin delivery systems: why are they not used more systematically? *J. Diabetes Sci. Technol.* 19322968241227976. https://doi.org/10.1177/19322968241227976.
83 Rodbard, D. (2016). Continuous glucose monitoring: a review of successes, challenges, and opportunities. *Diabetes Technol. Ther.* 18 Suppl 2 (Suppl 2): S3–S13. https://doi.org/10.1089/dia.2015.0417.
84 Yang, L., Hu, Z.M., Jiang, F.X., and Wang, W. (2022). Stem cell therapy for insulin-dependent diabetes: are we still on the road? *World J Stem Cells.* 14 (7): 503–512. https://doi.org/10.4252/wjsc.v14.i7.503.

7

Neuropeptide Y Receptor Ligands and Opportunities Within Diabetes and Obesity

Søren Østergaard

Novo Nordisk A/S, Therapeutic Discovery, Novo Nordisk Research Park, 2760 Maalov, Denmark

The Neuropeptide Y (NPY) Peptide and Receptor Family

Neuropeptide Y (NPY), peptide YY (PYY), and pancreatic polypeptide (PP) are 36-amino acid peptides that play vital roles in various physiological processes, including appetite regulation, stress response, and neuroprotection [1]. They are commonly called the NPY family of peptides, sharing high sequence similarity (Figure 7.1) and the same 3-dimensional structure (Figure 7.2), known as the PP-fold [4]. This family of neuropeptides binds to and activates G protein-coupled receptors (GPCRs), called the NPY1, NPY2, NPY4, and NPY5 receptors (Y_1R, Y_2R, Y_4R, and Y_5R), which control a wide range of biological functions [5, 6]. Another subtype, y_6R (where "y" indicates that a functional role has not been established), has been identified and produces a functional receptor in rabbits and mice but is a pseudogene in humans and pigs and is absent in rats [7].

Neuropeptides NPY, PYY, and PP

The NPY family of peptides is especially notable for its role in energy balance and feeding behavior. NPY1-36 is one of the most potent orexigenic peptides, promoting appetite and food intake [8]. It is mainly produced in the central nervous system (CNS), particularly in the hypothalamus, where it interacts with neuropeptides like agouti-related peptide (AgRP) to regulate hunger and satiety [9, 10]. Aside from its role in appetite control, NPY has been associated with various stress-related and neurodegenerative disorders, and it has also been shown to cause vasoconstriction [11].

PYY_{1-36} is secreted by the enteroendocrine L-cells located in the distal gut [12], particularly in response to food intake. The inhibition of food intake by peripheral administration of PYY in humans was demonstrated in the early 2000s [13]. This satiety effect of PYY is also observed in rodents and can be inhibited by specific Y_2R antagonists, but not by Y_1R or Y_4R antagonists [14]. Beyond its role in appetite

	1 10 20 30
NPY_{1-36}	YPSKPDNPGEDAPAEDMARYYSALRHYINLITRQRY-$CONH_2$
PYY_{1-36}	YPIKPEAPGEDASPEELNRYYASLRHYLNLVTRQRY-$CONH_2$
PP_{1-36}	APLEPVYPGDNATPEQMAQYAADLRRYINMLTRPRY-$CONH_2$

Figure 7.1 The primary structure of human NPY, PYY, and PP.

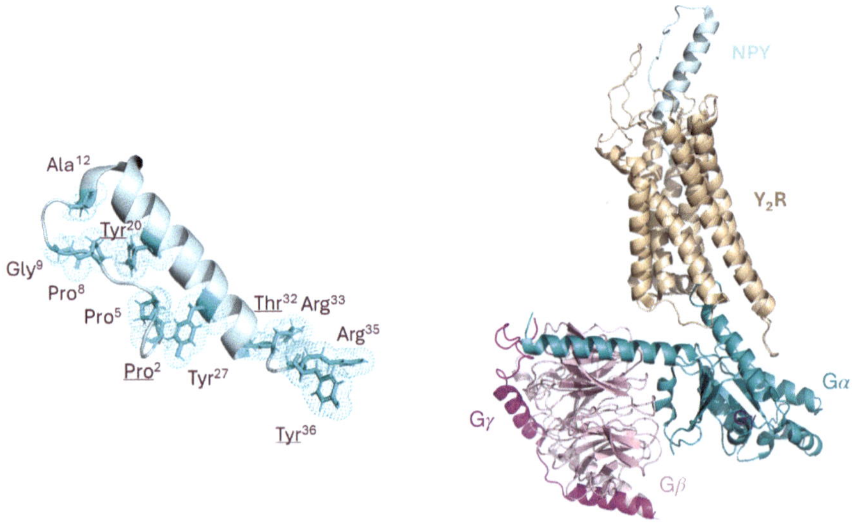

Figure 7.2 Structure of PYY_{1-36} (a) as measured by NMR, 2DEZ [2], and NPY in complex with Y_2R and its intracellular interaction with the G proteins (b), 7X9B [3]. Residues highlighted are conserved among all species in all three peptides NPY, PYY, and PP.

regulation, PYY has been implicated in various physiological processes, including gastrointestinal motility and bone metabolism. Like glucagon-like peptide-1 (GLP-1), it acts as an "ileal brake," slowing gastric emptying and enhancing nutrient absorption. This function is critical in energy balance, as it helps regulate the rate at which food leaves the stomach and enters the intestines, thereby influencing overall energy intake.

PP_{1-36} is primarily secreted by the F cells of the pancreatic islets of Langerhans [15]. Its biological functions are diverse and play a crucial role in regulating various physiological processes. One primary function of PP is to inhibit pancreatic exocrine secretion, reducing the release of digestive enzymes and modulating digestion. Additionally, PP has been shown to slow gastric emptying and decrease food intake, contributing to its role in controlling appetite and maintaining energy balance. Moreover, PP interacts with other hormones in the pancreatic environment, especially somatostatin and insulin. It has been documented that PP inhibits somatostatin secretion, which influences the release of insulin and glucagon [16]. This interaction indicates that PP is a key regulator of digestive function and plays an essential role in maintaining stable glucose levels by modulating the secretion of other pancreatic hormones.

All three peptides are characterized by a C-terminal amidation, which is crucial for their biological activity. Even minor changes to the C-terminus have a detrimental effect on the binding affinity. As NPY_{1-36} and PYY_{1-36} are structurally very similar, the binding specificity is also very similar, as both bind with high affinity to the Y_1R, Y_2R, and Y_5R but much less to Y_4R. However, as PYY_{1-36} rapidly gets cleaved to PYY_{3-36} by dipeptidylpeptidase IV (DPPIV), the affinity toward Y_1R is reduced by approximately two orders of magnitude. PP_{1-36}, on the other hand, is much more selective toward the Y_4R. All three peptides bind to their receptors via their highly conserved C-termini, which are deeply buried in a binding pocket [3]. However, as the peptides are homologous and share the same binding mode, clever amino acid substitutions can lead to altered, dual, or triple specificity by substituting key residues in the C-terminus that interact with the receptor [17].

NPY Receptors and Distribution

The sequence identity among NPY receptors is particularly fascinating, reflecting the evolutionary pressures that have shaped their functional roles. Despite their structural differences, Y_1R, Y_2R, and Y_5R have maintained essential functional features and all bind NPY with high affinity [3]. For 40 years, the NPY receptor family has been a significant focus of research in neurobiology and physiology, particularly for its role in various physiological processes. These receptors are found throughout the central and peripheral nervous systems, enabling these peptides to influence diverse functions such as energy balance, appetite, metabolic regulation, stress-related behaviors, and bone control [18].

The Y_1R is primarily located in the CNS, especially in the hypothalamus, which regulates food intake and energy balance. The arcuate nucleus of the hypothalamus is a critical area where NPY neurons produce and release NPY, which then acts on Y_1R to increase appetite and promote weight gain [8]. Additionally, the activation of Y_1R by NPY may also involve ghrelin, as this peptide hormone has been shown to stimulate NPY expression, adding complexity to the interaction between peptide hormones [19]. Furthermore, Y_1R is found in various brain regions, including the amygdala and hippocampus, where they are believed to influence anxiety and stress-related behaviors [20].

Y_2R is more widely distributed in the brain, as well as in sympathetic and parasympathetic nerve fibers. It is highly expressed in the hypothalamus, especially in the paraventricular nucleus (PVN) and other hypothalamic areas that regulate food intake and energy balance. In the periphery, Y_2R is present in adipose tissue, the intestine [21], and pancreatic islets.

The Y_4R is less well understood than the Y_1R and Y_2R receptors, but it is known to regulate feeding behavior and energy balance. Y_4R is expressed in the hypothalamus and is believed to interact with other neuropeptides to control appetite. However, Y_4R is primarily found in the periphery, such as the gastrointestinal tract, where it may affect gut motility and secretion [21, 22]. Therefore, the presence of Y_4R in both central and peripheral tissues indicates a complex role in energy regulation and metabolic processes.

Lastly, the Y_5R is mainly linked to the CNS, especially in areas involved in appetite control, like the hypothalamus [23]. Y_5R is thought to mediate the orexigenic effects of NPY, encouraging increased food consumption and weight gain [24]. Besides its role in appetite, Y_5R may also be involved in anxiety and stress responses, with research suggesting that its activation can affect emotions.

Knockout Studies in Rodents

Genetic studies using animal knockout models have also explored the importance of NPY receptors in feeding behavior, stress, and other CNS effects. These studies have involved knocking out peptide ligands (NPY, PYY, or PP) or one or more receptors. While some studies offer insights into biological functions, others challenge previous findings.

In some cases, the effects observed when ligands are administered to animals via intracerebroventricular (ICV) injection or peripheral administration do not correspond to those observed in the knockout model. For instance, it is well established that Y_1R agonism by NPY and analogs leads to orexigenic effects. However, studies with Y_1R knockout (KO) mice show a more complex story. While the knockout experiments demonstrate that elimination of the Y_1R can attenuate the effect of acutely administered NPY on food intake, only a modest reduction of daily food intake was observed in the Y_1R knockout mice [25].

In a PYY knockout mouse model, marked obesity was developed, which was reversed by exogenous PYY treatment [26]. Equally, another PYY knockout study in mice led to the development of hyperinsulinemia and obesity [27]. However, other studies have shown either no effect or the opposite effect. A germline Y_2R knockout in mice resulted in a modest increase in body weight [28]. In contrast, a conditional hypothalamus-specific Y_2R knockout showed a significant decrease in body weight but an increase in food intake [29]. However, in studies, the absence of peripheral Y_2R seemed to protect against high-fat diet-induced obesity [30]. Other KO studies demonstrated a synergistic attenuation of obesity in Y_2R and Y_4R double-knockout mice, ob/ob and normal, indicating that antagonizing Y_2R and Y_4R would reduce overweight [31, 32]. These findings contradict the current understanding that Y_2R agonism by peripheral administration of an Y_2R agonist reduces weight. While knockout animal studies have significantly advanced our knowledge of biology, they are thus not without limitations. The potential for compensatory mechanisms or developmental adaptations in knockout animals can complicate the interpretation of results. Furthermore, the above-described conflicting results between transgenic or knockout models and ligand administration must be considered when describing the physiological role of NPY peptides and their cognate receptors [33]. Additionally, the fact that NPY peptides have relatively poor selectivity further complicates the interpretation of results. For example, ICV injection of PYY_{1-36} shows that PYY can stimulate food intake rather than inhibit it [34], likely due to the poor selectivity of PYY_{1-36}, which binds to Y_1R, Y_5R, and Y_2R.

Y_1R/Y_5R Agonism

The discovery of peptide NPY dates back to 1982, when it was first isolated from the porcine brain and shown to be widely distributed in the CNS, serving as a neurotransmitter or neuromodulator [10, 35]. It has been shown to play a crucial role in various physiological processes, including appetite regulation, circadian rhythms, and stress response. This groundbreaking work identified NPY as a member of the NPY family, which also includes PYY and PP. The initial characterization of NPY revealed its significant sequence homology with other family members, indicating a highly conserved evolutionary function across species [9].

NPY has been extensively studied, focusing on its sequence, structure-activity relationships (SAR), and interactions with various NPY receptors. Understanding the structure of NPY and its binding mechanisms to these receptors has been essential for clarifying its interactions and providing insights into how PYY and PP also interact with the Y_2R and Y_4R, respectively. The introduction of the Fmoc (9-fluorenylmethyloxycarbonyl) solid-phase peptide synthesis (SPPS) method in 1981 by Atherton and Sheppard revolutionized peptide chemistry. It significantly increased interest in the synthesis of biologically active peptides [36]. The chemical synthesis of NPY peptides is relatively straightforward, and high-quality peptides can be produced via SPPS, due to their high proline content. Mild deprotection conditions make automation easier, allowing rapid and efficient synthesis of many peptides, thereby expanding the usefulness of SPPS to more laboratories than the previous Boc SPPS approach. From the late 1980s through the 1990s and into the early 2000s, numerous influential papers on the synthesis and pharmacological testing of NPY peptides were published, particularly by the Beck-Sickinger group, totaling over 150 publications on NPY SAR. By systematically modifying specific amino acid residues within the peptide backbone, researchers have identified several critical residues necessary for binding and activating each receptor subtype.

It was soon shown that both the N- and C-termini are essential for NPY's function when binding to the Y_1R [37]. In contrast, the central regions of NPY can be removed without losing potency [38], yielding effective analogs. Regarding the C-terminus, only a few residues can be substituted without losing activity, a trait shared by PYY and PP as well [39]. Using the chemical versatility of SPPS, many analogs have been created, highlighting the importance of specific residues and enabling the development of smaller analogs or those that selectively target particular receptor subtypes. For instance, some analogs have been designed to be more selective for the Y_1R than NPY itself [17].

The activation of Y_1R in the hypothalamus, especially within the arcuate nucleus, is crucial for NPY's orexigenic effects, which include increased food intake and energy expenditure [8]. Overexpression of NPY, particularly in the brain, has led to increased food consumption in rats on a high-calorie diet [40]. Furthermore, higher levels of NPY have been observed in the hypothalamus of diabetic rats, suggesting a potential role in the neuroendocrine dysfunction associated with insulin deficiency [41].

Studies have shown that NPY's effects on appetite are mediated not only through Y_1R but also through Y_5R [23, 24]. Both NPY_{1-36} and PYY_{1-36} exhibit similar affinity and are considered the main ligands for Y_5R. However, while PYY_{3-36} loses affinity about fivefold for Y_5R, the loss in affinity for NPY_{3-36} is around 100-fold, indicating that NPY and PYY interact differently with Y_5R [42, 43], with the former being the primary endogenous Y_5R ligand.

The affinity of PP_{1-36} for Y_1R is lower than that of NPY_{1-36} and PYY_{1-36}, which bind approximately slightly more than one order of magnitude less to Y_1R than NPY_{1-36} and PP_{1-36}. Interestingly, the low affinity of PP1-36 for Y_1R can be increased by substituting Pro^{34} with $NMeGln^{34}$, making PP's affinity comparable to that of the other two peptides [43]. The same improvement is not seen for $[Gln^{34}]PP$, indicating that cis/trans isomerization in peptide bond 34–35, along with the side chain of Gln^{34}, affects Y_1R interaction, as $NMeAla^{34}$ shows slightly lower affinity than $NMeGln^{34}$ toward Y_1R [43]. NPY_{1-36} can be made selective for Y_5R by replacing Ile^{31} and Thr^{32} with Ala^{31} and Aib^{32} [44]. As an Y_5R-selective agonist, this modified analog modestly increases food intake in a dose-dependent manner in acute settings, likely due to its moderate affinity for Y_5R relative to native NPY_{1-36} [45]. In the same study, another more potent Y_5R analog, $[cyclicPP_{1-7}, NPY_{19-23}, Ala^{31}, Aib^{32}, Gln^{34}]hPP_{1-36}$, was shown to stimulate food intake more effectively, suggesting that Y_5R could be an important target for increasing food intake and potentially useful in conditions like cachexia, with fewer side effects than Y_1R agonists. However, a unique biological role for a selective Y_5R remains poorly defined beyond its moderate orexigenic effect, and long-term treatment with an Y_5R-specific peptide has not yet been reported to fully explore the potential of Y_5R agonism.

Y_1R/Y_5R Antagonists for Diabetes or Obesity Treatment

The discovery that NPY stimulates food intake through Y_1R and Y_5R agonism also increased interest in its potential use in weight management by targeting these receptors with antagonists [46]. A rat study showed that the food-reducing effect of a specific Y_1R antagonist, administered directly into the hypothalamus, is more potent in fasted rats compared to NPY-treated, satiated rats [47]. Because NPY plays a complex role in many CNS effects, it is not surprising that CNS side effects could be expected from small-molecule Y_1R antagonists, which dampened interest in developing Y_1R antagonists for obesity treatment.

However, it has been shown that Y_1R signaling inhibits insulin release in β-cells, which could be exploited pharmacologically to increase insulin secretion [48]. Therefore, Y_1R antagonism might offer a new opportunity for treating type 2 diabetes mellitus (T2DM). Mechanistically, Y_1R signaling decreases cyclic adenosine monophosphate (cAMP) production in islets, thereby downregulating key enzymes involved in glycolysis and ATP generation. As a result, modulating Y_1R signaling in β-cells could provide a distinct therapeutic approach to address insulin deficiency seen in diabetes and during islet transplantation. Furthermore, increased levels of NPY and Y_1R mRNA in human islets are associated with reduced insulin secretion in human T2DM [49]. This suggests that Y_1R antagonism may help protect β-cells by improving their function and promoting better glycemic control in T2DM. For example, the Y_1R antagonist BIB03304 improved hyperglycemia and insulin sensitivity and preserved β-cell mass in low-dose streptozotocin (STZ)-induced and db/db T2DM mice [49]. In another study involving type 1 diabetic NOD mice, Y_1R antagonism with BIB03304 improved glycemic control after islet transplantation and delayed the onset of T1D [48]. The use of Y_1R antagonists should be limited to peripheral effects to avoid impacts on the CNS. For instance, BIB03304, administered intracerebroventricularly (ICV), inhibits NPY's anxiolytic effects via Y_1R in the central amygdala [50]. Therefore, for safety reasons, there may be potential for Y_1R antagonists that do not cross the blood–brain barrier and thus act solely in the periphery. However, BIB03304 has also been shown to lower blood pressure [51] and marginally increase bone mass in mice [52]. This suggests that peripheral Y_1R antagonism may affect physiological parameters beyond glucose metabolism. Another example is BMS-193885, a potent, selective, brain-penetrant Y_1R antagonist that has been shown to reduce food intake and body weight in animal models of obesity [53]. Whether Y1R antagonism will generate renewed interest in the treatment of diabetes or obesity remains to be seen.

Therefore, focus shifted to designing Y_5R antagonists (Figure 7.3) that could be shown to reduce food intake in rodents [54, 55], while CNS-related side effects might be fewer than those seen with Y_1R. However, other studies contradicted these results

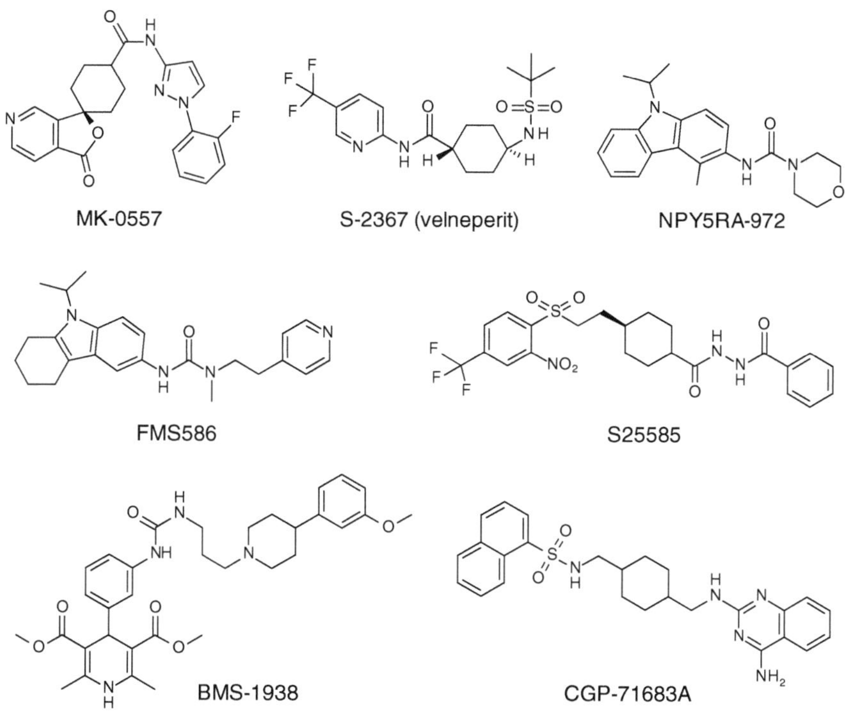

Figure 7.3 Overview of Y_5R antagonists used in clinical trials or animal studies.

regarding rodent food intake [56, 57]. Nonetheless, big pharma pursued Y_5R antagonists and advanced them into clinical trials. Sadly, Y_5R antagonists also failed to produce clinically significant weight loss in overweight adults [58, 59], and presently, no active Y_5R antagonists are in development for obesity.

PP and Y_4R Interaction

PP is the most selective of the NPY peptides as it binds with high affinity to only the Y_4R and orders of magnitude less to the Y_1R and Y_2R, while the binding to the Y_5R is on par with PYY_{3-36}. The F-cells of the pancreatic islets secrete it in response to food intake, and thus, it is believed to play a role in regulating appetite and energy balance [15]. Compared to NPY and PYY, PP is almost entirely localized in the intestinal tract, with more than 90% found in the pancreas [15]. It was shown early that PP given to children with Prader-Willi syndrome reduced their food intake [60]. Later, a key study by Batterham et al. in 2003 showed that intravenous administration of PP reduced appetite and food intake among regular participants. In obese subjects, short-term aerobic exercise training increased postprandial PP levels, suggesting that physical activity may enhance satiety signaling via the PP pathway [61].

In a study with transgenic mice, overexpression of PP, food intake, and body weight were reduced [62]. In another study, PP administered intraperitoneally (ip) reduced food intake in freely fed and fasted mice in a dose-dependent manner, and this effect is mediated through Y_4R, since it is greatly abolished in $Y_4R-/-$ mice [63]. Intriguingly, dual Y_4R and Y_2R agonism can be engineered rather easily. By substituting Pro^{34} in PP with Gln^{34}, a dual-acting Y_4R/Y_2R analog has been reported, albeit that the Y_4R binding was negatively affected by approximately one order of magnitude. Some of the earliest clinical exploration of NPY peptides for food-lowering was, in fact, an Y_2R/Y_4R dual agonist. 7TM Pharma in the mid-2000s developed two NPY peptides for obesity; a dual-acting Y_2R/Y_4R (TM303338) and a pure Y_4R agonist (TM30339). Both peptides were derivatized with a fatty acid (palmitic acid γGlu as in liraglutide), thus suitable for once-daily dosing only. Both peptides were found to be safe and well tolerated in phase I trials; however, they showed disappointing efficacy in humans, leading to the termination of both trials. Nevertheless, 7TM Pharma was pioneering the field as one of the first companies to recognize the potential of Y_2R or Y_4R agonism in obesity and to combine this with fatty acid (palmitic) derivatization technology to extend the half-life of a peptide drug suitable for once-daily dosing. While PP has been shown to decrease food intake, PYY is today considered a far more effective satiety hormone than PP, which is reflected by the fact that many more papers have shown weight or food-lowering effects by peripheral administration of PYY analogs than with PP analogs. As discussed later, an unrealized problem was the plasma instability of the C-terminus of PYY and, thus, the need for a fatty acid-derivatized $[Gln^{34}]$PP analog. However, some protection is obtained by fatty acid derivatization [64].

Still, Y_4R agonism is a relatively unexplored target and may still hold promise, maybe even in other indications. In a rat study, a peptide-based dual Y_1R

antagonist/Y_4R agonist elicited a dose-dependent surge of both luteinizing hormone (LH) and follicle-stimulating hormone (FSH) lasting up to six hours [65]. As a standalone, Y_1R antagonist could not elicit the same response, suggesting that the effect was mediated by Y_4R agonism. Recently, twice-daily injection of [Pro^3]PP was shown to improve beta-cell turnover and islet cell plasticity, thereby helping to preserve pancreatic islet architecture following STZ-induced metabolic stress [66]. Reduced-sized agonists, as well as antagonists, have been successfully applied, notably the Y_4R. Picomolar affinity has been obtained by small dimer peptides (modified pentapeptides) of the C-terminal [67]. In a recent study, a modified C-terminal peptide fragment (Arg-Tyr-Arg-Leu-Arg-Tyr) was subjected to various cyclizations, yielding a macrocycle agonist with picomolar affinity [68].

PYY and Y_2R Interaction

PYY is, without any doubt, the most studied and promising peptide from the NPY family of peptides that are being explored in obesity and diabetes. PYY has been known for three decades since its discovery in 1982 by Tatemoto and colleagues in 1982 [69]. PYY is cosecreted with GLP-1 by the L-cells of the gastrointestinal tract, particularly in the ileum and colon, in response to food intake [70–72]. L-cells are widely distributed throughout the gut, and it was initially thought they were primarily located in the distal gut. Still, it is established that the human duodenum contains L-cells that secrete PYY and GLP-1 in response to glucose stimuli [73]. PYY circulates in two forms, PYY_{1-36} and PYY_{3-36}, with the latter being more Y_2R-selective.

Regulator of Food Energy Homeostasis

For almost two decades, PYY was viewed primarily as an acting gut hormone that regulates gastric and pancreatic secretion [74, 75] and gastrointestinal (GI) motility [76]. The discovery of the impact of peripheral PYY administration on food intake was made in the early 2000s, notably in landmark papers by Batterham et al. They provided the first evidence that PYY_{3-36} effectively reduces food intake in animals and in obese humans [13, 77]. Albeit there was a transient controversy concerning the reproducibility of the PYY findings [78], it is now well established that PYY plays an essential role in energy homeostasis in mammals. Generally, circulating PYY levels are low, reaching a minimum in the fasted state. However, PYY levels increase rapidly and proportionally in response to the amount of caloric intake [79] and type of macronutrients [80].

By acting on the Y_2R in the hypothalamus, PYY_{3-36} inhibits the release of NPY, which, as described before, is a potent orexigenic factor. This inhibition plays a crucial role in the central regulation of appetite, as it counteracts NPY-mediated hunger signals, thereby promoting satiety [81]. This implies a complex interaction between the Y_1R and Y_2R signaling pathways, as this functional paradox underscores the intricate interplay between NPY and PYY in energy homeostasis.

Moreover, as previously mentioned, inhibiting Y_1R activation in beta cells with a selective Y_1R antagonist preserves beta cells and enhances glycemic control in T2DM. This highlights the potential need for Y_2R selective analogs to achieve optimal efficacy in a long-acting analog within a drug-design context.

Over the past few decades, substantial evidence has emerged supporting the role of PYY_{3-36} in energy metabolism. Although native PYY_{3-36} administered subcutaneously has not provided compelling data due to poor pharmacokinetic properties, in vivo studies demonstrate significant weight loss when PYY is infused via pump or when modified analogs with extended half-lives are used. Notably, weight loss results are even more critical when PYY is combined with agents such as GLP-1 receptor agonists, which will be further discussed in later sections, achieving weight reductions exceeding 25%.

Regulator of Glucose Homeostasis

While the role of peptide YY (PYY) in energy homeostasis has long been recognized, emerging research highlights its equally important role in regulating glucose homeostasis. Intriguingly, PYY is coexpressed with glucagon in pancreatic α-cells and somatostatin in δ-cells, suggesting its potential involvement in the paracrine regulation of insulin secretion alongside other peptide hormones [82].

The precise mechanisms by which PYY_{3-36} analogs exert their antidiabetic effects remain unclear. However, studies have demonstrated that PYY_{3-36} can enhance insulin sensitivity in mouse models of insulin resistance. These studies utilized the hyperinsulinemic-euglycemic clamp technique and indicated benefits beyond weight loss, even when measured acutely, even in weight-matched animals [83–86].

A recent study evaluated a highly Y_2R-selective agonist in ZSF rats. This agonist, when combined with the GLP-1 receptor agonist semaglutide, was more effective at reducing HbA1c levels than semaglutide alone [87]. Furthermore, the study reported a statistically significant reduction in triglycerides when compared to treatment with the GLP-1 receptor agonist semaglutide alone. The specific pathways through which PYY_{3-36} influences glucose uptake in muscle and adipose tissue are not yet well characterized, offering opportunities for further research.

Lessons from Bariatric Surgery Support the Critical Role of PYY

Bariatric surgery has become a vital intervention for managing obesity and its related health conditions, especially T2DM [88]. Many studies show that bariatric surgery can lead to remission of T2DM within a few days in many patients. The surgery includes various procedures, such as Roux-en-Y gastric bypass (RYGB), gastric banding, and sleeve gastrectomy, all of which have proven effective in promoting weight loss and improving metabolic health. The benefits of bariatric surgery go beyond just weight loss; it greatly affects the secretion and action of gut hormones, which are key to metabolic regulation after surgery. Patients experience changes in hormones like ghrelin, GLP-1, and PYY. Research shows that gastric bypass surgery significantly lowers ghrelin levels, a hormone mainly produced in the stomach that stimulates appetite, while increasing the secretion of GLP-1 and PYY [89]. Nutrients in the gut trigger PYY secretion, and levels are especially high after RYGB, where the rapid delivery of nutrients to the lower intestine stimulates its release. Studies suggest that PYY may help enhance insulin secretion, thus aiding in diabetes remission after bariatric surgery [90]. Some rodent research indicates that GLP-1 might not be as critical for the metabolic benefits observed after RYGB, as it was equally effective in rats lacking the GLP-1 receptor [91]. In another diabetic rat model, RYGB quickly reversed diabetes, but GLP-1 levels did not rise, unlike PYY. Furthermore, the positive effects of RYGB persisted even when a GLP-1 blocker was used [92]. In a different rat study, PYY appeared to activate earlier than GLP-1 and glucose-dependent insulinotropic polypeptide (GIP), suggesting a key role in regulating GLP-1 release [93]. These studies are in rodents, so it remains uncertain how they translate to humans. Nonetheless, this has led to speculation that PYY, rather than GLP-1, might be an underestimated factor in the quick T2DM remission seen after RYGB [90]. Although increased levels of GLP-1 and PYY after bariatric surgery offer clear benefits, the variability in hormonal responses among individuals suggests that more research is needed. For example, unlike gastric bypass, gastric banding does not impact PYY and GLP-1 levels [94]. Some studies indicate that not all patients experience the same hormonal changes or weight-loss outcomes, suggesting that genetics, environment, and behavior may influence the effectiveness of bariatric surgery [95].

SAR and Y_2R Selective Agonists

Since activation of Y_1R and Y_5R leads to increased food intake, and Y_1R activation may also stress β cells, having an Y_2R-selective analog could offer more effective and safer options by also avoiding unwanted CNS-related side effects. Because PYY_{3-36} is more Y2R-selective than PYY_{1-36}, it was relatively early shown that N-terminal truncated NPY could be made even more Y_2R-specific, though with a gradual reduction in Y_2R affinity [96]. Some of the first smaller Y_2R-selective analogs were designed based on NPY or PYY [97–99], although they were less potent on Y_2R than the parent NPY/PYY. Interestingly, some gain in Y_2R potency was observed in PYY_{25-36} when adding benzoic acid-derived groups to the N-terminus [100]. Similarly, PYY_{22-36} was extensively modified with noncanonical amino acids, resulting in selective and potent Y_2R agonists [101]. The C-terminus is highly sensitive to modifications, including peptide bonds. A SAR study of the C-terminal region of PYY revealed that altering peptide bonds also negatively impacts Y_2R potency [102, 103]. Adding a methyl group to the amide nitrogen (N-methylation) in this region is tolerated only at positions 34 and 35 without significantly reducing Y_2R affinity or potency [43]. Since N-methylation not only improves selectivity toward Y_2R but also enhances resistance to enzymatic degradation, *N*MeArg^{35} was considered to offer a dual advantage: protection against C-terminal degradation in vivo and improved selectivity for Y_2R over Y_1R, although with a moderate decrease in affinity [43]. Surprisingly, canonical amino acid substitutions can also achieve this dual function, sometimes even providing better selectivity and potency at the Y_2R. Recent studies have shown that Trp^{30} alone increases Y_2R selectivity over Y_1R and can prevent C-terminal degradation; when combined with Tyr^{28} and Leu^{31}, these modifications produced some of the most specific and potent Y_2R agonists [87].

The question arises about how necessary Y_2R selectivity is for safety and whether it provides any benefits in terms of increased effectiveness. In a combination study using native PYY_{3-36} and a Y_2R-selective analog [Trp^{30}, β-homoArg^{35}]PYY_{3-36} with semaglutide, the more selective analog led to greater weight loss [104]. However, the number of animals was too small to draw definitive conclusions, and the selective analog also had the benefit of being resistant to C-terminal inactivation. In another study with Y_5R knockout mice, exposure to PYY_{3-36} caused significantly greater weight loss than in wild-type mice [105], suggesting that activation of Y_5R (by the less selective PYY_{3-36}) might oppose the Y_2R agonist effect. These findings indicate that selectivity might be necessary, especially when designing long-acting analogs.

Half-Life Extension of PYY Analogs

Peptides generally have very short half-lives due to their smaller molecular size and susceptibility to enzymatic degradation, and PYY is no exception. PYY_{1-36} is quickly cleaved into PYY_{3-36} by dipeptidylpeptidase IV (DPPVI), which is then rapidly degraded into PYY_{3-34} [106, 107], an inactivated form of PYY. From a peptide drug design perspective, it is therefore crucial to prevent this cleavage to PYY_{3-34} if long-acting analogs are to be developed.

Attaching a fatty diacid, as used in the GLP-1 analog semaglutide, at position 30 of PYY_{3-36} can minimize cleavage to PYY_{3-34}, although this reduces Y_2R affinity [108]. Alternatively, substituting Arg^{35} with either *N*MeArg^{35} or β-homoArg^{35} can prevent cleavage to PYY_{3-34}. However, this also slightly decreases Y_2R affinity and potency, though replacing Leu^{30} with Trp^{30} can partially recover Y_2R affinity. Interestingly, such noncanonical amino acids are not even necessary for stabilizing the C-terminus, as recent reports indicate that Trp^{30} alone can protect the C-terminus from degradation [87]. More constrained analog designs have also been proposed, such as bridging the fatty acid between two Cys residues ($i, i+7$), which yields potent and long-lasting PYY analogs [109].

However, even when the backbone is stabilized, the half-life remains very short, reaching only approximately 30 minutes due to kidney clearance. To reduce this renal clearance, attaching a long polyoxyethylene chain (PEG) of 20–40 kDa, known as PEGylation, was one of the initial techniques used on PYY to extend the half-life of PYY analogs [110–112]. Interestingly, early on, a method called "transient PEGylation" was applied to PYY_{3-36} by conjugating it to the N-terminus via an Fmoc group. This method gradually releases the PEG unit in plasma and restores the free N-terminal in PYY [110]. However, these PEGylated analogs were designed based on the native PYY backbone and did not address C-terminal stabilization. As a result, while the analog might evade renal clearance, it would still be susceptible to degradation. Conjugating PYY_{3-36} and truncated PYY analogs to albumin also increases hydrodynamic volume [113, 114]. For example, a truncated PYY analog was stabilized at the C-terminus and conjugated to albumin. However, due to the small size of the peptide and its conjugation to a much larger protein, both affinity and potency were significantly reduced, which might explain the need for high doses to produce an effect. Additionally, vitamin B12 has been used to enhance the efficacy of native PYY_{3-36}. By conjugating vitamin B12 to the Lys residue at position 4, some improvements in weight loss were observed compared with native PYY [115].

Fatty diacid derivatization has successfully been used to extend the half-life of peptides like semaglutide and tirzepatide [116]. Unsurprisingly, this technology has also been applied to PYY analogs. However, the position of the modification can influence both potency and half-life in the context of native PYY_{3-36} [108]. The position is critical not only for half-life but also for Y_2R potency. When conjugating a moiety to PYY_{3-36} – whether it be a fatty acid, PEG chain, or albumin – positions 7 and 10 seem the most tolerated in preserving Y_2R potency.

Obinepitide (7TM pharma) was the first Y_2R/Y_4R dual agonist to be published (as a patent), essentially a PP analog with a Gln^{34}, derivatized with a fatty monoacid (palmitic acid) at position 13. This peptide was not stabilized at the C-terminus, and the fatty acid's position was not optimal in the backbone. Not being a fatty diacid might explain the lack of efficacy observed. Unlike fatty monoacid derivatization, fatty diacid derivatization yields more efficacious peptides due to lower hydrophobicity and much stronger binding to albumin [116]. PYY analogs suitable for a once-weekly dosing regimen that have reached clinical phase 2 trials are PYY1875 (Novo Nordisk) [87] and nisotirostide (LY 3457263, Eli Lilly). Both are derivatized with a fatty C18 diacid at position 7, and the C-terminus stabilized by Trp at position 30 (Figure 7.4).

Y_2R Agonism and Combinations with Other Peptide Agonists

Since GLP-1 and PYY are cosecreted from the L-cells in response to food intake, it is not surprising that human studies have been conducted to investigate any additive or synergistic effects of administering both GLP-1 and PYY. In fact, this is the case. Administering GLP-1 or oxyntomodulin together with PYY_{3-36} has an additive effect on reducing food intake and increasing energy expenditure in humans [117–119]. A triple combination of GLP-1, oxyntomodulin, and PYY demonstrated superior glucose regulation in obese pre- and diabetic individuals and was at least comparable to RYGB [120]. Animal studies have also demonstrated increased effectiveness when GLP-1 and PYY are combined. In two mouse models of obese T2DM, long-acting GLP-1 and PYY, both fused to the Fc domain, together led to restored glucose homeostasis, significant weight loss, and recovery of endogenous β-cell function [85]. Although these earlier studies used loose combinations,

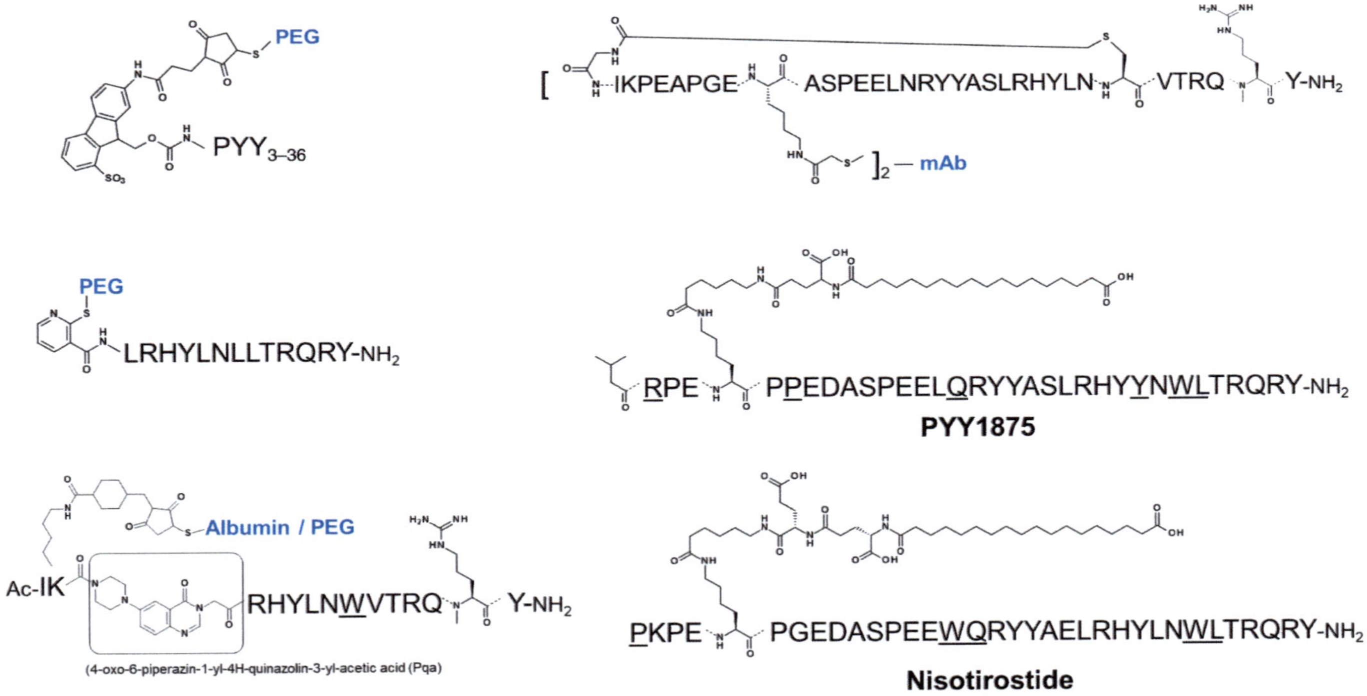

Figure 7.4 An overview of some of the various PYY analogs that have been modified to extend the half-life. Residues with an underline are different from native PYY_{3-36}.

subsequent reports describe single peptides with dual or triple receptor actions. By attaching the C-terminal part of PYY_{25-36} to exendin-4, a dual-acting GLP-1R and Y_2R agonist was developed [121], though its Y_2R affinity was moderate compared to native PYY_{3-36}. Conjugates between full-length GLP-1 and PYY_{3-36} analogs have also been created, showing increased efficacy in reducing food intake, body weight, and improving glucose regulation compared to GLP-1 alone [122–124]. Combining a dual-acting GLP-1/GIP peptide with the C-terminal part of PYY_{3-36} – featuring residues that enhance affinity and resist enzymatic degradation – has led to the development of triple agonists targeting GLP-1R, glucose-dependent insulinotropic polypeptide receptor (GIPR), and Y_2R [125]. Tri-agonists that incorporate Y_1R, Y_2R, and GLP-1R have also been reported. In this peptide, the C-terminal part of PYY_{25-36} was fused to a GLP-1 analog. Although including Y_1R may seem counterintuitive, given its orexigenic effects, weight loss was still observed [126]. Another tri-agonist designed to enhance energy expenditure is a GLP-1R/GCGR/Y_2R agonist [127]. Even quadruple (tetra-agonist) GLP-1R/GCGR/GIPR/Y_2R agonists have been reported [128].

The poly-agonists discussed earlier depend on attaching full-length PYY or PYY fragments to other hormones, such as GLP-1 or exendin-4. Although GLP-1 and PYY_{3-36} are not homologous, it is possible to engineer a dual-acting GLP-1 analog that includes specific residues from the C-terminus of PYY_{3-36}. These hybrids, matching the length of GLP-1, exhibit potency toward both Y_2R and the GLP-1 receptor that is nearly native-like, and in vivo, the dual-acting analog can quickly reduce food intake more than the individual counterparts [129].

While adding several features into one molecule might seem appealing, the question arises as to how necessary it really is. Is a dual agonist enough, and is it even essential to have triple or quadruple action? Although it is probably not required for most patients, triple (or even quadruple) action could offer some benefits for specific patient groups. Importantly, it is worth noting that including more pharmacological actions in a single molecule may also increase the risk.

Human Studies and Trials with PYY and Analogs

There is strong evidence that PYY_{3-36} or Y_2R agonists reduce food intake and enhance glucose metabolism in various animal studies, and importantly, this also applies to humans [13, 79, 118, 130]. This initially generated interest from the biotech and pharmaceutical industries in developing PYY analogs as effective drugs for obesity or diabetes. Since the interaction among the NPY receptor family and peptides is very complex, the selectivity profile and half-life are critical factors in designing an effective Y_2R peptide agonist. Additionally, safety, tolerability, suitable formulation properties, and scalability must be considered. However, the early human trials did not address these issues, as neither selectivity nor half-life extension was initially incorporated into the analogs tested.

Among the first reported clinical trials were the subcutaneous administration of a PYY_{3-36} by Amylin (USA) in 2004, followed shortly after by a collaboration between

Merck and Nastech (USA) in 2006 concerning the nasal delivery of PYY_{3-36} [131]. However, the disappointing outcomes of both clinical studies later led to Amylin and Merck discontinuing their programs. As mentioned earlier, 7TM Pharma (Denmark) announced a clinical trial in 2006 with a once-daily dual-acting Y_2R and Y_4R agonist (obinepitide, TM30338). The results showed that obinepitide was well tolerated, but its efficacy was disappointing. These studies all shared a standard limitation: their pharmacokinetic profiles and pharmacodynamic characteristics were not optimized despite their mutual dependence. As previously discussed, factors such as half-life and selectivity are crucial. For the Y_2R agonists mentioned above, enzymatic stability against C-terminal degradation was overlooked, which could have compromised both the half-life and efficacy, as well as the selectivity for the Y_2R.

In a recent human trial published in 2021 by Imperial College London and the spin-out company Zihipp Ltd in 2012 (later acquired by Metsera in 2023), a PYY analog called Y14 was tested over 28 days [130]. This analog was administered as a $ZnCl_2$ formulation, enabling a sustained-release approach. Although a specific mean half-life ($T^1/_2$) was not established, the estimated half-life was suitable for once-weekly dosing. The most common adverse events (AEs) included expected symptoms such as nausea, vomiting, and administration-site reactions, all mild and resolving over time. Over the 28 days, Y14 demonstrated weight loss and a significant reduction in food intake when dosed from 9 to 34 mg. Interestingly, the reduction in food intake observed on day 2 was similar to that recorded on day 30. Although direct comparisons are challenging due to differences in dosing regimens and participant characteristics, it is worth noting that Y14 achieved weight loss of similar magnitude over comparable time spans to semaglutide and tirzepatide. However, the clinical PYY program seems to have been discontinued, as Metsera is now focusing on ultra-long-acting GLP-1 agonists.

Another long-acting PYY analog, PYY1875 from Novo Nordisk, which is based on fatty diacid derivatization, has been in human clinical trials. This analog is a highly potent and very selective Y_2R agonist [87]. Interestingly, it consists entirely of L-amino acids, and the circulating half-life in humans was found to exceed 10 days due to a fatty diacid at position 7 and backbone modifications, allowing for once-weekly dosing. In a study as an add-on to semaglutide (2.4 mg per week) with dose escalation of PYY1875 at two-week intervals, the maximum tolerated dose was only 1 mg per week; at 2 mg per week, too many AEs, such as nausea and vomiting, occurred in this cohort. In the suboptimal dosing regimen of 1 mg per week, a 2.1% weight loss was observed in healthy obese adults, in addition to the weight loss already achieved with semaglutide [132]. Novo Nordisk has since halted the development of PYY1875 for obesity.

A standalone PYY analog, structurally very similar to PYY1875 and called nisotirostide, has been developed by Eli Lilly [133]. In March 2025, it entered phase 2 clinical trials with participants with T2DM who are on a stable dose of semaglutide or tirzepatide (NCT06897475). The biotech company CINRx Pharma has a PYY analog in clinical development and a dual-acting GLP-1/PYY receptor agonist in preclinical testing. Boehringer Ingelheim terminated their PYY program (BI 1820237, codeveloped with Gubra, Denmark). Boehringer Ingelheim now holds an Y_2R agonist in clinical development (BI 3034701), a tri-agonist peptide likely targeting GLP-1, GIP, and PYY. This tri-agonist includes the PYY C-terminus found in PYY1875, which provides increased stability against enzymatic degradation and improved Y_2R potency compared to the native PYY C-terminus. In July 2025, Roche decided to terminate their standalone PYY program (CT-173), acquired from Carmot Therapeutics, due to developability issues and a lack of competitiveness.

Prospects of Obesity and Diabetes Treatment with PYY

While PYY seems to be a promising candidate for T2DM and weight management by regulating appetite, its therapeutic use is limited by side effects such as nausea and vomiting [134, 135]. These effects mainly occur due to overstimulation of pathways that suppress appetite or induce aversion and vomiting responses. A key area involved in these responses is the area postrema (AP) in the hindbrain, which helps regulate both satiety and vomiting.

While similar AEs are also observed with GLP-1, these are often mitigated through slow titration, and for some patients, they tend to diminish over time. Although the side effects caused by PYY are also transient, it remains debatable how tolerable PYY is in humans and how slow the up-titration process needs to be. However, research has shown a dual benefit of using GIP receptor agonists. It is well established that combining GLP-1 with GIP receptor agonists, or having less GLP-1R β-arrestin recruitment, over an extended period can amplify the appetite-suppressing effects of GLP-1 receptor agonists in obese mice [136] as well as humans, as exemplified in tirzepatide [137, 138]. Interestingly, GIPR activation improves weight loss, prevents vomiting in animals, and reduces nausea-like behavior in both mice and rats [139, 140]. To PYY's rescue, studies have shown that a GIP agonist can also lessen nausea and discomfort caused by a long-acting PYY analog without affecting its ability to suppress appetite [141, 142]. Furthermore, it has been proposed that the pharmacokinetic profile of an Y_2R agonist might also influence emesis [143], although this is not entirely well established.

Success also depends on the accessibility of the compound. In other words, can the molecule be produced in the larger quantities needed? For the PYY analog Y14, doses around or exceeding 30 mg per week may be required for full efficacy. Serving 1–10 million patients would require the production of 1.5–15 tons annually. Since PYY is an amide, the most straightforward production method would be synthetic. However, producing more than 2–3 tons of synthetic peptides presents significant economic and manufacturing challenges, and to date, producing 15 tons of a single peptide has not been achieved. Moreover, PYY alone is not attractive, as its efficacy does not match that of GLP-1 agonists, not to mention dual or triple combinations like tirzepatide or retatrutide. Consequently, developing clinical programs with two molecules is quite complex. It is simpler with a single molecule that acts as a dual or even triple agonist. Additional challenges in developing a PYY treatment include other non-incretin-based combinations, such as amylin with GLP-1 (cagrisema) or dual agonists (amycretin), which are also in development and have demonstrated remarkable efficacy.

PYY shows potential as a treatment option for T2DM linked with obesity. Beyond tolerability concerns, improving patient access requires additional focus. The competitive landscape and possible advantages over current treatments like dual GLP-1/GIP, GLP-1/GCG, or GLP-1/amylin receptor dual agonists, along with emerging options such as small-molecule treatments, are crucial in assessing the investment potential of PYY-based therapies. Given existing production limitations and strategic decisions, PYY's future remains uncertain, but patient segmentation could uncover new opportunities.

References

1 Cabrele, C. and Beck-Sickinger, A.G. (2000). Molecular characterization of the ligand–receptor interaction of the neuropeptide Y family. *J. Pept. Sci.* 6: 97–122.

2 Nygaard, R., Nielbo, S., Schwartz, T.W., and Poulsen, F.M. (2006). The PP-fold solution structure of human polypeptide YY and human PYY_{3-36} as determined by NMR. *Biochemistry* 45: 8350–8357.

3 Tang, T., Tan, Q., Han, S. et al. (2022). Receptor-specific recognition of NPY peptides revealed by structures of NPY receptors. *Sci. Adv.* 8: eabm1232.

4 Blundell, T.L., Pitts, J.E., Tickle, I.J. et al. (1981). X-ray analysis (1. 4-Å resolution) of avian pancreatic polypeptide: small globular protein hormone. *Proc. Natl. Acad. Sci. USA* 78: 4175–4179.

5 Michel, M.C., Beck-Sickinger, A., Cox, H. et al. (1998). XVI. International union of pharmacology recommendations for the nomenclature of neuropeptide Y, peptide YY, and pancreatic polypeptide receptors. *Pharmacol. Rev.* 50: 143.

6 Larhammar, D. (1996). Evolution of neuropeptide Y, peptide YY and pancreatic polypeptide. *Regul. Pept.* 62: 1–11.

7 Starbäck, P., Wraith, A., Eriksson, H., and Larhammar, D. (2000). Neuropeptide Y receptor gene y6: multiple deaths or resurrections? *Biochem. Biophys. Res. Commun.* 277: 264–269.

8 Stanley, B.G. and Leibowitz, S.F. (1985). Neuropeptide Y injected in the paraventricular hypothalamus: a powerful stimulant of feeding behavior. *Proc. Natl. Acad. Sci. USA* 82: 3940–3943.

9 Larhammar, D., Ericsson, A., and Persson, H. (1987). Structure and expression of the rat neuropeptide Y gene. *Proc. Natl. Acad. Sci. USA* 84: 2068–2072.

10 Allen, Y.S., Adrian, T.E., Allen, J.M. et al. (1983). Neuropeptide Y distribution in the rat brain. *Science* 221: 877–879.

11 Maturi, M.F., Greene, R., Speir, E. et al. (1989). Neuropeptide-Y. A peptide found in human coronary arteries constricts primarily small coronary arteries to produce myocardial ischemia in dogs. *J. Clin. Invest.* 83: 1217–1224.

12 El-Salhy, M., Wilander, E., Grimelius, L. et al. (1982). The distribution of polypeptide YY (PYY)- and pancreatic polypeptide (PP)-immunoreactive cells in the domestic fowl. *Histochemistry* 75: 25–30.

13 Batterham, R.L., Cohen, M.A., Ellis, S.M. et al. (2003). Inhibition of food intake in obese subjects by peptide YY3–36. *New Engl. J. Med.* 349: 941–948.

14 Reidelberger, R., Haver, A., and Chelikani, P.K. (2013). Role of peptide YY(3–36) in the satiety produced by gastric delivery of macronutrients in rats. *Am. J. Physiol. Endocrinol. Metab.* 304: E944–E950.

15 Adrian, T.E., Bloom, S.R., Bryant, M.G. et al. (1976). Distribution and release of human pancreatic polypeptide. *Gut* 17: 940.

16 Kim, W., Fiori, J.L., Shin, Y.-K. et al. (2014). Pancreatic polypeptide inhibits somatostatin secretion. *FEBS Lett.* 588: 3233–3239.

17 Badia, X.P., Stichel, J., and Beck-Sickinger, A. (2013). Neuropeptide Y receptors: how to get subtype selectivity. *Front. Endocrinol.* 4: 5.

18 Lee, N.J. and Herzog, H. (2009). NPY regulation of bone remodelling. *Neuropeptides* 43: 457–463.

19 Shintani, M., Ogawa, Y., Ebihara, K. et al. (2001). Ghrelin, an endogenous growth hormone secretagogue, is a novel orexigenic peptide that antagonizes leptin action through the activation of hypothalamic neuropeptide Y/Y1 receptor pathway. *Diabetes* 50: 227–232.

20 Reichmann, F. and Holzer, P. (2016). Neuropeptide Y: a stressful review. *Neuropeptides* 55: 99–109.

21 Cox, H.M., Tough, I.R., Zandvliet, D.W.J., and Holliday, N.D. (2001). Constitutive neuropeptide Y Y4 receptor expression in human colonic adenocarcinoma cell lines. *Br. J. Pharmacol.* 132: 345–353.

22 Goumain, M., Voisin, T., Lorinet, A.-M., and Laburthe, M. (1998). Identification and distribution of mRNA encoding the Y1, Y2, Y4, and Y5 receptors for peptides of the PP-fold family in the rat intestine and colon. *Biochem. Biophys. Res. Commun.* 247: 52–56.

23 Gerald, C., Walker, M.W., Criscione, L. et al. (1996). A receptor subtype involved in neuropeptide-Y-induced food intake. *Nature* 382: 168–171.

24 Marsh, D.J., Hollopeter, G., Kafer, K.E., and Palmiter, R.D. (1998). Role of the Y5 neuropeptide Y receptor in feeding and obesity. *Nat. Med.* 4: 718–721.

25 Pedrazzini, T., Seydoux, J., Künstner, P. et al. (1998). Cardiovascular response, feeding behavior and locomotor activity in mice lacking the NPY Y1 receptor. *Nat. Med.* 4: 722–726.

26 Batterham, R.L., Heffron, H., Kapoor, S. et al. (2006). Critical role for peptide YY in protein-mediated satiation and body-weight regulation. *Cell Metab.* 4: 223–233.

27 Boey, D., Lin, S., Karl, T. et al. (2006). Peptide YY ablation in mice leads to the development of hyperinsulinaemia and obesity. *Diabetologia* 49: 1360–1370.

28 Naveilhan, P., Hassani, H., Canals, J.M. et al. (1999). Normal feeding behavior, body weight and leptin response require the neuropeptide Y Y2 receptor. *Nat. Med.* 5: 1188–1193.

29 Sainsbury, A., Schwarzer, C., Couzens, M. et al. (2002). Important role of hypothalamic Y2 receptors in body weight regulation revealed in conditional knockout mice. *Proc. Natl. Acad. Sci. USA* 99: 8938–8943.

30 Shi, Y.-C., Lin, S., Castillo, L. et al. (2011). Peripheral-specific Y2 receptor knockdown protects mice from high-fat diet-induced obesity. *Obesity* 19: 2137–2148.

31 Lee, N.J., Enriquez, R.F., Boey, D. et al. (2008). Synergistic attenuation of obesity by Y2- and Y4-receptor double knockout in ob/ob mice. *Nutrition* 24: 892–899.

32 Zhang, L., Riepler, S.J., Turner, N. et al. (2010). Y2 and Y4 receptor signaling synergistically act on energy expenditure and physical activity. *Am. J. Physiol. Regul. Integr. Comp. Physiol.* 299: R1618–R1628.

33 Lin, S., Boey, D., and Herzog, H. (2004). NPY and Y receptors: lessons from transgenic and knockout models. *Neuropeptides* 38: 189–200.

34 Morley, J.E., Levine, A.S., Grace, M., and Kneip, J. (1985). Peptide YY (PYY), a poteny orexigenic agent. *Brain Res.* 341: 200–203.

35 Tatemoto, K., Carlquist, M., and Mutt, V. (1982). Neuropeptide Y – a novel brain peptide with structural similarities to peptide YY and pancreatic polypeptide. *Nature* 296: 659–660.

36 Atherton, E., Logan, C.J., and Sheppard, R.C. (1981). Peptide synthesis. Part 2. Procedures for solid-phase synthesis using Nα-fluorenylmethoxycarbonylamino-acids on polyamide supports. Synthesis of substance P and of acyl carrier protein 65–74 decapeptide. *J. Chem. Soc. Perkin Trans.* 1: 538–546.

37 Danho, W., Triscari, J., Vincent, G. et al. (1988). Synthesis and biological evaluation of pNPY fragments. *Int. J. Pept. Protein Res.* 32: 496–505.

38 Michel, M.C., Gaida, W., Beck-Sickinger, A.G. et al. (1992). Further characterization of neuropeptide Y receptor subtypes using centrally truncated analogs of neuropeptide Y: evidence for subtype-differentiating effects on affinity and intrinsic efficacy. *Mol. Pharmacol.* 42: 642–648.

39 Beck-Sickinger, A.G., Weland, H.A., Wittneben, H. et al. (1994). Complete L-alanine scan of neuropeptide Y reveals ligands binding to Y1 and Y2 receptors with distinguished conformations. *Eur. J. Biochem.* 225: 947–958.

40 Kaga, T., Inui, A., Okita, M. et al. (2001). Modest overexpression of neuropeptide Y in the brain leads to obesity after high-sucrose feeding. *Diabetes* 50: 1206–1210.

41 Williams, G., Lee, Y.C., Ghatei, M.A. et al. (1989). Elevated neuropeptide Y concentrations in the central hypothalamus of the spontaneously diabetic BB/E wistar rat. *Diabet. Med.* 6: 601–607.

42 McCrea, K., Wisialowski, T., Cabrele, C. et al. (2000). 2-36(K4,RYYSA19-23)PP a novel Y5-receptor preferring ligand with strong stimulatory effect on food intake. *Regul. Pept.* 87: 47–58.

43 Østergaard, S., Kofoed, J., Paulsson, J.F. et al. (2018). Design of Y2 receptor selective and proteolytically stable PYY3–36 analogues. *J. Med. Chem.* 61: 10519–10530.

44 Cabrele, C., Langer, M., Bader, R. et al. (2000). The first selective agonist for the neuropeptide YY5 receptor increases food intake in rats. *J. Biol. Chem.* 275: 36043–36048.

45 Lecklin, A., Lundell, I., Salmela, S. et al. (2003). Agonists for neuropeptide Y receptors Y1 and Y5 stimulate different phases of feeding in guinea pigs. *Br. J. Pharmacol.* 139: 1433–1440.

46 MacNeil, J.D. (2007). NPY Y1 and Y5 receptor selective antagonists as anti-obesity drugs. *Curr. Top. Med. Chem.* 7: 1721–1733.

47 Balasubramaniam, A., Dhawan, V.C., Mullins, D.E. et al. (2001). Highly selective and potent neuropeptide Y (NPY) Y1 receptor antagonists based on [Pro30, Tyr32, Leu34]NPY(28-36)-NH2 (BW1911U90). *J. Med. Chem.* 44: 1479–1482.

48 Loh, K., Shi, Y.-C., Walters, S. et al. (2017). Inhibition of Y1 receptor signaling improves islet transplant outcome. *Nat. Commun.* 8: 490.

49 Yang, C.-H., Ann-Onda, D., Lin, X. et al. (2022). Neuropeptide Y1 receptor antagonism protects β-cells and improves glycemic control in type 2 diabetes. *Mol. Metab.* 55: 101413.

50 Kornhuber, J. and Zoicas, I. (2021). Neuropeptide Y reduces social fear in male mice: involvement of Y1 and Y2 receptors in the dorsolateral septum and central amygdala. *Int. J. Mol. Sci.* 22 (18): 10142. https://doi.org/10.3390/ijms221810142.

51 Gruber, K.A., Fan, W., Akerberg, H. et al. (2009). Neuropeptide Y and gamma-melanocyte stimulating hormone (γ-MSH) share a common pressor mechanism of action. *Endocrine* 35: 312–324.

52 Sousa, D.M., Baldock, P.A., Enriquez, R.F. et al. (2012). Neuropeptide Y Y1 receptor antagonism increases bone mass in mice. *Bone* 51: 8–16.

53 Antal-Zimanyi, I., Bruce, M.A., Leboulluec, K.L. et al. (2008). Pharmacological characterization and appetite suppressive properties of BMS-193885, a novel and selective neuropeptide Y1 receptor antagonist. *Eur. J. Pharmacol.* 590: 224–232.

54 Criscione, L., Rigollier, P., Batzl-Hartmann, C. et al. (1998). Food intake in free-feeding and energy-deprived lean rats is mediated by the neuropeptide Y5 receptor. *J. Clin. Invest.* 102: 2136–2145.

55 Kakui, N., Tanaka, J., Tabata, Y. et al. (2006). Pharmacological characterization and feeding-suppressive property of FMS586 [3-(5,6,7,8-tetrahydro-9-isopropyl-carbazol-3-yl)-1-methyl-1-(2-pyridin-4-yl-ethyl)-urea hydrochloride], a novel, selective, and orally active antagonist for neuropeptide Y Y5 receptor. *J. Pharmacol. Exp. Ther.* 317: 562.

56 Turnbull, A.V., Ellershaw, L., Masters, D.J. et al. (2002). Selective antagonism of the NPY Y5 receptor does not have a major effect on feeding in rats. *Diabetes* 51: 2441–2449.

57 Della-Zuana, O., Revereault, L., Beck-Sickinger, A. et al. (2004). A potent and selective NPY Y5 antagonist reduces food intake but not through blockade of the NPY Y5 receptor. *Int. J. Obes.* 28: 628–639.

58 Erondu, N., Gantz, I., Musser, B. et al. (2006). Neuropeptide Y5 receptor antagonism does not induce clinically meaningful weight loss in overweight and obese adults. *Cell Metab.* 4: 275–282.

59 Oda, S., Manaka, K., Kakiya, K. et al. (2015). Development of an optimized synthetic and purification process of S-2367 (velneperit), a novel neuropeptide Y (NPY) Y5 receptor antagonist. *Org. Process. Res. Dev.* 19: 531–536.

60 Berntson, G.G., Zipf, W.B., O'Dorisio, T.M. et al. (1993). Pancreatic polypeptide infusions reduce food intake in Prader-Willi syndrome. *Peptides* 14: 497–503.

61 Kanaley, J.A., Heden, T.D., Liu, Y. et al. (2014). Short-term aerobic exercise training increases postprandial pancreatic polypeptide but not peptide YY concentrations in obese individuals. *Int. J. Obes.* 38: 266–271.

62 Ueno, N., Inui, A., Iwamoto, M. et al. (1999). Decreased food intake and body weight in pancreatic polypeptide-overexpressing mice. *Gastroenterology* 117: 1427–1432.

63 Lin, S., Shi, Y.-C., Yulyaningsih, E. et al. (2010). Critical role of arcuate Y4 receptors and the melanocortin system in pancreatic polypeptide-induced reduction in food intake in mice. *PLoS One* 4: e8488.

64 Bellmann-Sickert, K., Elling, C.E., Madsen, A.N. et al. (2011). Long-acting lipidated analogue of human pancreatic polypeptide is slowly released into circulation. *J. Med. Chem.* 54: 2658–2667.

65 Raposinho, P.D., Broqua, P., Hayward, A. et al. (2000). Stimulation of the gonadotropic axis by the neuropeptide Y receptor Y1 antagonist/ Y4 agonist 1229U91 in the male rat. *Neuroendocrinology* 71: 2–7.

66 Zhu, W., Tanday, N., Flatt, P.R., and Irwin, N. (2025). The beneficial impact of a novel pancreatic polypeptide analogue on islet cell lineage. *Int. J. Mol. Sci.* 26 (9): 4215. https://doi.org/10.3390/ijms26094215.

67 Balasubramaniam, A., Mullins, D.E., Lin, S. et al. (2006). Neuropeptide Y (NPY) Y4 receptor selective agonists based on NPY(32–36): development of an anorectic Y4 receptor selective agonist with picomolar affinity. *J. Med. Chem.* 49: 2661–2665.

68 Konieczny, A., Conrad, M., Ertl, F.J. et al. (2021). N-terminus to arginine side-chain cyclization of linear peptidic neuropeptide Y Y4 receptor ligands results in picomolar binding constants. *J. Med. Chem.* 64: 16746–16769.

69 Tatemoto, K. and Neuropeptide, Y. (1982). Complete amino acid sequence of the brain peptide. *Proc. Natl. Acad. Sci. USA* 79: 5485.

70 Adrian, T.E., Bacarese-Hamilton, A.J., Smith, H.A. et al. (1987). Distribution and postprandial release of porcine peptide YY. *J. Endocrinol.* 113: 11–14.

71 Greeley, G.H.J., Hashimoto, T., Izukura, M. et al. (1989). Acomparison of intraduodenally and intracolonically administered nutrients on the release of peptide-YY in the dog. *Endocrinology* 125: 1761–1765.

72 Gribble, F.M. (2012). The gut endocrine system as a coordinator of postprandial nutrient homoeostasis. *Proc. Nutr. Soc.* 71: 456–462.

73 Kim, B.-J., Carlson, O.D., Jang, H.-J. et al. (2005). Peptide YY is secreted after oral glucose administration in a gender-specific manner. *J. Clin. Endocrinol. Metab.* 90: 6665–6671.

74 Naruse, S., Kitagawa, M., Ishiguro, H., and Hayakawa, T. (2002). Feedback regulation of pancreatic secretion by peptide YY. *Peptides* 23: 359–365.

75 Yang, H. (2002). Central and peripheral regulation of gastric acid secretion by peptide YY. *Peptides* 23: 349–358.
76 Imamura, M. (2002). Effects of surgical manipulation of the intestine on peptide YY and its physiology. *Peptides* 23: 403–407.
77 Batterham, R.L., Cowley, M.A., Small, C.J. et al. (2002). Gut hormone PYY3-36 physiologically inhibits food intake. *Nature* 418: 650–654.
78 Tschöp, M., Castañeda, T.R., Joost, H.G. et al. (2004). Does gut hormone PYY3–36 decrease food intake in rodents? *Nature* 430: 1–3.
79 le Roux, C.W., Batterham, R.L., Aylwin, S.J.B. et al. (2006). Attenuated peptide YY release in obese subjects is associated with reduced satiety. *Endocrinology* 147: 3–8.
80 Essah, P.A., Levy, J.R., Sistrun, S.N. et al. (2007). Effect of macronutrient composition on postprandial peptide YY levels. *J. Clin. Endocrinol. Metab.* 92: 4052–4055.
81 Karra, E., Chandarana, K., and Batterham, R.L. (2009). The role of peptide YY in appetite regulation and obesity. *J. Physiol.* 587: 19–25.
82 Sam, A.H., Gunner, D.J., King, A. et al. (2012). Selective ablation of peptide YY cells in adult mice reveals their role in beta cell survival. *Gastroenterology* 143: 459–468.
83 van den Hoek, A.M., Heijboer, A.C., Corssmit, E.P.M. et al. (2004). PYY3–36 reinforces insulin action on glucose disposal in mice fed a high-fat diet. *Diabetes* 53: 1949–1952.
84 van den Hoek, A.M., Heijboer, A.C., Voshol, P.J. et al. (2007). Chronic PYY3–36 treatment promotes fat oxidation and ameliorates insulin resistance in C57BL6 mice. *Am. J. Physiol. Endocrinol. Metab.* 292: E238–E245.
85 Boland, B.B., Laker, R.C., O'Brien, S. et al. (2021). Peptide-YY3-36/glucagon-like peptide-1 combination treatment of obese diabetic mice improves insulin sensitivity associated with recovered pancreatic β-cell function and synergistic activation of discrete hypothalamic and brainstem neuronal circuitries. *Mol. Metab.* 55: 101392.
86 Pittner, R.A., Moore, C.X., Bhavsar, S.P. et al. (2004). Effects of PYY[3–36] in rodent models of diabetes and obesity. *Int. J. Obes.* 28: 963–971.
87 Østergaard, S., Jessen, C., Paulsson, J.F. et al. (2025). Variant screening of PYY3–36 leads to potent long-acting PYY analogs with superior Y2 receptor selectivity. *Sci. Transl. Med.* 17: eadq6392.
88 Arterburn, D.E., Telem, D.A., Kushner, R.F., and Courcoulas, A.P. (2020). Benefits and risks of bariatric surgery in adults: a review. *JAMA* 324: 879–887.
89 Chan, J.L., Mun, E.C., Stoyneva, V. et al. (2006). Peptide YY levels are elevated after gastric bypass surgery. *Obesity* 14: 194–198.
90 Guida, C., Stephen, S.D., Watson, M. et al. (2019). PYY plays a key role in the resolution of diabetes following bariatric surgery in humans. *EBioMedicine* 40: 67–76.
91 Ye, J., Hao, Z., Mumphrey, M.B. et al. (2014). GLP-1 receptor signaling is not required for reduced body weight after RYGB in rodents. *Am. J. Physiol. Regul. Integr. Comp. Physiol.* 306: R352–R362.

92 Ramracheya, R.D., McCulloch, L.J., Clark, A. et al. (2016). PYY-dependent restoration of impaired insulin and glucagon secretion in type 2 diabetes following Roux-en-Y gastric bypass surgery. *Cell Rep.* 15: 944–950.

93 Camacho-Ramírez, A., Prada-Oliveira, J.A., Ribelles-García, A. et al. (2020). The leading role of peptide tyrosine tyrosine in glycemic control after Roux-en-Y gastric bypass in rats. *Obes. Surg.* 30: 697–706.

94 Bose, M., Machineni, S., Oliván, B. et al. (2010). Superior appetite hormone profile after equivalent weight loss by gastric bypass compared to gastric banding. *Obesity* 18: 1085–1091.

95 Lampropoulos, C., Alexandrides, T., Tsochatzis, S. et al. (2021). Are the changes in gastrointestinal hormone secretion necessary for the success of bariatric surgery? A critical review of the literature. *Obes. Surg.* 31: 4575–4584.

96 Leban, J.J., Heyer, D., Landavazo, A. et al. (1995). Novel modified carboxy terminal fragments of neuropeptide Y with high affinity for Y2-type receptors and potent functional antagonism at the Y1-type receptor. *J. Med. Chem.* 38: 1150–1157.

97 Beck-Sickinger, A.G., Grouzmann, E., Hoffmann, E. et al. (1992). A novel cyclic analog of neuropeptide Y specific for the Y2 receptor. *Eur. J. Biochem.* 206: 957–964.

98 Beck, A., Jung, G., Gaida, W. et al. (1989). Highly potent and small neuropeptide Y agonist obtained by linking NPY 1–4 via spacer to α-helical NPY 25–36. *FEBS Lett.* 244: 119–122.

99 Beck-Sickinger, A.G., Hoffmann, E., Gaida, W. et al. (1993). Novel Y2-selective, reduced-size agonists of neuropeptide Y. *Bioorg. Med. Chem. Lett.* 3: 937–942.

100 DeCarr, L.B., Buckholz, T.M., Coish, P.D.G. et al. (2007). Identification of selective neuropeptide Y2 peptide agonists. *Bioorg. Med. Chem. Lett.* 17: 538–541.

101 Nishizawa, N., Niida, A., Masuda, Y. et al. (2017). Antiobesity effect of a short-length peptide YY analogue after continuous administration in mice. *ACS Med. Chem. Lett.* 8: 628–631.

102 Balasubramaniam, A., Tao, Z., Zhai, W. et al. (2000). Structure-activity studies including a Psi(CH(2)-NH) scan of peptide YY (PYY) active site, PYY(22-36), for interaction with rat intestinal PYY receptors: development of analogues with potent in vivo activity in the intestine. *J. Med. Chem.* 43: 3420–3427.

103 Albertsen, L., Andersen, J.J., Paulsson, J.F. et al. (2013). Design and synthesis of peptide YY analogues with C-terminal backbone amide-to-ester modifications. *ACS Med. Chem. Lett.* 4: 1228–1232.

104 Oertel, M., Ziegler, C.G., Kohlhaas, M. et al. (2024). GLP-1 and PYY for the treatment of obesity: a pilot study on the use of agonists and antagonists in diet-induced rats. *Endocr. Connect.* 13: e230398.

105 Shi, Y.C., Ip, C.K., Reed, F. et al. (2017). Y5 receptor signalling counteracts the anorectic effects of PYY3-36 in diet-induced obese mice. *J. Neuroendocrinol.* 29: e12483.

106 Toräng, S., Veedfald, S., Rosenkilde, M.M. et al. (2015). The anorexic hormone peptide YY3–36 is rapidly metabolized to inactive Peptide YY3–34 in vivo. *Physiol. Rep.* 3: 1–8.

107 Olsen, J., Kofoed, J., Østergaard, S. et al. (2016). Metabolism of peptide YY 3-36 in Gottingen mini-pig and rhesus monkey. *Peptides* 78: 59–67.

108 Østergaard, S., Paulsson, J.F., Kofoed, J. et al. (2021). The effect of fatty diacid acylation of human PYY_{3-36} on Y_2 receptor potency and half-life in minipigs. *Sci. Rep.* 11: 21179.

109 Lear, S., Pflimlin, E., Zhou, Z. et al. (2020). Engineering of a potent, long-acting NPY2R agonist for combination with a GLP-1R agonist as a multi-hormonal treatment for obesity. *J. Med. Chem.* 63: 9660–9671.

110 Shechter, Y., Tsubery, H., Mironchik, M. et al. (2005). Reversible PEGylation of peptide YY3-36 prolongs its inhibition of food intake in mice. *FEBS Lett.* 579: 2439–2444.

111 DeCarr, L.B., Buckholz, T.M., Milardo, L.F. et al. (2007). A long-acting selective neuropeptide Y2 receptor PEGylated peptide agonist reduces food intake in mice. *Bioorg. Med. Chem. Lett.* 17: 1916–1919.

112 Ortiz, A.A., Milardo, L.F., DeCarr, L.B. et al. (2007). A novel long-acting selective neuropeptide Y2 receptor polyethylene glycol-conjugated peptide agonist reduces food intake and body weight and improves glucose metabolism in rodents. *J. Pharmacol. Exp. Ther.* 323: 692–700.

113 Baraboi, E.D., Michel, C., Smith, P. et al. (2010). Effects of albumin-conjugated PYY on food intake: the respective roles of the circumventricular organs and vagus nerve. *Eur. J. Neurosci.* 32: 826–839.

114 Ehrlich, G.K., Michel, H., Truitt, T. et al. (2013). Preparation and characterization of albumin conjugates of a truncated peptide YY analogue for half-life extension. *Bioconjug. Chem.* 24: 2015–2024.

115 Henry, K.E., Elfers, C.T., Burke, R.M. et al. (2015). Vitamin B12 conjugation of peptide-YY_{3-36} decreases food intake compared to native peptide-YY_{3-36} upon subcutaneous administration in male rats. *Endocrinology* 156: 1739–1749.

116 Kurtzhals, P., Østergaard, S., Nishimura, E., and Kjeldsen, T. (2022). Derivatization with fatty acids in peptide and protein drug discovery. *Nat. Rev. Drug Discov.* 22: 59–80.

117 De Silva, A., Salem, V., Long, C.J. et al. (2011). The gut hormones PYY 3-36 and GLP-1 7-36 amide reduce food intake and modulate brain activity in appetite centers in humans. *Cell Metab.* 14: 700–706.

118 Schmidt, J.B., Gregersen, N.T., Pedersen, S.D. et al. (2014). Effects of PYY3–36 and GLP-1 on energy intake, energy expenditure, and appetite in overweight men. *Am. J. Physiol. Endocrinol. Metab.* 306: E1248–E1256.

119 Field, B.C., Wren, A.M., Peters, V. et al. (2010). PYY3-36 and oxyntomodulin can be additive in their effect on food intake in overweight and obese humans. *Diabetes* 59: 1635–1639.

120 Behary, P., Tharakan, G., Alexiadou, K. et al. (2019). Combined GLP-1, oxyntomodulin, and peptide YY improves body weight and glycemia in obesity and prediabetes/type 2 diabetes: a randomized, single-blinded, placebo-controlled study. *Diabetes Care* 42: 1446–1453.

121 Chepurny, O.G., Bonaccorso, R.L., Leech, C.A. et al. (2018). Chimeric peptide EP45 as a dual agonist at GLP-1 and NPY2R receptors. *Sci. Rep.* 8: 3749.

122 Yang, Q., Tang, W., Sun, L. et al. (2022). Design of xenopus GLP-1-based long-acting dual GLP-1/Y2 receptor agonists. *J. Med. Chem.* 65: 14201–14220.

123 Xu, J., Wang, S., Wu, H. et al. (2023). Engineering a potent and long-acting GLP-1/Y2 receptor dual agonist as a multi-agonist therapy for diabetes and obesity. *Peptides* 169: 171073.

124 Liu, J., Lu, W., Wu, H. et al. (2025). Rational design of dual-agonist peptides targeting GLP-1 and NPY2 receptors for regulating glucose homeostasis and body weight with minimal nausea and emesis. *Eur. J. Med. Chem.* 287: 117320.

125 Haebel, P.W., Augustin, R., Madsen, C.S. et al. (2024). GLP1/GIP/NPY2 recptor triple agonists. WO2024133382A1 Boehringer Ingelheim Gmbh.

126 Chichura, K.S., Elfers, C.T., Salameh, T.S. et al. (2023). A peptide triple agonist of GLP-1, neuropeptide Y1, and neuropeptide Y2 receptors promotes glycemic control and weight loss. *Sci. Rep.* 13: 9554.

127 Yuan, Y., Yan, Z., Lao, Q. et al. (2022). Discovery of a potent and long-acting xenopus GLP-1-based GLP-1/glucagon/Y2 receptor triple agonist. *Eur. J. Med. Chem.* 247: 115036.

128 Dinsmore, T.C., Cortigiano, J.E., Xiang, S. et al. (2025). Molecular design of unimolecular tetra-receptor agonists. *J. Am. Chem. Soc.* 147 (24): 20819–20832.

129 Østergaard, S., Paulsson, J.F., Kjærgaard Gerstenberg, M., and Wulff, B.S. (2021). The design of a GLP-1/PYY dual acting agonist. *Angew. Chem. Int. Ed.* 60: 8268–8275.

130 Tan, T.M.M., Minnion, J., Khoo, B. et al. (2021). Safety and efficacy of an extended-release peptide YY analogue for obesity: a randomized, placebo-controlled, phase 1 trial. *Diabetes Obes. Metab.* 23: 1471–1483.

131 Gantz, I., Erondu, N., Mallick, M. et al. (2007). Efficacy and safety of intranasal peptide YY3–36 for weight reduction in obese adults. *J. Clin. Endocrinol. Metab.* 92: 1754–1757.

132 Wulff, B.S., Chambers, A.P., Contreras, C.K.O. et al. (2025). Long-acting PYY3–36 analogue with semaglutide for obesity: from preclinical assessment through randomized clinical studies. *Obesity* 33: 1457–1474.

133 Briere, D.A., Lopes, D.C., and Muppidi, A. (2020). Protein tyrosine-tyrosine analogs and methods of using the same. WO20200921981A1 Eli Lilly.

134 Degen, L., Oesch, S., Casanova, M. et al. (2005). Effect of peptide YY3–36 on food intake in humans. *Gastroenterology* 129: 1430–1436.

135 le Roux, C.W., Borg, C.M., Murphy, K.G. et al. (2008). Supraphysiological doses of intravenous PYY_{3-36} cause nausea, but no additional reduction in food intake. *Ann. Clin. Biochem.* 45: 93–95.

136 Zhang, Q., Delessa, C.T., Augustin, R. et al. (2021). The glucose-dependent insulinotropic polypeptide (GIP) regulates body weight and food intake via CNS-GIPR signaling. *Cell Metab.* 33: 833–844.e835.

137 Frias, J.P., Nauck, M.A., Van, J. et al. (2020). Efficacy and tolerability of tirzepatide, a dual glucose-dependent insulinotropic peptide and glucagon-like peptide-1 receptor agonist in patients with type 2 diabetes: a 12-week, randomized, double-blind, placebo-controlled study to evaluate different dose-escalation regimens. *Diabetes Obes. Metab.* 22: 938–946.

138 Coskun, T., Sloop, K.W., Loghin, C. et al. (2018). LY3298176, a novel dual GIP and GLP-1 receptor agonist for the treatment of type 2 diabetes mellitus: from discovery to clinical proof of concept. *Mol. Metab.* 18: 3–14.

139 Borner, T., Geisler, C.E., Fortin, S.M. et al. (2021). GIP receptor agonism attenuates GLP-1 receptor agonist–induced nausea and emesis in preclinical models. *Diabetes* 70: 2545–2553.

140 Costa, A., Ai, M., Nunn, N. et al. (2022). Anorectic and aversive effects of GLP-1 receptor agonism are mediated by brainstem cholecystokinin neurons, and modulated by GIP receptor activation. *Mol. Metab.* 55: 101407.

141 Samms, R.J., Cosgrove, R., Snider, B.M. et al. (2022). GIPR agonism inhibits PYY-induced nausea-like behavior. *Diabetes* 71: 1410–1423.

142 Asami, T., Nishizawa N., Niida A., Kanematsu Y., Adachi M., Takekawa S., Mrimoto T. et al. (2018). Gip receptor activating peptide. WO2018181864A.

143 Rangwala, S.M., D'Aquino, K., Zhang, Y.-M. et al. (2019). A long-acting PYY3–36 analog mediates robust anorectic efficacy with minimal emesis in nonhuman primates. *Cell Metab.* 29: 837–843.

8

PrRP-GPR10 Signaling and Metabolism

Claire H. Feetham, Amy A. Worth, Sam Groom, and Simon M. Luckman

University of Manchester, Faculty of Biology, Medicine and Health, Oxford Road, Manchester M13 9PT, UK

Modified PrRP Peptides as a New Pharmacological Tool

Prolactin-releasing peptide (PrRP; gene name *Prlh*), unlike as suggested by its name, is not involved in prolactin secretion but, instead, has an important role in the physiological regulation of appetite and body weight [1]. It is a brain peptide found in very discrete populations of neurons, and binds to its receptor, GPR10 [2] (now known as PRLHR). As will be discussed later, a number of groups have described lipidated analogs of the PrRP peptide that can reduce body weight when administered systemically to diet-induced obese rodents [3–6]. It may be premature to call agonists of the receptor PRLHRA, for example as we call agonists of the glucagon-like peptide-1 (GLP-1) hormone receptor, GLP1RA, since PrRP binds with high affinity to at least one other known receptor; neuropeptide FF receptor 2 (NPFFR2).

The weight-reducing effects of PrRP analogs are impressive, though they may not be as efficacious as GLP1RA in comparable rodent models. Based only on this, PrRP analogs might be unlikely to undergo further development, as new clinical drugs need to be better (or safer) than those already available. That said, the mechanism of action of systemically administered PrRP analogs has not been elucidated. GLP1RA cause hypophagia but can also have detrimental off-target effects, the most notable being gastric malaise, nausea, and lean-mass loss. GLP1RA effects are probably due to the engagement of central receptors that are not normally exposed to naturally circulating GLP-1. To date, there are no reports of aversion with systemically administered PrRP analogs, and, in fact, native brain PrRP acts as expected for a true satiety factor without causing nausea [7]. Initial mechanistic studies on lipidated PrRP were very limited and reported an effect on cumulative food intake – though actually the results are not convincing. The fact that native PrRP can act in the brain to increase energy expenditure in addition to causing hypophagia suggested that further investigation was warranted, including whether PrRP analogs might be useful adjuncts to other obesity treatments. In fact, the most recent research suggests PrRP analogs administered systemically cause significant weight loss mainly through sustained fatty acid oxidation rather than major effects on food intake, and can do so without causing aversion or lean-mass loss [4].

This review will consider only the functions of PrRP in mammalian metabolism, though reference will be made to other work when it is relevant to the discussion.

The Discovery of GPR10 and PrRP

One can tell by the eponymous number that GPR10 was one of the first G protein-coupled receptors to be described [8, 9] and, in fact, it was also one of the first to be deorphanized by reverse pharmacology [2]. Of other GPCRs, beyond receptors for its immediate RF-amide family, GPR10 (also previously known as UHR1 or hGR3) has most similarity with neuropeptide Y receptor 1 (31% sequence homology overall and 46% in the transmembrane domains) and may have evolved as a redundant neuropeptide Y receptor [10]. Northern blot and *in situ* hybridization histology revealed that the highest expression of *Gpr10/Prlhr* mRNA in rat tissues is in the anterior pituitary, suggesting a potential role in the regulation of hormone secretion [2]. The receptor then was expressed in a heterologous cell system and extracts of bovine tissues used to identify putative binding activity, which could then be separated by chromatography. In this way, two peptide ligands were isolated from bovine hypothalamus. Complementary DNA analysis indicated that a precursor protein gives rise to two peptides of 31 and 20 amino acids, respectively. Interestingly, although mRNA was highest in the brainstem, peptide levels were highest in the hypothalamus. The two peptides were synthesized and found to induce prolactin secretion from cultured lactotrophs, with a similar potency to thyrotropin-releasing hormone, but without significant effect on the release of other anterior pituitary hormones [2]. Thus, the peptides were christened prolactin-releasing peptide (PrRP31 and the truncated PrRP20).

Subsequent localization of immunoreactive PrRP, as measured by enzyme-linked immunosorbent assay, confirmed that the highest concentrations of mature peptide are in the brain and pituitary [11]. In descending order, wet tissue concentrations in fmol/g were from the hypothalamus 1800 ± 320, midbrain 720 ± 110, neurohypophysis 530 ± 63, medulla oblongata 330 ± 82, thalamus 220 ± 30, striatum 140 ± 53, adenohypophysis 100 ± 29, cortex 94 ± 45, cerebellum 64 ± 8, and spinal cord 6 ± 1. The adrenal medulla has 62 ± 15 fmol/g, while no other tissue has above 4 fmol/g. Both PrRP31 and PrRP20 are present in the hypothalamus, but only PrRP31 is present in the adrenal medulla. Similar distributions of mature mRNA were detected by Northern analysis [12]. Plasma concentrations of PrRP are the same in male (0.13 ± 0.01 fmol/ml) and female (0.14 ± 0.01 fmol/ml) rats. All immunoreactive PrRP in the plasma appears to be PrRP31 [11]. Although *Gpr10/Prlhr* mRNA is greatest in the anterior pituitary, it is also present in the hypothalamus, thalamus, brainstem, spinal cord, adrenal medulla, testis, and epididymis [2, 12, 13].

Prolactin-Releasing Hormone – A Misnomer?

The finding that PrRP can stimulate prolactin release, but not the release of other hormones, from cultured rat pituitary cells *in vitro* was repeated in several early experiments [2, 14, 15]. However, later studies have found either no or mixed effects [16–18]. Since a barrier lies between the brain and the anterior pituitary (communication is achieved through the median eminence and portal blood system), the best proxy for an *in vivo* hypophysiotropic effect should be to administer the peptide intravenously rather than into the brain. Results have generally favored an effect of intravenous PrRP on prolactin secretion in female rats, dependent on stage of the estrous cycle [15, 19, 20]. By comparison, injection of PrRP into the ventricles of the brain does not mimic a true hypophysiotropic effect. Some such studies have noted an increase in the secretion of several anterior pituitary hormones, not limited to prolactin [16, 21–23]. In contrast, others have found no effect of centrally administered PrRP on prolactin secretion, including in the lactating rat [20, 24].

Our own interest in PrRP started with the supposition that a true prolactin secretagogue would be expressed in the "hypophysiotropic" hypothalamus and median eminence, and would be upregulated during lactation when prolactin secretion is required for milk production [7]. Thus, we were surprised that the expression of PrRP in cell bodies (demonstrated by both immunohistochemistry and *in situ* hybridization histology) was restricted to three brain regions not normally associated with the regulation of pituitary secretion: the dorsomedial nucleus of the hypothalamus (DMH) and two regions in the brainstem: the nucleus of the tractus solitarius (NTS) and the ventrolateral medulla oblongata (VLM) [7, 25–31]. Immunoreactive fibers were noted in the medulla oblongata, the parabrachial nucleus (PBN), bed nucleus of the stria terminalis (BNST), preoptic area, supraoptic and paraventricular hypothalamic nuclei, basolateral amygdala, septal nucleus, thalamus, internal median eminence, and posterior pituitary, but importantly not the external median eminence [26, 29, 31], as might have been expected for a hypophysiotropic hormone.

Perhaps the clearest evidence that PrRP is not a releasing factor for prolactin, at least during female reproduction, is that the expression of mRNA for the peptide in the female rat DMH, NTS, and VLM is clearly downregulated during lactation [7]. Lactating mothers are under negative energy balance due to the extreme metabolic cost of milk production. This led us to investigate other similar sequelae. Indeed, we found reduced mRNA expression in both female and male rats following fasting and in male homozygous Zucker rats, which lack leptin receptors and hence perceive that they are in negative energy balance. These findings, together with the fact that the central administration of PrRP reduced food intake and increased body temperature, led us to propose an alternative role for PrRP in metabolic regulation [7, 25, 32].

Classically, hypophysiotropic messengers were usually named as factors when initially discovered, were "converted" to hormones if found to circulate, and then to peptides (rather than "nuclear" hormones) if a protein structure was determined. In fact, though it is found in the circulation, there is little evidence that PrRP is a hormone at all: it has no certain role in regulating prolactin release and, to date, is known only to function as a neuropeptide. Perhaps due to potential confusion with prion protein, the newly proposed gene name for PrRP is prolactin-releasing hormone (*PRLH*), while the receptor gene is *PRLHR*, which might seem a rather retrograde step and does lead to further confusion in the literature. For reference, see the IUPHAR/BPS Guide to Pharmacology (https://www.guidetopharmacology.org) and the HUGO Gene Nomenclature Committee (https://www.genenames.org).

For the remainder of this review, the terms PrRP and GPR10 will be used generally, while *Prlh* and *Prlhr* will be used where specificity is appropriate, for example, in naming genes and transgenic animals.

Central Metabolic Effects of PrRP

As demonstrated first in rats [7, 25], *Prlh* mRNA is decreased in the DMH and NTS of fasted animals. *Prlh* mRNA is also decreased in fasted mice but, conversely, it is increased in diet-induced obese (DIO) mice [33]. Furthermore, intracerebroventricular administration of PrRP reduced both normal, nighttime feeding and fast-induced food intake, while increasing core body temperature (a surrogate measure for increased adaptive thermogenesis, which requires energy expenditure), leading to our hypothesis that PrRP functions centrally to control body weight [7, 25, 32, 34]. These effects are not due to peptide "leakage" from the brain into the circulation as the same doses do not cause metabolic effects if administered systemically [32]. More direct evidence that central PrRP causes energy expenditure through adaptive thermogenesis was provided by the demonstration that it increased oxygen consumption in rats at thermoneutrality [35], and increased uncoupling protein 1 (*Ucp1*) gene expression in brown adipose tissue [34]. Doses of PrRP that cause anorexia and energy expenditure when given into the lateral ventricle increase the expression of the cellular activity marker, FOS protein, in the forebrain (hypothalamus, thalamus, and amygdala) and brainstem (NTS, VLM, and area postrema [AP]), suggesting potential sites of action. Seal and colleagues [36] found that direct injection of PrRP into the parenchyma of the DMH caused a reduction in food intake. Interestingly, PrRP injected into the fourth ventricle or directly into the NTS parenchyma also affects both food intake and body temperature [37], suggesting an additional direct metabolic action at the caudal brainstem (see discussion below).

Receptor Coupling and Distribution

PrRP is a member of the RF-amide family of peptides, many of which have a conserved role in feeding regulation [38]. Thus, it is important to acknowledge the potential for interaction between the peptides and other family member receptors. GPR10 is very ligand-selective and only binds with high affinity to PrRP. Other RF-amide peptides, such as neuropeptide FF (NPFF), bind only with low affinity [39, 40]. Human and rat PrRP31 and PrRP20 all display high affinity/potency and are full agonists at GPR10. Functional responses are blocked by thapsigargin, indicating mobilization of intracellular Ca^{2+} stores [2, 39, 41]. Other studies suggest potential downstream coupling with CREB, extracellular signal-regulated kinase (ERK), Jnk, and Akt [42–45]. There is some evidence from the literature suggesting that GPR10 may be part of a family of related sequences [9], thus it is possible that PrRP has more than one endogenous receptor. This is further supported by evidence from chemical cross-linking studies that indicate that PrRP has different binding sites in the hypothalamus compared to the cardiac and skeletal muscle, and northern blot analysis indicates that *Prlhr* mRNA in these regions also differ in size [46]. However, it is clear that PrRP also binds NPFFR2 and to a lesser extent NPFFR1 [39, 47, 48]. NPFF and PrRP both displace [^{125}I]-26RFa binding in brain regions enriched with NPFF2 receptor [49]. NPFF receptors exhibit complex pharmacology as they can bind many of the RF-amide peptides. Three similar peptides, NPFF and RF-amide-related peptides 1 and 2, along with PrRP, have affinity for NPFF receptors. NPFF and PrRP have high affinity for NPFFR2 in *in vitro* binding studies [39]. While there is much uncertainty, NPFFR2 and NPFFR1 are thought to be endogenous receptors for NPFF and RFRP-1, respectively. RFRP-3 has a high affinity for NPFFR1, but there is still some dispute whether it also acts through NPFFR2 (for summary, see [40]). Stimulation of NPFF receptors seems to not mobilize intracellular calcium release. Instead, RF-amide peptides are able to dose-dependently inhibit accumulation of forskolin-stimulated cyclic adenosine monophosphate (cAMP) in different cell lines transfected with NPFFR2 as full receptor agonists [47, 50–52]. Thus, it appears that NPFFR2 may couple with pertussis toxin-sensitive Gi/o proteins to inhibit adenylyl cyclase and activate MAPK/ERK pathways [53].

Northern analysis identified strong *Prlhr* mRNA expression in the hypothalamus, thalamus, brainstem, and spinal cord [2, 12]. *In situ* hybridization histology located *Prlhr* more specifically in the reticular nucleus of the thalamus (RT), the DMH, paraventricular (PVH), and periventricular (PeV) nuclei of the hypothalamus, and the NTS and AP in the dorsal medulla oblongata [7, 12, 54]. This matches binding for rat [^{125}I]-PrRP31 or human [^{125}I]-PrRP20 to rat brain sections [55]. To date, there have been relatively few histological studies to identify individual cell types that express GPR10, though limited dual immunohistochemistry or dual *in situ* hybridization studies have described colocalization with corticotrophin-releasing hormone in the BNST and central amygdala (CeA), enkephalin in the PBN, and γ-aminobutyric acid in the RT [56, 57]. Finally, other studies have reported *Gpr10/Prlhr* expression in the rat anterior pituitary, adrenal medulla, muscle, testis and epididymis, placenta, and decidua [12, 13, 46, 58–60]. There are high densities of NPFF binding to NPFFR2 in the thalamus, hypothalamus, amygdala, substantia nigra, ventral hippocampus, and brainstem, including in the A5 noradrenergic cell group, spinal trigeminal nucleus, and dorsal vagal complex [61]. Interestingly, RNAScope analysis reveals a high level of *Npffr2* mRNA, particularly in the motor nucleus of the vagus [62].

Early distribution studies for NPFF itself may be misleading because of antibody cross reactivity [63]. Thus, suggestions that NPFF is expressed in the hypothalamus between the DMH and ventromedial nucleus of the hypothalamus (VMH) are probably due to cross reactivity with pyroglutamylated RF-amide (QRFP) and/or RFRP-3. Using a more selective antibody, we have found strong cell body staining for NPFF in the brainstem NTS, immediately abutting the AP, with notable fiber staining in the PBN, dorsal motor nucleus of the vagus (DMV), and VLM all within the brainstem (paper in prep.), corroborating the published immunohistochemical data from other groups [64, 65]. Similarly, studies have mapped the expression of *Npff* mRNA to the "sub-postrema" (SubP) region of the NTS, but not to other parts of the brain [62, 66–68]. It should be noted that NPFF is highly expressed within the dorsal horn of the spinal cord, along with binding sites [65], presumably related to a role for NPFF in nociception [69]. To date, no role for NPFF or PrRP in the spinal cord related to metabolism has been put forward.

Prlh and *Prlhr* Knockout Mouse Models

Takayanagi *et al.* [70] generated a PrRP (*Prlh*$^{-/-}$) null mouse, the males of which became obese on either chow or high-energy diet (HED). The obesity was due, apparently, solely to increased food intake (with no obvious difference in food preference). *Prlh*$^{-/-}$ null mice pair-fed to their wild-type littermates did not put on weight, and no differences were recorded in energy expenditure, body temperature, or locomotor activity. In the same paper, wild-type mice injected with a PrRP neutralizing antibody ate more and had a reduced response to the satiety hormone, cholecystokinin (CCK), but again there was no change in their energy expenditure. However, in a follow-up paper, the same *Prlh*$^{-/-}$ null mice had lower expression of UCP1 in brown adipose tissue [71]. We found a similar phenotype in a conditional PrRP knockout model, in which a loxSTOPlox codon was inserted upstream of the *Prlh* promoter [33]. These LSL-*Prlh* mice put on more weight than wild-type littermates when on chow or HED, but the effect was greater in females than in males. The mice had higher food intake and lower core-body temperature. Interestingly, the phenotype could be reversed by crossing with Cre-recombinase-expressing mice to re-instate the expression of *Prlh* in different parts of the brain [33], providing evidence for different roles for brainstem and forebrain PrRP neuron populations in energy intake and expenditure (see sections below).

Two GPR10 (*Prlhr*$^{-/-}$) null mice have been reported in the literature, both of which display late-onset obesity, but with slight differences in the level of adiposity reached by the two sexes [72, 73]. Interestingly, neither model was hyperphagic. In one model, obese female (but not male) mice had lower respiratory exchange ratio (RER), as expected for an obese animal. However, they also had slightly lower energy expenditure [72]. We have found that *Prlhr*$^{-/-}$ null mice have low oxygen consumption but normal food intake, before they become obese, suggesting that the adult phenotype is due to reduced energy expenditure rather than intake [74]. The primacy of GPR10 over other potential RF-amide peptide receptors in PrRP's actions is supported by the fact that deletion of *Prlhr* completely abolished PrRP binding to isolated hypothalamic cell membranes [73] and the hypophagic effect of the native peptide [75].

Natural Polymorphisms in the *PRLHR* Gene

The Otsuka Long-Evans Tokushima Fatty (OLETF) rat strain has a natural deletion in the *Cck1r* gene, which leads to a deficit in the expression of the cholecystokinin receptor 1 in the gastrointestinal tract, vagus and brain. This was long assumed as the reason for the increased meal size and hyperphagia in this rodent model of obesity and type 2 diabetes [76]. However, the critical mutant deletion in OLETF rats occurs in a 570 kb region which contains the *Prlhr* gene [77]. Importantly, PrRP is ineffective at suppressing food intake in OLETF rats but does in congenic rats that have the wild-type *Prlhr* sequence. It is noteworthy that there are some cardiovascular effects evoked by PrRP, which remain in OLETF rats but are blocked by an NPFFR2 receptor antagonist, suggesting that these additional effects of PrRP may not be mediated by GPR10 [78].

Rare single nucleotide polymorphisms (SNPs) have been found in the coding region of the human *GPR10* (*PRLHR*) gene that associate with high body mass index and/or low blood pressure [74, 79, 80]. In a comprehensive study, in collaboration with the Cambridge group led by Sadaf Farooqi, we demonstrated that the most common of the mutant gene variants could recapitulate the obesity phenotype in a humanized mouse model [74]. Twenty variants were found in people with severe obesity or in normal weight controls. In cell expression studies, the majority of variants led to an impairment of PrRP binding and a loss of G protein-dependent signaling. We went on to introduce the most common variant, which leads to an amino acid substitution, *Prlhr*^{P193S}, into the genome of a transgenic mouse. This humanized mouse gained excessive weight due to a decrease in energy expenditure rather than a change in energy intake [74], reiterating the disparate mechanism by which PRLHR and PRLH mutations alter energy balance.

Genetic Mutations Affecting NPFF Signaling Related to Metabolism

Npff$^{-/-}$ null mice do not have an obvious metabolic phenotype when on normal chow or HED, other than small changes in wheel running and water intake [81]. However, higher adaptive thermogenesis is revealed if the mice are maintained at thermoneutrality [68]. Interestingly, while *Npff*$^{-/-}$ null mice respond the same as wild-type controls during a 24 h fast, they have significantly greater weight regain during a subsequent 48 h refeeding period. RER in male *Npff*$^{-/-}$ null mice showed a significant decrease during the last 6 h of fasting – indicative of greater lipid oxidation, and a significant increase in RER during refeeding – indicative of greater usage of carbohydrate as energy stores are being replenished. This substrate flexibility during fast-induced refeeding suggests that NPFF may play a key role in regulating oxidative fuel utilization during changes in energy balance. This is interesting since *Npff* mRNA expression in the SubP is upregulated under energy deficit [67], the opposite of what is seen with *Prlh* mRNA [7, 33].

Homozygous knockout of the *Npffr2* receptor gene also has little effect on phenotype when mice are maintained on chow. However, when placed on HED, null *Npffr2*$^{-/-}$ mice showed exacerbated fat gain, due to impaired adaptive thermogenesis and lower energy expenditure [67]. Interestingly, cold-induced thermogenesis was not affected. A potential role for NPFF signaling on glucose regulation may be complicated by the expression of receptors in both the brain and in peripheral tissues. Zhang *et al.* [62, 68] found that null *Npffr2*$^{-/-}$ mice have improved glucose tolerance, while Karnosova *et al.* [82] report that another null model exhibits severe glucose intolerance. Finally, we are aware of only one study in humans, which describes SNPs in the *NPFFR2* gene that are associated with body mass index (BMI) and suggest they may be protective against the development of obesity [83].

Brainstem PrRP^{NTS} Neurons

As already mentioned, PrRP is expressed in three populations of neuron within the rodent brain: the DMH, NTS, and VLM. To date, no definitive role for PrRP^{VLM} neurons has been described, so here we will concentrate on the two populations which we know most about [1]. The strongest expressions of *Prlh* mRNA and PrRP protein are in the soma and projections of brainstem PrRP^{NTS} neurons [26, 29, 31]. The fact that *Prlh* mRNA is downregulated in negative energy balance and that central injection of PrRP causes anorexia without causing aversion, first alerted us to a potential role in appetite regulation [7, 25, 32]. The NTS is a relay where information from peripheral organs reaches the brain. Gut-derived vagal sensory afferents terminate in the posterior NTS, at a level just rostral of the AP to just caudal of the AP. Feedback loops engaging descending vagal efferents that emanate from the adjacent dorsal motor nucleus regulate digestion, while ascending PrRP projections to the hind-, mid-, and forebrain integrate with indirect regulators of feeding and body weight. Thus, PrRP^{NTS} neurons are activated by administration of the enteroendocrine satiety hormone CCK [32, 75] or by refeeding fasted mice [70], suggesting they respond to vagal afferents and are involved in normal satiation. Indeed, germline knockout of *Prlhr* blocks the hypophagia induced by administration of exogenous CCK [75], while mice injected with a PrRP-neutralizing antibody are hyperphagic and also have a reduced response to CCK [70]. The activation of PrRP^{NTS} neurons following direct infusion of nutrients into the stomach can be blocked by pre-administration of the CCK receptor antagonist, devazepide, confirming the role of these neurons in satiety signaling [84].

We made use of differential gene expression in PrRP^{NTS} neurons versus PrRP^{DMH} neurons to examine the relative importance of these two populations in body-weight regulation. PrRP^{NTS} neurons are noradrenergic and, therefore, express the genes for the catecholamine synthetic enzymes, tyrosine hydroxylase (*Th*) and dopamine ß hydroxylase (*Dbh*) [85]. By comparison, PrRP^{DMH} neurons do not express catecholamine markers but, unlike PrRP^{NTS} neurons, they instead express the gene for the leptin receptor (*Lepr*) [33]. Using our aforementioned LSL-*Prlh* mouse model, we demonstrated that conditional knockout of PrRP causes obesity [33]. Furthermore, LSL-*Prlh* mice do not respond to CCK to reduce food intake. Crossing this mouse with other Cre-recombinase-expressing lines permits excision of the loxSTOPlox transcriptional block and rescues the expression of PrRP. Thus, crossing the LSL-*Prlh* mouse with a *Th*-Cre rescued expression of PrRP only in the brainstem, whereas crossing it with a *nestin*-Cre mouse restored PrRP expression in all brain sites. Interestingly, both crosses reestablished the response to CCK and reversed the obesity of LSL-*Prlh* mice [33], demonstrating the sufficiency of brainstem PrRP to regulate feeding behavior and body weight. Collectively, the literature suggests that PrRP^{NTS} neurons respond to nutrients within the gut following the activation of vagal afferents. However, Blouet *et al.* have demonstrated that PrRP^{NTS} neurons are also directly sensitive to the amino acid, leucine, and through this have an additional role in the satiating effect of dietary protein [86].

Rinaman and colleagues [87] measured FOS activity in nontrained rats after voluntary first-time intake of an unrestricted, satiating volume of the liquid nutritional supplement, Ensure. DBH-positive A2 neurons within the caudal NTS were progressively recruited to express FOS in rats that consumed progressively larger volumes of Ensure. Among these DBH-positive neurons, the PrRP-positive subset was more sensitive to feeding-induced activation than the PrRP-negative subset. Notably, significant activation of preproglucagon (GCG; GLP-1-positive) neurons occurred only in rats that consumed the largest volumes of Ensure, corresponding to nearly 5% of their body weight, and indicated that GCG neurons respond mainly to volume [87, 88]. This difference in behavior of these two distinct populations of NTS neurons is interesting when considering their known physiology [89]. For example, we have found that PrRP neurons are activated by lipid gavage (an effect blocked by pre-administration of a CCK receptor antagonist) and not by the nausea-inducing compound, lithium chloride, whereas the opposite is true for GCG neurons ([32] and unpublished). The comparison of these two adjacent populations of NTS neuron has been further analyzed using fiber photometry [84]. In a very elegant paper, Knight and colleagues confirmed that infusion of nutrients directly into the stomach leads to the activation of both PrRP^{NTS} and GCG^{NTS} neurons over a period of minutes and depending on the amount infused, which would appear congruent with vagally mediated satiation. However, unlike PrRP^{NTS} neurons, the GCG^{NTS} neurons do not respond to nutrient content but rather to volume, and they are equally responsive to nonnutrient stimuli such as stretch of the stomach with mannitol or air. More interestingly, PrRP^{NTS} neuron activity can also track licking behavior and the taste of nutrients in the mouth. Thus, PrRP^{NTS} neurons respond immediately (within seconds) to nutrients in the mouth and longer term (tens of minutes) to nutrients in the gut [84].

Finally, the role for PrRP^{NTS} neurons in mediating satiety signaling has been further supported using *Prlh*^{Cre} mice. Acute activation of PrRP^{NTS} neurons using either chemogenetic or optogenetic models is sufficient to reduce food intake without causing an aversive response [84, 90]. Importantly, genetically silencing PrRP^{NTS} neurons either by expressing tetanus toxin in NTS *Prlh*^{Cre} mice [90] or by blocking the production of PrRP in NTS neurons in the conditional knockout mouse [33] produces hyperphagia and obesity.

Hypothalamic PrRP^{DMH} Neurons

One of our early discoveries was that, in addition to hypophagia, central administration of PrRP increases core-body temperature [7]. Coadministration of PrRP and leptin also had additive effects to reduce nighttime feeding and increase core-body temperature, leading to greater body weight loss [25]. Furthermore, *Prlh* mRNA expression is reduced in both fasted rats and obese Zucker rats, which lack *Lepr*, suggesting that PrRP neurons form part of the leptin-sensitive circuitry [7, 25]. Leptin is considered mainly as a permissive hormone, and its action to increase core-body temperature is thought to be pyrexic rather than thermogenic [91]. That is leptin increases core-body temperature by modifying blood flow to the tail to decrease heat loss rather than causing nonshivering adaptive thermogenesis. Contrary to our initial immunohistochemical evidence [25], *Lepr* is expressed in only one population of PrRP neuron, those in the dorsomedial hypothalamus, and only this population is activated by administration of leptin [33]. Crossing a *Prlh*^{Cre} and *Lepr*$^{flox/flox}$ mice produces offspring that lack *Lepr* on hypothalamic PrRP^{DMH} neurons [33]. These mice are not hyperphagic, but they do have lower energy expenditure and temperature, and they are obese compared with littermates. Accordingly, animals with selective deletion of either the leptin receptor or PrRP knocked specifically from PrRP^{DMH} neurons alone do not respond to exogenous leptin administration, but they do still respond to the satiating effect of CCK.

Although leptin's effects are mainly pyrexic [91], we did find that wild-type mice treated with leptin had a twofold increase in the expression of uncoupling protein-1 (*Ucp1*) mRNA in brown adipose tissue, an indirect measure of adaptive thermogenesis, but which did not occur in *Prlh*^{Cre}:*Lepr*$^{flox/flox}$ mice [33]. In fact, using calorimetry, we have shown that central administration of PrRP causes an increase in oxygen consumption/energy expenditure in both rats [35] and in mice (unpublished). Thus, although further investigation is required, PrRP and specifically PrRP^{DMH} neurons appear to mediate both pyrexia and adaptive thermogenesis.

Systemically Administered PrRP Analogs

We have described the use of a PrRP analog to reduce body weight when administered systemically and suggested its development as a possible treatment for obesity [4]. Four other groups have published on the use of modified PrRP peptides, but they have provided only very limited data on mode of action. They tested lipidated analogs which are designed to increase the half-life of the peptide and its lipid solubility, though it is not known whether these analogs penetrate the brain. As with native PrRP [39, 47, 48], the first lipidated analogs produced by the academic group at the Prague Institute of Organic Chemistry and Biochemistry [5, 92, 93] and by the Biotech company, Gubra [3], have high affinity for both GPR10 and NPFFR2 and cause weight loss when administered systemically. An almost identical lipidated analog has been reported by one group to have an anorectic effect in mice but does not appear to act through either GPR10 or NPFFR2 [94]. Instead, the anorectic effect of this molecule appears to be linked to off-target effects that cause immobilization. Interestingly, a PrRP analog from the nonprofit research company, Calibr at Scripps, has low affinity for NPFFR2 which is matched by a relatively poor effect on body weight [6].

Subcutaneous administration of lipidated PrRP analogs to DIO mice reduces cumulative food intake (though most of the effect is in the first few days) and body weight [5, 95, 96]. As expected with sufficient weight loss, several metabolic parameters, including glucose tolerance and circulating triglyceride levels, are improved. There is no definitive evidence for an action of these analogs on energy expenditure. In one study, weight loss was lower in pair-fed mice but *Ucp-1* mRNA expression in brown adipose tissue was unaffected [5], while in another study an increase in *Ucp-1* expression was recorded [96].

By comparison, our studies using a further modified PrRP analog, NN501, demonstrate relatively small effects on food intake, but with a sustained effect to increase fatty acid oxidation, which produces weight loss comparable to a GLP1R agonist [4]. NN501 does not cause aversion, lean-mass loss, or rebound overfeeding when treatment is stopped. Thus, NN501 can have an additive effect when coadministered with a GLP1R agonist. The route by which NN501 increases fatty acid oxidation and body weight reduction has not been fully characterized though it does depend on the expression of both GPR10 and NPFFR2.

Peripheral administration of some of the other lipidated PrRP analogs induces a pattern of FOS expression in the brain [97, 98], which is similar to the engagement of brain circuits activated by central injection of native PrRP [32, 75]. However, this is not convincing evidence that these PrRP analogs can penetrate the brain. The neuronal activation may instead be secondary to metabolic changes or due to unrelated peripheral effects. Indeed, we found that palm^{11}-PrRP31 has poor solubility and can cause skin irritation after repeated dosing (unpublished observations). Instead, we have direct evidence that fluorescently tagged NN501 has access to the brain, though this is limited to circumventricular organs [4]. Furthermore, we found that activation of brain regions by systemic NN501 is different from that produced by central injection of PrRP, again suggesting a different mode of action. On this point, it also is noteworthy that weight loss is achieved with repeated administration of NN501 systemically, yet repeated central injection of native PrRP leads to rapid tolerance [34].

Conclusions

PrRP peptide, PrRP neurons, and GPR10 are still relatively understudied even though they arguably constitute the best described endogenous system mediating satiety signaling in the brain. Importantly, knockout of PrRP in the dorsomedial hypothalamus or leptin receptors selectively from PrRP^{DMH} neurons has similar weight-increasing consequences as knocking out leptin receptors in either the arcuate or ventromedial hypothalamic nuclei [33, 99, 100]. Thus, the signaling system appears critical for body weight regulation, including in humans [74]. Preclinical experiments in rodents using modified PrRP peptides have produced promising effects to ameliorate diet-induced obesity. However, further in-depth studies are required to elucidate completely their mode of action. The PrRP analog, NN501, administered systemically can access the brain, to reduce body weight, with a moderate effect on food intake but a sustained effect on fatty acid oxidation [4]. Furthermore, it appears to do so without causing aversion or lean-mass loss, and without rebound feeding when treatment stops. We must bear in mind that, even though PrRP/GPR10 signaling is important in the regulation of human body weight [74], there may be species differences in response to PrRP analogs. Therefore, future studies using models other than rodents will be required to confirm safety and long-term efficacy, before we can realize the true translational potential of this fascinating peptide system.

References

1 Dodd, G.T. and Luckman, S.M. (2013). Physiological roles of GPR10 and PrRP signaling. *Front. Endocrinol. (Lausanne)* 4: 20.
2 Hinuma, S., Habata, Y., Fujii, R. et al. (1998). A prolactin-releasing peptide in the brain. *Nature* 393 (6682): 272–276.
3 Alexopoulou, F., Bech, E.M., Pedersen, S.L. et al. (2022). Lipidated PrRP31 metabolites are long acting dual GPR10 and NPFF2 receptor agonists with potent body weight lowering effect. *Sci. Rep.* 12 (1): 1696.
4 Feetham, C.H., Groom, S., John, L.M. et al. (2026). Analog of prolactin-releasing peptide reduces body weight primarily through sustained fatty acid oxidation rather than hypophagia. *Cell Metab.*: https://doi.org/10.1016/j.cmet.2025.10.021 38: 100–114.e6.
5 Maletinska, L., Nagelova, V., Ticha, A. et al. (2015). Novel lipidized analogs of prolactin-releasing peptide have prolonged half-lives and exert anti-obesity effects after peripheral administration. *Int. J. Obes.* 39 (6): 986–993.
6 Pflimlin, E., Lear, S., Lee, C. et al. (2019). Design of a long-acting and selective MEG-fatty acid stapled prolactin-releasing peptide analog. *ACS Med. Chem. Lett.* 10 (8): 1166–1172.
7 Lawrence, C.B., Celsi, F., Brennand, J., and Luckman, S.M. (2000). Alternative role for prolactin-releasing peptide in the regulation of food intake. *Nat. Neurosci.* 3 (7): 645–646.
8 Marchese, A., Heiber, M., Nguyen, T. et al. (1995). Cloning and chromosomal mapping of three novel genes, GPR9, GPR10, and GPR14, encoding receptors related to interleukin 8, neuropeptide Y, and somatostatin receptors. *Forensic Genomics* 29 (2): 335–344.
9 Welch, S.K., O'Hara, B.F., Kilduff, T.S., and Heller, H.C. (1995). Sequence and tissue distribution of a candidate G-coupled receptor cloned from rat hypothalamus. *Biochem. Biophys. Res. Commun.* 209 (2): 606–613.
10 Lagerstrom, M.C., Fredriksson, R., Bjarnadottir, T.K. et al. (2005). Origin of the prolactin-releasing hormone (PRLH) receptors: evidence of coevolution between

PRLH and a redundant neuropeptide Y receptor during vertebrate evolution. *Forensic Genom.* 85 (6): 688–703.

11 Matsumoto, H., Murakami, Y., Horikoshi, Y. et al. (1999). Distribution and characterization of immunoreactive prolactin-releasing peptide (PrRP) in rat tissue and plasma. *Biochem. Biophys. Res. Commun.* 257 (2): 264–268.

12 Fujii, R., Fukusumi, S., Hosoya, M. et al. (1999). Tissue distribution of prolactin-releasing peptide (PrRP) and its receptor. *Regul. Pept.* 83 (1): 1–10.

13 Nieminen, M.L., Brandt, A., Pietila, P., and Panula, P. (2000). Expression of mammalian RF-amide peptides neuropeptide FF (NPFF), prolactin-releasing peptide (PrRP) and the PrRP receptor in the peripheral tissues of the rat. *Peptides* 21 (11): 1695–1701.

14 Kawamata, Y., Fujii, R., Fukusumi, S. et al. (2000). Analyses for susceptibility of rat anterior pituitary cells to prolactin-releasing peptide. *Endocrine* 12 (3): 215–221.

15 Matsumoto, H., Noguchi, J., Horikoshi, Y. et al. (1999). Stimulation of prolactin release by prolactin-releasing peptide in rats. *Biochem. Biophys. Res. Commun.* 259 (2): 321–324.

16 Samson, W.K., Keown, C., Samson, C.K. et al. (2003). Prolactin-releasing peptide and its homolog RFRP-1 act in hypothalamus but not in anterior pituitary gland to stimulate stress hormone secretion. *Endocrine* 20 (1–2): 59–66.

17 Samson, W.K., Resch, Z.T., Murphy, T.C., and Chang, J.K. (1998). Gender-biased activity of the novel prolactin releasing peptides: comparison with thyrotropin releasing hormone reveals only pharmacologic effects. *Endocrine* 9 (3): 289–292.

18 Swinnen, E., Boussemaere, M., and Denef, C. (2005). Stimulation and inhibition of prolactin release by prolactin-releasing peptide in rat anterior pituitary cell aggregates. *J. Neuroendocrinol.* 17 (6): 379–386.

19 Tokita, R., Nakata, T., Katsumata, H. et al. (1999). Prolactin secretion in response to prolactin-releasing peptide and the expression of the prolactin-releasing peptide gene in the medulla oblongata are estrogen dependent in rats. *Neurosci. Lett.* 276 (2): 103–106.

20 Yuan, Z.F., Yang, S.C., and Pan, J.T. (2002). Effects of prolactin-releasing peptide on tuberoinfundibular dopaminergic neuronal activity and prolactin secretion in estrogen-treated female rats. *J. Biomed. Sci.* 9 (2): 112–118.

21 Iijima, N., Matsumoto, Y., Yano, T. et al. (2001). A novel function of prolactin-releasing peptide in the control of growth hormone via secretion of somatostatin from the hypothalamus. *Endocrinology* 142 (7): 3239–3243.

22 Matsumoto, H., Maruyama, M., Noguchi, J. et al. (2000). Stimulation of corticotropin-releasing hormone-mediated adrenocorticotropin secretion by central administration of prolactin-releasing peptide in rats. *Neurosci. Lett.* 285 (3): 234–238.

23 Seal, L.J., Small, C.J., Kim, M.S. et al. (2000). Prolactin releasing peptide (PrRP) stimulates luteinizing hormone (LH) and follicle stimulating hormone (FSH) via a hypothalamic mechanism in male rats. *Endocrinology* 141 (5): 1909–1912.

24 Jarry, H., Heuer, H., Schomburg, L., and Bauer, K. (2000). Prolactin-releasing peptides do not stimulate prolactin release in vivo. *Neuroendocrinology* 71 (4): 262–267.

25 Ellacott, K.L., Lawrence, C.B., Rothwell, N.J., and Luckman, S.M. (2002). PRL-releasing peptide interacts with leptin to reduce food intake and body weight. *Endocrinology* 143 (2): 368–374.

26 Iijima, N., Kataoka, Y., Kakihara, K. et al. (1999). Cytochemical study of prolactin-releasing peptide (PrRP) in the rat brain. *Neuroreport* 10 (8): 1713–1716.

27 Kalliomaki, M.L., Pertovaara, A., Brandt, A. et al. (2004). Prolactin-releasing peptide affects pain, allodynia and autonomic reflexes through medullary mechanisms. *Neuropharmacology* 46 (3): 412–424.

28 Lee, Y., Yang, S.P., Soares, M.J., and Voogt, J.L. (2000). Distribution of prolactin-releasing peptide mRNA in the rat brain. *Brain Res. Bull.* 51 (2): 171–176.

29 Maruyama, M., Matsumoto, H., Fujiwara, K. et al. (1999). Immunocytochemical localization of prolactin-releasing peptide in the rat brain. *Endocrinology* 140 (5): 2326–2333.

30 Minami, S., Nakata, T., Tokita, R. et al. (1999). Cellular localization of prolactin-releasing peptide messenger RNA in the rat brain. *Neurosci. Lett.* 266 (1): 73–75.

31 Yamakawa, K., Kudo, K., Kanba, S., and Arita, J. (1999). Distribution of prolactin-releasing peptide-immunoreactive neurons in the rat hypothalamus. *Neurosci. Lett.* 267 (2): 113–116.

32 Lawrence, C.B., Ellacott, K.L., and Luckman, S.M. (2002). PRL-releasing peptide reduces food intake and may mediate satiety signaling. *Endocrinology* 143 (2): 360–367.

33 Dodd, G.T., Worth, A.A., Nunn, N. et al. (2014). The thermogenic effect of leptin is dependent on a distinct population of prolactin-releasing peptide neurons in the dorsomedial hypothalamus. *Cell Metab.* 20 (4): 639–649.

34 Ellacott, K.L., Lawrence, C.B., Pritchard, L.E., and Luckman, S.M. (2003). Repeated administration of the anorectic factor prolactin-releasing peptide leads to tolerance to its effects on energy homeostasis. *Am. J. Physiol. Regul. Integr. Comp. Physiol.* 285 (5): R1005–R1010.

35 Lawrence, C.B., Liu, Y.L., Stock, M.J., and Luckman, S.M. (2004). Anorectic actions of prolactin-releasing peptide are mediated by corticotropin-releasing hormone receptors. *Am. J. Physiol. Regul. Integr. Comp. Physiol.* 286 (1): R101–R107.

36 Seal, L.J., Small, C.J., Dhillo, W.S. et al. (2001). PRL-releasing peptide inhibits food intake in male rats via the dorsomedial hypothalamic nucleus and not the paraventricular hypothalamic nucleus. *Endocrinology* 142 (10): 4236–4243.

37 Davis, X.S. and Grill, H.J. (2018). The hindbrain is a site of energy balance action for prolactin-releasing peptide: feeding and thermic effects from GPR10 stimulation of the nucleus tractus solitarius/area postrema. *Psychopharmacology* 235 (8): 2287–2301.

38 Bechtold, D.A. and Luckman, S.M. (2007). The role of RFamide peptides in feeding. *J. Endocrinol.* 192 (1): 3–15.

39 Engstrom, M., Brandt, A., Wurster, S. et al. (2003). Prolactin releasing peptide has high affinity and efficacy at neuropeptide FF2 receptors. *J. Pharmacol. Exp. Ther.* 305 (3): 825–832.

40 Quillet, R., Ayachi, S., Bihel, F. et al. (2016). RF-amide neuropeptides and their receptors in mammals: pharmacological properties, drug development and main physiological functions. *Pharmacol. Ther.* 160: 84–132.

41 Langmead, C.J., Szekeres, P.G., Chambers, J.K. et al. (2000). Characterization of the binding of [(125)I]-human prolactin releasing peptide (PrRP) to GPR10, a novel G protein coupled receptor. *Br. J. Pharmacol.* 131 (4): 683–688.

42 Hayakawa, J., Ohmichi, M., Tasaka, K. et al. (2002). Regulation of the PRL promoter by Akt through cAMP response element binding protein. *Endocrinology* 143 (1): 13–22.

43 Kimura, A., Ohmichi, M., Tasaka, K. et al. (2000). Prolactin-releasing peptide activation of the prolactin promoter is differentially mediated by extracellular signal-regulated protein kinase and c-Jun N-terminal protein kinase. *J. Biol. Chem.* 275 (5): 3667–3674.

44 Maixnerova, J., Spolcova, A., Pychova, M. et al. (2011). Characterization of prolactin-releasing peptide: binding, signaling and hormone secretion in rodent pituitary cell lines endogenously expressing its receptor. *Peptides* 32 (4): 811–817.

45 Nanmoku, T., Takekoshi, K., Fukuda, T. et al. (2005). Stimulation of catecholamine biosynthesis via the PKC pathway by prolactin-releasing peptide in PC12 rat pheochromocytoma cells. *J. Endocrinol.* 186 (1): 233–239.

46 Satoh, F., Smith, D.M., Gardiner, J.V. et al. (2000). Characterization and distribution of prolactin releasing peptide (PrRP) binding sites in the rat--evidence for a novel binding site subtype in cardiac and skeletal muscle. *Br. J. Pharmacol.* 129 (8): 1787.

47 Elhabazi, K., Humbert, J.P., Bertin, I. et al. (2013). Endogenous mammalian RF-amide peptides, including PrRP, kisspeptin and 26RFa, modulate nociception and morphine analgesia via NPFF receptors. *Neuropharmacology* 75: 164–171.

48 Gouarderes, C., Mazarguil, H., Mollereau, C. et al. (2007). Functional differences between NPFF1 and NPFF2 receptor coupling: high intrinsic activities of RFamide-related peptides on stimulation of [35S]GTPgammaS binding. *Neuropharmacology* 52 (2): 376–386.

49 Bruzzone, F., Lectez, B., Alexandre, D. et al. (2007). Distribution of 26RFa binding sites and GPR103 mRNA in the central nervous system of the rat. *J. Comp. Neurol.* 503 (4): 573–591.

50 Elshourbagy, N.A., Ames, R.S., Fitzgerald, L.R. et al. (2000). Receptor for the pain modulatory neuropeptides FF and AF is an orphan G protein-coupled receptor. *J. Biol. Chem.* 275 (34): 25965–25971.

51 Hinuma, S., Shintani, Y., Fukusumi, S. et al. (2000). New neuropeptides containing carboxy-terminal RFamide and their receptor in mammals. *Nat. Cell Biol.* 2 (10): 703–708.

52 Mollereau, C., Mazarguil, H., Marcus, D. et al. (2002). Pharmacological characterization of human NPFF(1) and NPFF(2) receptors expressed in CHO cells by using NPY Y(1) receptor antagonists. *Eur. J. Pharmacol.* 451 (3): 245–256.

53 Bray, L., Froment, C., Pardo, P. et al. (2014). Identification and functional characterization of the phosphorylation sites of the neuropeptide FF2 receptor. *J. Biol. Chem.* 289 (49): 33754–33766.

54 Roland, B.L., Sutton, S.W., Wilson, S.J. et al. (1999). Anatomical distribution of prolactin-releasing peptide and its receptor suggests additional functions in the central nervous system and periphery. *Endocrinology* 140 (12): 5736–5745.

55 Ellacott, K.L., Donald, E.L., Clarkson, P. et al. (2005). Characterization of a naturally-occurring polymorphism in the UHR-1 gene encoding the putative rat prolactin-releasing peptide receptor. *Peptides* 26 (4): 675–681.

56 Lin, S.H., Arai, A.C., Espana, R.A. et al. (2002). Prolactin-releasing peptide (PrRP) promotes awakening and suppresses absence seizures. *Neuroscience* 114 (1): 229–238.

57 Lin, S.H., Leslie, F.M., and Civelli, O. (2002). Neurochemical properties of the prolactin releasing peptide (PrRP) receptor expressing neurons: evidence for a role of PrRP as a regulator of stress and nociception. *Brain Res.* 952 (1): 15.

58 Reis, F.M., Vigano, P., Arnaboldi, E. et al. (2002). Expression of prolactin-releasing peptide and its receptor in the human decidua. *Mol. Hum. Reprod.* 8 (4): 356–362.

59 Takahashi, K., Totsune, K., Murakami, O. et al. (2002). Expression of prolactin-releasing peptide and its receptor in the human adrenal glands and tumor tissues of adrenocortical tumors, pheochromocytomas and neuroblastomas. *Peptides* 23 (6): 1135–1140.

60 Yasui, Y., Yamaguchi, M., Jikihara, H. et al. (2001). Expression of prolactin-releasing peptide in human placenta and decidua. *Endocr. J.* 48 (3): 397–401.

61 Bonini, J.A., Jones, K.A., Adham, N. et al. (2000). Identification and characterization of two G protein-coupled receptors for neuropeptide FF. *J. Biol. Chem.* 275 (50): 39324–39331.

62 Zhang, L., Koller, J., Gopalasingam, G. et al. (2022). Central NPFF signalling is critical in the regulation of glucose homeostasis. *Mol. Metab.* 62: 101525.

63 Panula, P., Aarnisalo, A.A., and Wasowicz, K. (1996). Neuropeptide FF, a mammalian neuropeptide with multiple functions. *Prog. Neurobiol.* 48 (4–5): 461–487.

64 Jhamandas, J.H., Jhamandas, A., and Harris, K.H. (2001). New central projections of neuropeptide FF: colateral branching pathways in the brainstem and hypothalamus in the rat. *J. Chem. Neuroanat.* 21 (2): 171–179.

65 Kivipelto, L. and Panula, P. (1991). Comparative distribution of neurons containing FLFQPQRFamide-like (morphine-modulating) peptide and related neuropeptides in the rat brain. *Eur. J. Neurosci.* 3 (2): 175–185.

66 Vilim, F.S., Aarnisalo, A.A., Nieminen, M.L. et al. (1999). Gene for pain modulatory neuropeptide NPFF: induction in spinal cord by noxious stimuli. *Mol. Pharmacol.* 55 (5): 804–811.

67 Zhang, L., Ip, C.K., Lee, I.J. et al. (2018). Diet-induced adaptive thermogenesis requires neuropeptide FF receptor-2 signalling. *Nat. Commun.* 9 (1): 4722.

68 Zhang, L., Koller, J., Gopalasingam, G., and Herzog, H. (2022). NPFF signalling is critical for thermosensory and dietary regulation of thermogenesis. *Neuropeptides* 96: 102292.

69 Yang, H.Y., Tao, T., and Iadarola, M.J. (2008). Modulatory role of neuropeptide FF system in nociception and opiate analgesia. *Neuropeptides* 42 (1): 1–18.

70 Takayanagi, Y., Matsumoto, H., Nakata, M. et al. (2008). Endogenous prolactin-releasing peptide regulates food intake in rodents. *J. Clin. Invest.* 118 (12): 4014–4024.

71 Mochiduki, A., Takeda, T., Kaga, S., and Inoue, K. (2010). Stress response of prolactin-releasing peptide knockout mice as to glucocorticoid secretion. *J. Neuroendocrinol.* 22 (6): 576–584.

72 Bjursell, M., Lenneras, M., Goransson, M. et al. (2007). GPR10 deficiency in mice results in altered energy expenditure and obesity. *Biochem. Biophys. Res. Commun.* 363 (3): 633–638.

73 Gu, W., Geddes, B.J., Zhang, C. et al. (2004). The prolactin-releasing peptide receptor (GPR10) regulates body weight homeostasis in mice. *J. Mol. Neurosci.* 22 (1–2): 93–104.

74 Talbot, F., Feetham, C.H., Mokrosinski, J. et al. (2023). A rare human variant that disrupts GPR10 signalling causes weight gain in mice. *Nat. Commun.* 14 (1): 1450.

75 Bechtold, D.A. and Luckman, S.M. (2006). Prolactin-releasing peptide mediates cholecystokinin-induced satiety in mice. *Endocrinology* 147 (10): 4723–4729.

76 Bi, S. and Moran, T.H. (2016). Obesity in the Otsuka Long Evans Tokushima fatty rat: mechanisms and discoveries. *Front. Nutr.* 3: 21.

77 Watanabe, T.K., Suzuki, M., Yamasaki, Y. et al. (2005). Mutated G-protein-coupled receptor GPR10 is responsible for the hyperphagia/dyslipidaemia/obesity locus of Dmo1 in the OLETF rat. *Clin. Exp. Pharmacol. Physiol.* 32 (5–6): 355–366.

78 Ma, L., MacTavish, D., Simonin, F. et al. (2009). Prolactin-releasing peptide effects in the rat brain are mediated through the Neuropeptide FF receptor. *Eur. J. Neurosci.* 30 (8): 1585–1593.

79 Bhattacharyya, S., Luan, J., Challis, B. et al. (2003). Association of polymorphisms in GPR10, the gene encoding the prolactin-releasing peptide receptor with blood pressure, but not obesity, in a U.K. Caucasian population. *Diabetes* 52 (5): 1296–1299.

80 Franks, P.W., Bhattacharyya, S., Luan, J. et al. (2004). Association between physical activity and blood pressure is modified by variants in the G-protein coupled receptor 10. *Hypertension* 43 (2): 224–228.

81 Zhang, L., Koller, J., Ip, C.K. et al. (2021). Lack of neuropeptide FF signalling in mice leads to reduced repetitive behavior, altered drinking behavior, and fuel type selection. *FASEB J.* 35 (11): e21980.

82 Karnosova, A., Strnadova, V., Zelezna, B. et al. (2023). NPFFR2-deficient mice fed a high-fat diet develop strong intolerance to glucose. *Clin. Sci. (Lond.)* 137 (10): 847–862.

83 Hunt, S.C., Hasstedt, S.J., Xin, Y. et al. (2011). Polymorphisms in the NPY2R gene show significant associations with BMI that are additive to FTO, MC4R, and NPFFR2 gene effects. *Obesity (Silver Spring)* 19 (11): 2241–2247.

84 Ly, T., Oh, J.Y., Sivakumar, N. et al. (2023). Sequential appetite suppression by oral and visceral feedback to the brainstem. *Nature* 624 (7990): 130–137.

85 Chen, C., Dun, S.L., Dun, N.J., and Chang, J.K. (1999). Prolactin-releasing peptide-immunoreactivity in A1 and A2 noradrenergic neurons of the rat medulla. *Brain Res.* 822 (1–2): 276–279.

86 Tsang, A.H., Nuzzaci, D., Darwish, T. et al. (2020). Nutrient sensing in the nucleus of the solitary tract mediates non-aversive suppression of feeding via inhibition of AgRP neurons. *Mol. Metab.* 42: 101070.

87 Kreisler, A.D., Davis, E.A., and Rinaman, L. (2014). Differential activation of chemically identified neurons in the caudal nucleus of the solitary tract in non-entrained rats after intake of satiating vs. non-satiating meals. *Physiol. Behav.* 136: 47–54.

88 Kreisler, A.D. and Rinaman, L. (2016). Hindbrain glucagon-like peptide-1 neurons track intake volume and contribute to injection stress-induced hypophagia in meal-entrained rats. *Am. J. Physiol. Regul. Integr. Comp. Physiol.* 310 (10): R906–R916.

89 Luckman, S.M. and Lawrence, C.B. (2003). Anorectic brainstem peptides: more pieces to the puzzle. *Trends Endocrinol. Metab.* 14 (2): 60–65.

90 Cheng, W., Ndoka, E., Maung, J.N. et al. (2021). NTS Prlh overcomes orexigenic stimuli and ameliorates dietary and genetic forms of obesity. *Nat. Commun.* 12 (1): 5175.

91 Fischer, A.W., Hoefig, C.S., Abreu-Vieira, G. et al. (2016). Leptin raises defended body temperature without activating thermogenesis. *Cell Rep.* 14 (7): 1621–1631.

92 Karnosova, A., Strnadova, V., Hola, L. et al. (2021). Palmitoylation of prolactin-releasing peptide increased affinity for and activation of the GPR10, NPFF-R2 and NPFF-R1 receptors: in vitro study. *Int. J. Mol. Sci.* 22: 8904.

93 Mrazikova, L., Neprasova, B., Mengr, A. et al. (2021). Lipidized prolactin-releasing peptide as a new potential tool to treat obesity and type 2 diabetes mellitus: preclinical studies in rodent models. *Front. Pharmacol.* 12: 779962.

94 Wang, Y., Qiu, W., Kernodle, S. et al. (2025). Roles for Prlhr/GPR10 and Npffr2/GPR74 in feeding responses to PrRP. *Mol. Metab.* 92: 102093.

95 Holubova, M., Zemenova, J., Mikulaskova, B. et al. (2016). Palmitoylated PrRP analog decreases body weight in DIO rats but not in ZDF rats. *J. Endocrinol.* 229 (2): 85–96.

96 Prazienkova, V., Holubova, M., Pelantova, H. et al. (2017). Impact of novel palmitoylated prolactin-releasing peptide analogs on metabolic changes in mice with diet-induced obesity. *PLoS One* 12 (8): e0183449.

97 Pirnik, Z., Kolesarova, M., Zelezna, B., and Maletinska, L. (2018). Repeated peripheral administration of lipidized prolactin-releasing peptide analog induces c-fos and FosB expression in neurons of dorsomedial hypothalamic nucleus in male C57 mice. *Neurochem. Int.* 116: 77–84.

98 Pirnik, Z., Zelezna, B., Kiss, A., and Maletinska, L. (2015). Peripheral administration of palmitoylated prolactin-releasing peptide induces Fos expression in hypothalamic neurons involved in energy homeostasis in NMRI male mice. *Brain Res.* 1625: 151–158.

99 Balthasar, N., Coppari, R., McMinn, J. et al. (2004). Leptin receptor signaling in POMC neurons is required for normal body weight homeostasis. *Neuron* 42 (6): 983–991.

100 Dhillon, H., Zigman, J.M., Ye, C. et al. (2006). Leptin directly activates SF1 neurons in the VMH, and this action by leptin is required for normal body-weight homeostasis. *Neuron* 49 (2): 191–203.

9

The Becoming of Dasiglucagon

Ditte Riber[1], Jesper M. Mathiesen[1], Lise Giehm[1], Francesca Macchi[1,2], Mikael Elander[1], and Jesper S. Villadsen[1]

[1] *Zealand Pharma A/S, Sydmarken 11, Soeborg 2860, Denmark*
[2] *Gubra A/S, Hoersholm Kongevej 11B, Hoersholm 2970, Denmark*

The Becoming of Dasiglucagon

The Discovery of Glucagon and Its Physiological Effects

The relation between diabetes mellitus and the pancreas was established in the late 1890s [1], and the discovery was followed by attempts to administer pancreatic extracts both orally as well as parenterally to treat diabetes mellitus [1]. Insulin from ox pancreatic extract was successfully administered to diabetic patients in 1921 to control blood glucose, and in 1922 a hyperglycemic fraction of the extract was discovered [2]. However, it was not until 1953 before glucagon was purified and crystallized [1, 3].

The physiological effects of glucagon are presented in Figure 9.1. Glucagon is secreted from the α-cells of pancreatic islets and is central in the regulation of glucose homeostasis, opposing the action of insulin in its effects on blood glucose levels. Glucagon stimulates hepatic glycogenolysis and gluconeogenesis in hypoglycemic states to restore glucose homeostasis and has been shown to exert effects on lipid metabolism, energy balance, and body adipose tissue mass [4–6]. In addition, glucagon administration produces positive inotropic and chronotropic effects on the heart, exerts spasmolytic effects on gastrointestinal smooth muscle, and stimulates growth hormone release [7–10]. Glucagon also increases glomerular filtration rate (GFR) and decreases food intake [11, 12].

Glucagon stimulates insulin release indirectly via the increase in blood glucose (and presumably directly via glucagon receptors on beta-cells in the pancreas), whereas insulin inhibits glucagon release [13, 14].

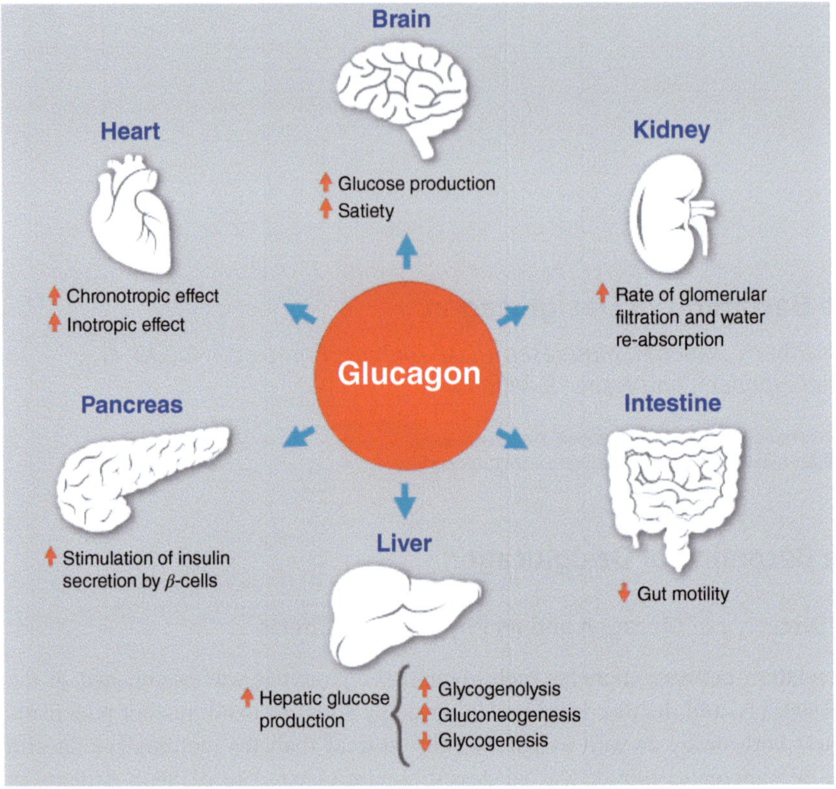

Figure 9.1 Physiological effects of glucagon receptor (GCGR) agonism. Released from pancreatic α-cells glucagon is central for the regulation of glucose homeostasis by activation of the GCGR. In the liver, GCGR activation stimulates hepatic glycogenolysis and gluconeogenesis. Glucagon has many additional effects across a number of tissues.

Medical Use of Glucagon as a Rescue Treatment for Insulin Induced Hypoglycemia in Diabetes Mellitus

The glucose-lowering effect of parenterally administered insulin inherently leads to a risk of hypoglycemic episodes. Mild hypoglycemia can be corrected by oral consumption of carbohydrates, whereas severe hypoglycemia, characterized by severe cognitive impairment requiring assistance from another person for recovery, can be treated with glucagon or administration of intravenous (IV) glucose [15–18]. For patients with type 1 or type 2 diabetes mellitus who rely on insulin for daily management, severe hypoglycemia is one of the most-feared adverse events (AEs) associated with insulin therapy. For these patients, hypoglycemia most often results from an imbalance between near-term insulin demands and dosing due to miscounting of carbohydrate loads or misjudgment of immediate requirements, and/or unanticipated exercise-induced insulin-independent glucose transport into skeletal muscles [19].

Subcutaneous administration of glucagon leads to a rapid increase in blood glucose and is thus suitable for rescuing severe hypoglycemia. However, the drug-like

Amino acid																												
1	2	3	4	5	6	7	8	9	10	11	12	13	14	15	16	17	18	19	20	21	22	23	24	25	26	27	28	29
H	S	Q	G	T	F	T	S	D	Y	S	K	Y	L	D	S	R	R	A	Q	D	F	V	Q	W	L	M	N	T

Figure 9.2 The amino acid sequence of human glucagon.

properties of native glucagon are poor as it has a low solubility in the pH range of 4–8 due to its isoelectric point of around pH 7.

The solubility of native glucagon increases under acidic or alkaline conditions, but at these conditions it is not stable. The first glucagon products developed by Eli Lilly and Novo Nordisk were therefore supplied as "hypo kit" products [20, 21], for which reconstitution of the drug product is required immediately prior to administration, and the drug product must be administered directly after reconstitution. The need for a lyophilized glucagon product is thus a consequence of glucagon's intrinsic tendency to form peptide aggregates and the chemical instability in aqueous solutions [22–24].

Rational Design of Dasiglucagon

Dasiglucagon (ZP4207) is a glucagon analog developed by Zealand Pharma and disclosed for the first time in WO 2014/016300. Dasiglucagon was developed with the aim of identifying a glucagon analog with improved solubility and physiochemical properties around neutral pH, while retaining pharmacokinetic (PK) and pharmacodynamic (PD) properties equivalent to human glucagon, enabling a "ready-to-use" product. Dasiglucagon was approved as Zegalogue® in 2021 in the United States as a treatment for severe hypoglycemia in adults and children above six years of age with diabetes. Zegalogue® injection is a clear, colorless solution supplied as a prefilled syringe or an autoinjector at a concentration of 0.6 mg dasiglucagon/0.6 ml, pH 6.5.

Basis for the Chemical and Physical Instability of Native Glucagon

Human glucagon consists of 29 amino acid residues (Figure 9.2). The chemical instability of glucagon is mainly due to isomerization and cleavage of aspartic acid residues, deamidation of glutamine and asparagine residues, and oxidation of methionine [23].

Generally, Asn and Gln deamidation occurs at high and low pH, but also with significant rates at neutral pH. The deamidation occurs via a cyclic imide ring formation opening to L-Asp and L-Iso-Asp and to L-Glu and L-Iso-Glu, respectively, with a small amount of the corresponding D-isomers indicating a slow racemization of the cyclic imide. Thus, from Asn and Gln, a family of five degradation products may be generated at significant rates (see Figure 9.3) [25]. In addition, the adjacent amino acid sequence influences the deamidation kinetics, where residues such as Xxx-Gly, Xxx-Thr, and Xxx-Ser (Xxx = Asn or Gln) are more susceptible to deamidation, due to the smaller amino acid side chain allowing for easier cyclic imide formation [25]. The intramolecular cyclization to an imide occurs to a larger extent with Asn and Asp than the longer side-chain analogs Gln and Glu due to the formation of a five-membered ring, which is energetically more favored [25].

At pH below physiological conditions, the deamidation of Asn and Gln is slowed down, but the formation of a cyclic imide from Asp and Glu and hence isomerization

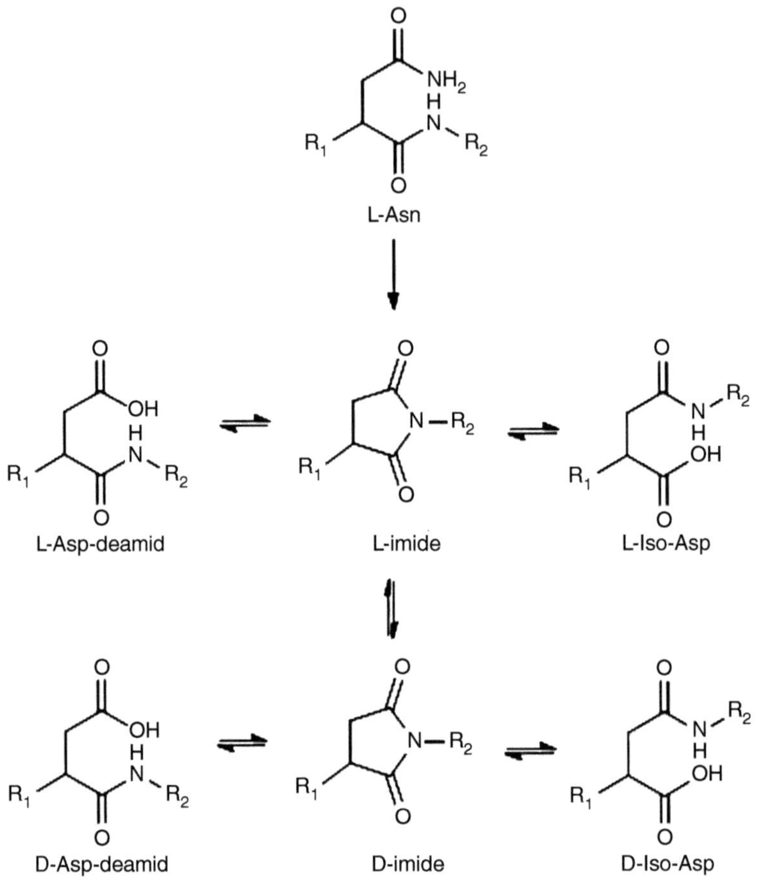

Figure 9.3 Pathways for deamidation, isomerization, and racemization for asparagine in peptides.

is increased with decreasing pH and is optimal at pH 4–6 [26]. Below pH 4, deamidation increases again as a result of direct acid-catalyzed deamidation.

Thus, stabilizing a peptide containing especially Asn/Gln and/or Asp as a drug product is often a challenge. This is so even for lyophilized drug products because the lyophilized drug product has an intermediate process step as a liquid formulation. Thus, eliminating Asn/Gln and/or Asp in the glucagon sequence (Figure 9.2) increases the potential for obtaining a stabilized drug product.

The physical stability of glucagon is decreased due to an increased propensity to form amyloid fibrils at low and high pH [27]. The literature mainly describes how different additives [28], glucagon concentration [29, 30], different temperatures [30], and degree of agitation affect the aggregation kinetics and fibril morphology [29, 30]. Literature also provides a mechanistic insight into the aggregation process of glucagon [31] and which amino acids in the glucagon sequence promote fibrillation [27]. The fibrillation propensity of glucagon at low pH (pH 2.5, 50 mM glycine buffer) has been investigated by Ala-scan with 15 different point mutations. This study indicated that Phe6, Tyr10, Val23, and Met27 were particularly important for the fibrillation propensity of glucagon, which highlights hydrophobic amino acids as important amino acids for fibrillation [27]. In contrast, it appeared from literature that residues in the middle part of glucagon are less important for fibrillation at low pH.

Design Strategy and Assays

By rational design of amino acid substitutions in the sequence of glucagon, the feasibility of producing a glucagon analog suitable for liquid formulation at neutral pH with increased chemical and physical stability was assessed.

The key objectives of the designs were to:

1) Preserve the potency at the human glucagon receptor (GCGR).
2) Improve the solubility in aqueous buffers at neutral pH.
3) Increase the chemical stability.
4) Minimize the tendency to form amyloid fibrils.
5) Retain the native glucagon-like PK and PD properties in established preclinical models.

To optimize the chemical and physical stability of glucagon, iterative design rounds were made with a focus on substitutions of chemically unstable amino acids, disrupting hydrophobic regions, and increasing α-helicity.

Initially, a critical review of the available literature was performed to identify key amino acids responsible for maintaining the high-potency binding and intrinsic activity at the glucagon receptor. The domains responsible for the unfortunate propensities toward peptide aggregation, and chemical instability that characterize human glucagon, limiting its utility as a therapeutic were also investigated [23, 27]. To display the effects of known substitutions, a "map" was created to highlight domains of interest for guiding which native glucagon residues to substitute and which to preserve (see Figure 9.4). From the review, it was also clear that the N-terminal region including histidine in position 1 of native glucagon is important to maintain the agonistic intracellular signaling properties and the rapid clearance from the blood via enzymatic degradation [33]. Consequently, no substitutions were made to the N-terminal residues 1–14 although some residues affecting chemical (Gln3, Asp9) and physical (Phe6, Tyr10, Tyr13) stability are present in this region. Additionally, it has been shown that human glucagon (hGCG) (1–27) has a significantly reduced potency [34], and therefore full-length hGCG (1–29) was used as starting point for the designs.

For evaluation of the designed glucagon analogs, several assays were performed. For all analogous synthesized, an in vitro cell signaling assay was performed to test the agonist potency toward the GCGR. To determine the potency of an analog, HEK293 cells overexpressing the GCGR were stimulated with increasing peptide concentrations. The accumulation of the second messenger cyclic adenosine monophosphate (cAMP) was quantified and plotted against the peptide concentration, followed by nonlinear regression to estimate the EC_{50} as a measure of peptide potency. Solubility was investigated by a solubility screen pH range 4–7.5

	Amino acid																												
	1	2	3	4	5	6	7	8	9	10	11	12	13	14	15	16	17	18	19	20	21	22	23	24	25	26	27	28	29
Chem	H	S	Q	G	T	F	T	S	D	Y	S	K	Y	L	D	S	R	R	A	Q	D	F	V	Q	W	L	M	N	T
Phys	H	S	Q	G	T	F	T	S	D	Y	S	K	Y	L	D	S	R	R	A	Q	D	F	V	Q	W	L	M	N	T
Potency	H	S	Q	G	T	F	T	S	D	Y	S	K	Y	L	D	S	R	R	A	Q	D	F	V	Q	W	L	M	N	T

Figure 9.4 Literature-derived AAs in the sequence of human glucagon affecting chemical stability, physical stability, and/or potency on the GCGR. Red = amino acids impacting the chemical and physical stability. Green = amino acids that when mutated to Ala do not significantly impact the potency of glucagon at the human glucagon receptor [23, 27, 32].

(selected analogs) using turbidity measurements at 325 nm to estimate whether analogs were in solution in different buffer systems. Chemical stability was investigated by stress degradation (pH 4, 7 and 9, and oxidative stress) for 15 days (40 °C) and 28 days (25 °C), and based on LC–MS analysis on selected analogs, the major degradation pathways were identified. The knowledge on the major degradation pathways was used to optimize the peptide sequence, and labile amino acids were substituted. Physical stability (fibrillation) was investigated by measuring Thioflavin T emission at 485 nm (ex 450) over 96 h at 40 °C with continuous agitation at pH 7.4 (selected analogs soluble to a concentration of ≥1 mg/ml). The best candidates also underwent in vivo testing to assess PK and PD properties.

1st Design: Exploring Substitution of Residues Susceptible for Isomerization, Cleavage, and Oxidation

Initially, single amino acid substitutions of Asp15, Asp21, and Met27 of human glucagon were explored to obtain structure–activity relationship data of these positions for the subsequent design of chemically and physically stabilized glucagon analogs. Representative amino acids from the following groups were chosen: a polar amino acid (Ser or Asn), an acidic amino acid (Glu), or a basic amino acid (Lys). No hydrophobic amino acids were chosen as they potentially could further induce or enhance aggregation. The substitution of Asp15 with Asn (a polar amino acid of the same size as Asp) was not considered the optimal choice due to the deamidation propensity of Asn as described above but was implemented in the design in case none of the other substitutions led to acceptable activity in the in vitro assay.

The above considerations resulted in synthesis of nine peptides listed in Table 9.1. The conservative substitution of Asp to Glu in position 15 preserved activity on the GCGR. Peptides even with nonconservative substitutions in positions 21 and 27 were also highly active, except for Lys27, and provided the basis for further design of a soluble and nonaggregating glucagon analog.

2nd Design: Exploring Substitution of Potential Deamidation Sites and Disruption of an Aggregation Prone Hydrophobic Region

In the 2nd design, substitutions of Gln, Met, and Asn in positions 20, 24, 27, and 28 were explored to avoid deamidation sites and avoid oxidation of methionine. Furthermore, the isoelectric point was altered to increase the solubility at pH 7, and the hydrophobic region between amino acids 22–27 was disrupted to possibly decrease the propensity for aggregation.

Table 9.1 Sequences of 1st design.

Peptide	Amino acid number															EC50 (nM) hGCGR
	1–14	15	16	17	18	19	20	21	22	23	24	25	26	27	28	29	
Glucagon[a)]	HSQGTFTSDYSKYL	D	S	R	R	A	Q	D	F	V	Q	W	L	M	N	T	0.02
1	HSQGTFTSDYSKYL	**E**	S	R	R	A	Q	D	F	V	Q	W	L	M	N	T	0.03
2	HSQGTFTSDYSKYL	**S**	S	R	R	A	Q	D	F	V	Q	W	L	M	N	T	0.26
3	HSQGTFTSDYSKYL	**K**	S	R	R	A	Q	D	F	V	Q	W	L	M	N	T	39.30
4	HSQGTFTSDYSKYL	**N**	S	R	R	A	Q	D	F	V	Q	W	L	M	N	T	0.50
5	HSQGTFTSDYSKYL	D	S	R	R	A	Q	**S**	F	V	Q	W	L	M	N	T	0.03
6	HSQGTFTSDYSKYL	D	S	R	R	A	Q	**K**	F	V	Q	W	L	M	N	T	0.03
7	HSQGTFTSDYSKYL	D	S	R	R	A	Q	D	F	V	Q	W	L	**S**	N	T	0.05
8	HSQGTFTSDYSKYL	D	S	R	R	A	Q	D	F	V	Q	W	L	**K**	N	T	0.21
9	HSQGTFTSDYSKYL	D	S	R	R	A	Q	D	F	V	Q	W	L	**E**	N	T	0.005

hGCGR: human glucagon receptor; Bold AA: changes compared to human glucagon.

a) Human glucagon.

To decrease the aggregation propensity of the peptides compared to native glucagon, preferably charged (Arg, Lys, Glu), polar (Ser), and/or α-helix stabilizing amino acids (Ala, Leu, Glu, Lys) were introduced at the specified positions in the specified combinations. This was hypothesized to disturb the hydrophobic region in positions 22–27 and enhance physical stability. The Glu and Lys substitutions in positions 20, 24, and 28 also introduced potential (i, $i+4$) salt bridges to further enhance α-helix formation, while simultaneously minimizing the propensity to form β-pleated sheets that can promote peptide fibrillation.

To increase the solubility of the peptides around pH 7.5 compared to native glucagon, the peptides were designed to have a theoretical pI lower than 6 or higher than 9.

The substitution of Met27 with Glu, which was found to retain GCGR potency in the previous design, is considered a very attractive substitution for many reasons as it lowers pI, disrupts the aggregation-prone region with a charged amino acid, removes the oxidation-prone methionine, introduces an α-helix stabilizing amino acid and is a nonconservative substitution, which may be attractive from an intellectual property (IP) perspective. Consequently, further substitutions at this position were explored, including Leu, which despite its hydrophobic nature, is also an α-helix stabilizing amino acid and expected to be highly active in vitro, as well as Arg to explore if another basic residue at this position was not tolerated as an effort to decrease aggregation propensity and raise pI.

The substitution of Arg17 with Ala was performed to lower pI. Likewise, the substitution of Asp21 with Ser was used to raise pI and avoid degradation of Asp21.

The above design considerations resulted in synthesis of 16 peptides listed in Table 9.2.

Interestingly, most of the nonconservative substitutions in positions 20, 24, 27, and 28 retained potency on the GCGR. With these modifications, it appeared easier to increase the solubility at neutral pH by lowering the pI than to raise it, as introduction of several basic residues, and in particular in position 27 as also shown in the 1st design, appeared to lower potency or not improve solubility, whereas substitutions to lower pI, such as by, e.g., introducing Glu, were better tolerated and increased solubility.

Only peptide 17 of the ones tested, with expected improvement of α-helix formation in the hydrophobic region due to a potential salt bridge network between residues Glu20, Lys24, and Glu27, displayed no fibrillation. However, the potency was reduced by a factor of 6 compared to native glucagon.

Likewise, only peptide 13 from the 2nd design displayed a chemical stability above 90%, but unfortunately the physical stability of this compound was very poor.

The overall conclusion was that further modifications were necessary to obtain both an acceptable chemical and physical stability.

3rd Design: Combining the Learnings from Previous SAR Rounds

In the 3rd design, focus was on the combination of 1st design active substitutions with selected peptides from the 2nd design having a good physical stability and/or solubility to further improve the chemical stability.

Table 9.2 Sequences of 2nd design.

Peptide	Amino acid number[a]															EC50 (nM) hGCGR	Solubility[c] (mg/ml)	Physical stability[d]	Chemical Stability (%)[e]
	15	16	17	18	19	20	21	22	23	24	25	26	27	28	29				
Peptides with a theoretical pI lower than 6																			
Glucagon[b]	D	S	R	R	A	Q	D	F	V	Q	W	L	M	N	T	0.02	<1	—	—
10	D	S	R	R	A	**E**	D	F	V	**S**	W	L	**E**	**S**	T	0.09	≥1	FD	83
11	D	S	R	R	A	**E**	D	F	V	**A**	W	L	**E**	**S**	T	0.02	≥1	—	—
12	D	S	R	R	A	**E**	D	F	V	**S**	W	L	**L**	**S**	T	0.02	≥1	—	—
13	D	S	R	R	A	**K**	D	F	V	**E**	W	L	**E**	**S**	T	0.04	≥1	FD	91
14	**E**	S	R	R	A	**K**	D	F	V	**E**	W	L	**L**	**E**	T	0.07	≥1	—	—
15	D	S	R	R	A	**A**	D	F	V	**E**	W	L	**E**	**K**	T	0.03	—	FD	82
16	D	S	**A**	R	A	**E**	D	F	V	**A**	W	L	**E**	**R**	T	0.58	≥1	—	—
17	D	S	**A**	R	A	**E**	D	F	V	**K**	W	L	**E**	**S**	T	0.11	≥1	FND	86
18	D	S	R	R	A	**K**	D	F	**L**	**E**	W	L	**E**	**S**	T	0.18	≥1	—	—
Peptides with a theoretical pI higher than 9																			
19	D	S	R	R	A	**R**	D	F	V	**A**	W	L	**S**	**R**	T	0.05	≥1	FD	84
20	D	S	R	R	A	**A**	D	F	V	**R**	W	L	**R**	**S**	T	0.27	—	—	—
21	D	S	R	R	A	**R**	D	F	V	**A**	W	L	**L**	**R**	T	0.04	<1	—	85
22	D	S	R	R	A	**K**	**S**	F	V	**E**	W	L	**L**	**K**	T	0.07	<1	—	83
23	D	S	R	R	A	**K**	**S**	F	V	**E**	W	L	**R**	**S**	T	0.78	≥1	—	—
24	D	S	R	R	A	**E**	D	F	V	**K**	W	L	**R**	**S**	T	0.93	—	—	—
25	D	S	R	R	A	**K**	D	F	V	**L**	W	L	**E**	**R**	T	0.08	≥1	FD	84

hGCGR: human glucagon receptor; Bold AA: changes compared to human glucagon; —: no data.

a) AA 1–14 = HSQGTFTSDYSKYL.

b) Human glucagon.

c) Solubility in phosphate buffer pH 7.0.

d) Physical stability was evaluated at pH 7.0 by an accelerated fibrillation assay (40 °C, 96 h continuous agitation) using Thioflavin T (ThT), FD (fibrillation detected), and FND (fibrillation not detected).

e) 15 days chemical stability pH 7 (% remaining of original peptide).

The 1st design revealed that substitutions Asp15Glu, Asp21Ser/Lys, and Met27Ser/Glu were all highly active in the GCGR cAMP assay with EC_{50}s below 0.2 nM (see Table 9.1). These substitutions were combined among these three positions (peptides 26–34) and also with promising sequences from the 2nd design. Additionally, the amino acid substitutions Asp21Glu and Met27Leu were also included for combination as these had previously shown to retain in vitro activity.

Despite its reduced in vitro potency, peptide 17 from the 2nd design was chosen as a starting point since it displayed excellent solubility and physical stability. To increase the chemical stability and to keep the pI low, Asp in positions 15 and 21 was substituted with Glu to give peptide 35. To explore which substitutions in peptide 17 were responsible for the good solubility and physical stability, it was attempted to reverse the salt bridge between position 20 and 24 to give peptide 36 and likewise to exchange the substitutions in positions 27 and 28, while substituting both Asp15 and 21 with Glu.

Peptides 13, 19, and 22 from 2nd design were also chosen as starting points for further modifications since they all had acceptable solubility and potency. To increase the chemical stability of peptide 13 and keep pI low, Asp15 and 21 were substituted with Glu to give peptide 38. In the case of peptides 19 and 22, having a high pI, Asp15 was substituted with Glu, but Asp21 was substituted with Ser to increase pI further leading to peptide 39 and 40, respectively.

Two additional peptide 19 analogs were also part of the 3rd design. To increase both the chemical stability and pI further, Asp15 was substituted with Glu and Asp21 with Lys to give peptide 41. For the second analog, both Asp15 and Asp21 were substituted with Glu, but the C-terminal was amidated, leading to peptide 42.

The above design hypotheses resulted in the synthesis of the 17 peptides listed in Table 9.3.

Unfortunately, all peptides tested in the ThT assay indicated reduced physical stability (Table 9.3), likely due to the substitution of Asp in position 15 with Glu that was introduced in all the 3rd design peptides to improve the chemical stability. Indeed, all tested peptides showed improved chemical stability, presumably due to the prevention of aspartimide formation at positions 15 and 21 as the chemical stability at pH 4 in particular was increased (data not shown). The SAR round also provided insights into combinations of substitutions that retained in vitro activity.

4th Design

The starting point for the 4th design was also chosen to be predominantly based on the sequence of peptide 17 from the 2nd design, as the peptides from the 3rd design did not have the desired improvements when substituting Asp15 with Glu. The particular motif of Asp followed by Ser is known to be very prone to degradation and even fragmentation of the peptide bond between the two amino acids, as previously described. As an alternative to substituting Asp15 with Glu to remove the liability completely, the Ser16 can be substituted to reduce the propensity of aspartate degradation.

In the 4th design, Aib was thus introduced in position 16. Aib (1-aminoisobutyric acid) is a rare, nonproteinogenic bulky amino acid. The hypothesis was that this

Table 9.3 Sequences of 3rd design.

Peptide	Amino acid number[a]															EC50 (nM) hGCGR	Solubility[c] (mg/ml)	Physical stability[d]	Chemical stability (%)[e]
	15	16	17	18	19	20	21	22	23	24	25	26	27	28	29				
Glucagon[b]	D	S	R	R	A	Q	D	F	V	Q	W	L	M	N	T	0.02	<1	—	—
26	**E**	S	R	R	A	Q	**E**	F	V	Q	W	L	**E**	N	T	0.03	≥1	FD	87
27	**E**	S	R	R	A	Q	**E**	F	V	Q	W	L	**S**	N	T	0.10	—	—	—
28	**E**	S	R	R	A	Q	**E**	F	V	Q	W	L	**L**	N	T	0.02	—	—	—
29	**E**	S	R	R	A	Q	**S**	F	V	Q	W	L	**E**	N	T	—	—	—	—
30	**E**	S	R	R	A	Q	**S**	F	V	Q	W	L	**S**	N	T	0.59	—	—	—
31	**E**	S	R	R	A	Q	**E**	F	V	Q	W	L	**E**	N	T	0.05	—	—	93
32	**E**	S	R	R	A	Q	**K**	F	V	Q	W	L	**E**	N	T	0.10	≥1	FD	—
33	**E**	S	R	R	A	Q	**K**	F	V	Q	W	L	**S**	N	T	0.46	≥1	FD	—
34	**E**	S	R	R	A	Q	**K**	F	V	Q	W	L	**L**	N	T	0.09	—	—	—
35	**E**	S	**A**	R	A	**E**	**E**	F	V	**K**	W	L	**E**	**S**	T	0.30	≥1	FD	98
36	**E**	S	**A**	R	A	**K**	**E**	F	V	**E**	W	L	**E**	**S**	T	0.15	<1	—	—
37	**E**	S	**A**	R	A	**E**	**E**	F	V	**K**	W	L	**S**	**E**	T	0.91	≥1	FD	96
38	**E**	S	R	R	A	**K**	**E**	F	V	**E**	W	L	**E**	**S**	T	0.04	—	—	85
39	**E**	S	R	R	A	**R**	**S**	F	V	**A**	W	L	**S**	**R**	T	1.43	—	—	—
40	**E**	S	R	R	A	**K**	**S**	F	V	**E**	W	L	**L**	**K**	T	0.14	≥1	FD	87
41	**E**	S	R	R	A	**R**	**K**	F	V	**A**	W	L	**S**	**R**	T	3.50	—	—	—
42	**E**	S	R	R	A	**R**	**E**	F	V	**A**	W	L	**S**	**R**	T	0.06	≥1	FD	82

hGCGR: human glucagon receptor; Bold AA: changes compared to human glucagon; —: no data.

a) AA 1–14 = HSQGTFTSDYSKYL.

b) Human glucagon.

c) Solubility in phosphate buffer pH 7.0.

d) Physical stability evaluated by an accelerated fibrillation assay (40 °C, 96 h, continuous agitation) using Thioflavin T (ThT), FD (fibrillation detected), and FND (fibrillation not detected).

e) 15 days chemical stability pH 7 (% remaining original peptide).

sterically hindered amino acid would prevent the backbone nitrogen between position 15 and 16 to participate in ring closure with the side chain of Asp in position 15 to generate an aspartimide moiety. Furthermore, Aib is known to favor a helical conformation as well as inducing beta-sheet disruption, so this substitution was anticipated to also increase the physical stability. Glu, Lys, and Leu in position 16 were also explored.

Again, inspired by peptide 17, Glu and Lys substitutions were introduced along some or all the positions 16, 20, 24, and 28 to create $(i, i+4)$ salt bridges expected to enhance α-helix formation. The negatively charged amino acid Glu in position 27 is envisioned to disrupt the hydrophobic area responsible for poor physical stability and may also form a $(i, i+3)$ salt bridge to position 24 and is therefore kept in many of the sequences or placed in position 28 instead, retaining the possibility of a salt bridge to a positive-charged amino acid in position 24.

To increase the chemical stability, the chemical labile Asp in position 21 was substituted to Ser or Glu known to retain GCGR activity, and although disappointing results regarding physical stability were obtained in the 3rd design when substituting Asp in position 15 with Glu, this substitution was introduced again in other sequences.

The substitution of Arg17 with Ala was previously found to maintain activity in the GCGR cAMP assay as well as lowering pI and increasing solubility and was therefore introduced in most of the sequences of the 4th design.

Additionally, a few peptides were made to examine the effect of truncating from the C-terminus, and this resulted in the synthesis of 25 peptides listed in Table 9.4.

Although a majority of the presumed $(i, i+4)$ salt bridge stabilized peptides did not fibrillate, there were also exceptions, and no clear conclusions to the best combination could be made, besides the combination already found from peptide 17 appeared to be superior. The introduction of Aib, in position 16 did indeed prevent fibrillation in the ThT assay (peptides 52 and 56), as was also the case for the two peptides with a Glu in this position (peptides 47 and 55). Interestingly, these four peptides also displayed good chemical stability of equal to or above 90%, but peptides with Aib in position 16 retained GCGR in vitro potency to a larger extent.

Peptide 56 displaying excellent potency, chemical and physical stability, and thus fulfilling all the preset criteria was selected for further analysis and long-term studies. Unfortunately, peptide 56 was subsequently shown to precipitate at low temperature, and a further design was therefore made.

Of note, due to its high solubility and in vitro potency, the peptide 65 was subsequently used as a full agonistic and soluble glucagon analog and enabled determination of the cryo-electron microscopy structure of the GCGR in complex with its cognate G protein [35]. Together with another cryo-electron microscopy study using native glucagon [36], these studies support our initial reasoning of not modifying the N-terminal part of the glucagon peptide as this is deeply engaged in interactions with the GCGR, to stabilize the receptor in an active and native signaling conformation.

5th Design

The fifth and final design focused on peptide 56 analogs, as this peptide was very promising apart from precipitation noted at low temperature as described above.

Table 9.4 Sequences of 4th design.

Peptide	Amino acid number[a)]															EC50 (nM) hGCGR	Solubility[c)] (mg/ml)	Physical stability[d)]	Chemical stability (%)[e)]
	15	16	17	18	19	20	21	22	23	24	25	26	27	28	29				
Glucagon[b)]	D	S	R	R	A	Q	D	F	V	Q	W	L	M	N	T	0.020	<1	—	—
43	D	S	**A**	R	A	**E**	**S**	F	V	**K**	W	L	**E**	**S**	T	0.066	≥1	FD	86
44	D	S	**A**	R	A	**E**	D	F	V	**K**	W	L	**E**	**E**	T	0.174	≥1	FND	86
45	D	**K**	**A**	R	A	**E**	D	F	V	**K**	W	L	**E**	**S**	T	0.033	≥1	FD	87
46	D	S	**A**	R	A	**E**	D	F	V	**A**	W	L	**E**	**S**	T	0.340	≥1	FND	85
47	D	**E**	**A**	R	A	**K**	D	F	V	**E**	W	L	**E**	**K**	T	0.168	≥1	FND	90
48	D	S	**A**	R	A	**E**	D	F	V	**E**	W	L	**E**	**S**	T	0.869	≥1	—	—
49	**E**	S	**A**	R	A	**E**	D	F	V	**K**	W	L	**E**	**S**	T	0.376	≥1	FD	—
50	D	S	**A**	R	A	**E**	**E**	F	V	**K**	W	L	**E**	**S**	T	0.031	≥1	FD	—
51	D	S	**A**	R	A	**E**	D	F	V	**S**	W	L	**E**	**S**	T	0.299	≥1	FND	—
52	D	**Aib**	**A**	R	A	**E**	D	F	V	**K**	W	L	**E**	**S**	T	0.030	≥1	FND	91
53	D	S	**A**	R	A	**E**	D	F	V	**K**	W	L	**E**	**S**		0.068	≥1	FD	89
54	D	S	**A**	R	A	**E**	D	F	V	**K**	W	L	**E**			9.881	≥1	FND	—
55	D	**E**	**A**	R	A	**E**	D	F	V	**K**	W	L	**E**	**S**	T	0.155	≥1	FND	92
56	D	**Aib**	**A**	R	A	**E**	**S**	F	V	**K**	W	L	**E**	**S**	T	0.025	≥1	FND	89
57	**E**	S	**A**	R	A	**E**	**S**	F	V	**K**	W	L	**E**	**S**	T	0.347	—	—	—
58	D	**L**	**A**	R	A	**E**	D	F	V	**K**	W	L	**E**	**S**	T	0.029	≥1	FD	88

Table 9.4 (Continued)

Peptide	Amino acid number[a]															EC50 (nM) hGCGR	Solubility[c] (mg/ml)	Physical stability[d]	Chemical stability (%)[e]
	15	16	17	18	19	20	21	22	23	24	25	26	27	28	29				
59	D	S	**A**	R	A	**E**	D	F	V	**K**	W	L	**S**	**E**	T	0.221	≥1	FND	86
60	D	S	**A**	R	A	**E**	D	F	V	**K**	W	L	**S**	**E**	T	0.189	≥1	FND	85
61	D	**E**	**A**	R	A	**K**	D	F	V	**E**	W	L	**S**	**K**	T	0.361	—	—	—
62	D	S	R	R	A	**E**	D	F	V	**E**	W	L	**E**	**S**	T	0.135	≥1	FND	83
63	D	S	R	R	A	**E**	D	F	V	**A**	W	L	**E**	**S**	T	0.034	≥1	FD	—
64	D	**K**	R	R	A	**E**	D	F	V	**S**	W	L	**E**	**S**	T	0.026	≥1	FD	—
65	D	S	R	R	A	**E**	D	F	V	**K**	W	L	**E**	**S**	T	0.008	≥1	FD	80
66	**E**	S	R	R	A	**R**	**E**	F	V	**A**	W	L	**S**	**R**	T	0.169	≥1	FD	—
67	**E**	S	R	R	A	**K**	**S**	F	V	**E**	W	L	**L**	**K**	T	0.320	—	—	—

hGCGR: human glucagon receptor; Aib: 1-aminoisobutyric acid; Bold AA: changes compared to human glucagon; —: no data.

a) AA 1–14 = HSQGTFTSDYSKYL.
b) Human glucagon.
c) Solubility in phosphate buffer pH 7.0.
d) Physical stability evaluated by an accelerated fibrillation assay (40 °C, 96 h, continuous agitation) using Thioflavin T (ThT), FD (fibrillation detected), and FND (fibrillation not detected).
e) 14 days chemical stability pH 7.0–7.5 (% remaining original peptide).

To explore whether the properties of peptide 56 could be further improved, several strategies were pursued.

To prevent the degradation of Asp in position 15, other substitutions than Aib in position 16 were investigated. This included introduction of the sterically hindered amino acid Val to possibly increase the chemical stability or the introduction of Glu to lower pI further and thus increase the solubility. The direct substitution of Asp in position 15 to Glu to increase the chemical stability was avoided as this appeared to have a negative impact on the physical stability as seen from the result of the 3rd design.

It was also explored if the peptide could be further stabilized by additional salt bridges or α-helix stabilizing amino acids. Thus, Glu and Lys were introduced in position 16 and 28, respectively, and the salt bridge between positions 20 and 24 was reversed. Also, substitution of Thr in position 29 with the more α-helix-stabilizing amino acid Ala was performed.

To further lower the overall charge of the peptide, Glu was introduced in position 16 or 21.

Following synthesis and testing of the 7 peptides shown in Table 9.5, it was seen that the introduction of Val and Glu in position 16 was nicely tolerated with respect to in vitro potency and solubility. Aib in position 16 still appeared to lead to superior physical stability, when compared to Glu in position 16, comparing peptide 73 to 71. Peptide 68 was not tested for physical or chemical stability.

Introducing the potential for formation of additional salt bridges and/or reversal of salt bridges as in peptides 71, 72, and 73 also gave highly active peptides with improved solubility compared to glucagon; however, they did not lead to further improvements compared to peptide 56. Neither did substitution of Ala in position 29.

In contrast, the introduction of Glu in position 21 in peptide 69, which lowers pI further as well as introduce the possibility of salt bridges between positions 18, 21, and 24, resulted in superior solubility (data not shown) and chemical stability compared to peptide 56. This substitution also improved the potency even further compared to peptide 56, while having an excellent physical stability, and peptide 69 was thus selected as lead candidate.

In summary, the reiterative design and in vitro functional assessment process led to the selection of dasiglucagon (peptide 69), which fulfilled the predefined criteria for potency, solubility, and physical and chemical stability. Through this process, 7 out of 14 amino acids in the C-terminal region in glucagon were substituted. These were Ser in position 16 to Aib, Arg in position 17 to Ala, Gln in position 20 to Glu, Asp in position 21 to Glu, Gln in position 24 to Lys, Met in position 27 to Glu, and Asn in position 28 to Ser. The corresponding increases in chemical stability that were achieved can be seen from Figure 9.5. Dasiglucagon was chosen as the candidate that moved forward into clinical testing as this peptide displayed excellent solubility (150 mg/ml in water) and physical and chemical stability, enabling a "ready-to-use" aqueous formulation while retaining in essence the same potency and pharmacodynamic profile as human glucagon (see Figure 9.10).

Table 9.5 Sequences of 5th design.

Peptide	Amino acid number[a)]															EC50 (nM) hGCGR	Solubility[c)] (mg/ml)	Physical stability[d)]	Chemical stability (%)[e)]
	15	16	17	18	19	20	21	22	23	24	25	26	27	28	29				
Glucagon[b)]	D	S	R	R	A	Q	D	F	V	Q	W	L	M	N	T	0.02	<1	—	—
68	D	**V**	**A**	R	A	**E**	**S**	F	V	**K**	W	L	**E**	**S**	T	0.054	≥1	—	—
69	D	**Aib**	**A**	R	A	**E**	**E**	F	V	**K**	W	L	**E**	**S**	T	0.0095	≥1	FND	94
70	D	**Aib**	R	R	A	**E**	**S**	F	V	**K**	W	L	**E**	**S**	T	0.0066	≥1	FND	90
71	D	**E**	**A**	R	A	**K**	**S**	F	V	**E**	W	L	**E**	**K**	T	0.063	≥1	FD	—
72	D	**E**	**A**	R	A	**K**	**S**	F	V	**E**	W	L	**E**	**S**	T	0.035	≥1	FD	—
73	D	**Aib**	**A**	R	A	**K**	**S**	F	V	**E**	W	L	**E**	**K**	T	0.023	≥1	FND	92
74	D	**Aib**	**A**	R	A	**E**	**S**	F	V	**K**	W	L	**E**	**S**	**A**	0.016	≥1	FND	91

hGCGR: human glucagon receptor; Aib: 1-aminoisobutyric acid; Bold AA: changes compared to human glucagon; —: no data.

a) AA 1–14 = HSQGTFTSDYSKYL.

b) Human glucagon.

c) Solubility in phosphate buffer pH 7.0.

d) Physical stability evaluated by an accelerated fibrillation assay (40 °C, 96 h, continuous agitation) using Thioflavin T (ThT), FD (fibrillation detected), and FND (fibrillation not detected).

e) 14 days chemical stability pH 7–7.5 (% remaining original peptide).

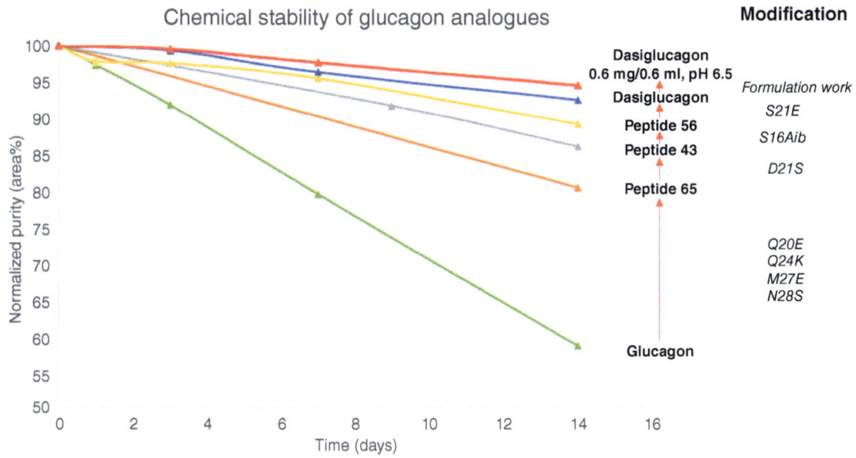

Figure 9.5 The contribution from amino acid substitutions and formulation development to chemical stability. Chemical stability was tested at 40 °C.

Characterization of Dasiglucagon

Physical and Chemical Stability of Dasiglucagon

The formulation development for dasiglucagon was based on the knowledge of the isoelectric point (pI = 5.0) and the pH degradation profile (Figure 9.6).

The pI for dasiglucagon is around pH 5.0, and the optimal pH for chemical stability is in the range from pH 5.5–6.5. Different buffers were screened in this pH range, and tris(hydroxymethyl)aminomethane (TRIS) buffer was found to be a suitable buffer. Different tonicity agents were tested, and NaCl was found to be a suitable tonicity agent.

The fibrillation tendency of dasiglucagon in different formulations was evaluated in a 14-day study where samples were exposed to 40 °C temperature and vigorous shaking in the presence and absence of Thioflavin T (ThT), which is known to bind specifically to amyloid-like fibrillar structures. Reconstituted GlucaGen® rescue kit (contains human glucagon) was run head-to-head with dasiglucagon in the GlucaGen® vehicle and in the commercial dasiglucagon formulation (0.6 mg dasiglucagon/0.6 ml, pH 6.5). All conditions were tested in three replica wells on a 96-well plate. The results show that fibril formation under these heavily stressed conditions only occurs for GlucaGen®, while dasiglucagon is stable for 14 days under strong agitation at 40 °C in both formulations. The native glucagon samples start fibrillating after three hours, as shown by the significant increase in fluorescence signal, which follows the classic sigmoidal shape as expected during fibril formation (see Figure 9.7).

Rotation Study – Simulating Real Use by Patients

Zegalogue® can be stored at room temperature for up to one year to provide patients and caregivers with a portable and convenient treatment option, allowing flexibility in their everyday life while ensuring immediate access to a ready-to-use treatment

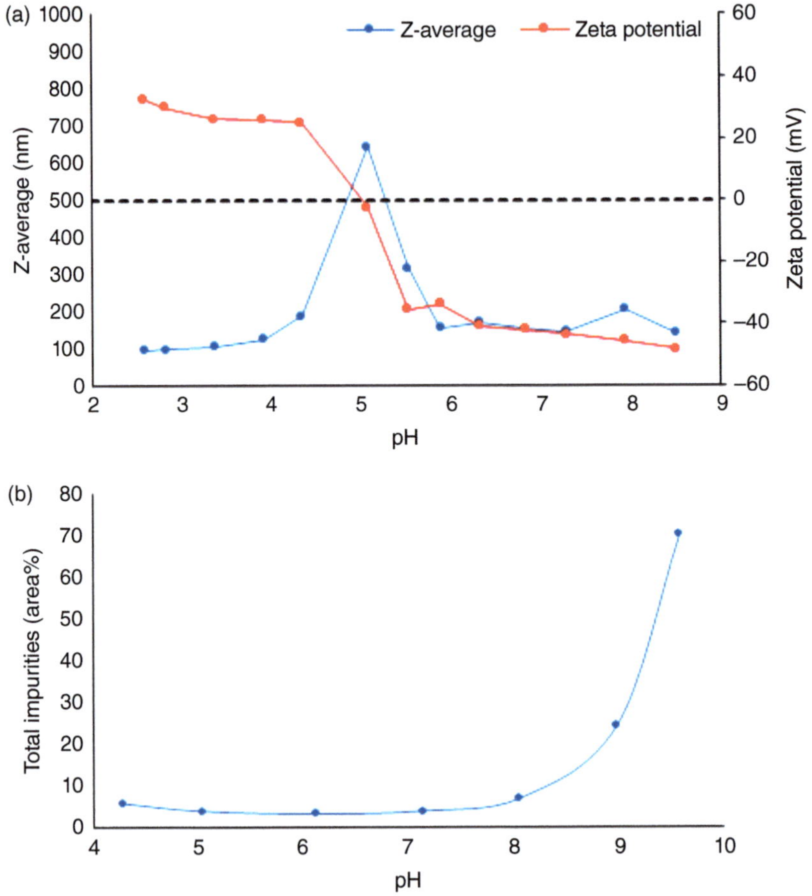

Figure 9.6 Dasiglucagon pI (a) and pH dependent degradation profile (b).

for episodes of severe hypoglycemia. In practice, this means that the product could be subjected to mechanical stress during this "in-use" period. The mechanical stress could be a result of the product being stored in a handbag, backpack, or similar over a period of one year. A study was set up to examine if continuous mechanical stress would impact the chemical and physical stability of dasiglucagon. Prefilled syringes with 0.6 mg dasiglucagon/0.6 ml, pH 6.5 was wrapped in aluminum foil and placed on a tube rotator machine at room temperature. The rotation machine was set to 10 rpm. The stability was followed by HPLC (chemical degradation) and DLS (dynamic light scattering, physical stability) over 52 weeks. The data was compared to control samples that were stored under the same conditions, but no rotation was applied. The data is presented in Figure 9.8 and Table 9.6.

There is no difference between rotated and nonrotated samples in terms of HPLC purity and DLS data over 52 weeks at 25 °C. This supports that dasiglucagon is unaffected by extensive mechanical stress (see Table 9.6 and Figure 9.8).

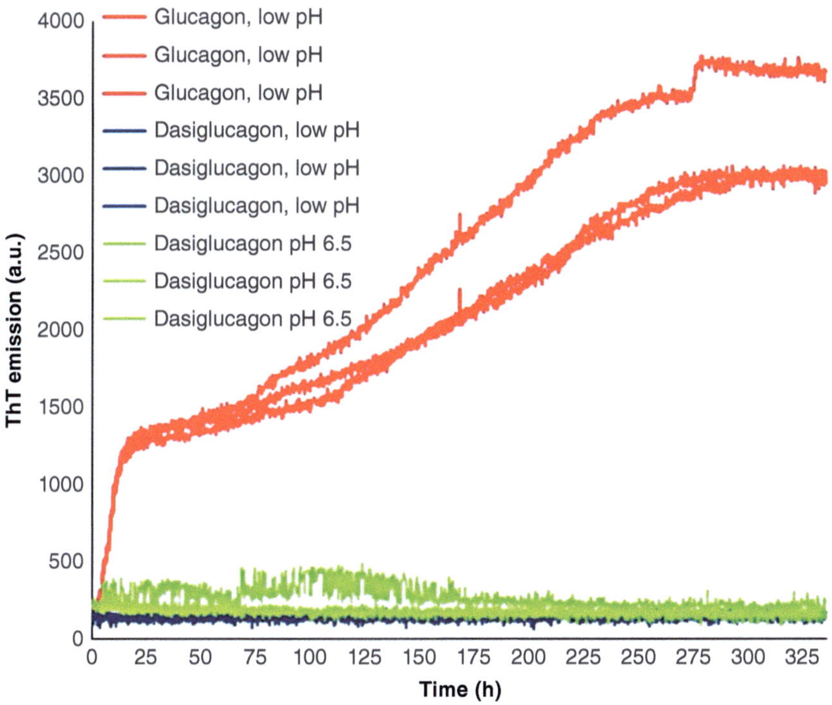

Figure 9.7 ThT assay (triple determination) with glucagon (pH 2.5–3.5, 1 mg/ml, 107 mg/ml lactose), dasiglucagon (pH 2.5–3.5, 1 mg/ml, 107 mg/ml lactose) and 0.6 mg dasiglucagon/0.6 ml, pH 6.5.

Table 9.6 DLS data on 0.6 mg dasiglucagon/0.6 ml, pH 6.5 at room temperature.

Time (weeks)	0	4	8	17	26	39	52
DLS data				z-average (nm)			
Dasiglucagon – no rotation	1.4	1.3	1.3	1.3	1.3	1.2	1.9
Dasiglucagon – rotation	1.4	1.5	1.5	1.3	1.3	1.6	1.4

DLS, dynamic light scattering.

Structural Characterization by Circular Dichroism

The secondary structure was characterized using circular dichroism (CD). The data shows that 0.6 mg dasiglucagon/0.6 ml, pH 6.5 has a largely random coil secondary structure, as expected for a short and flexible peptide mostly in the monomeric/dimeric state (see Figure 9.9). Furthermore, the data obtained for the different storage conditions are identical, indicating that storage at higher temperatures have no impact on the peptide conformation.

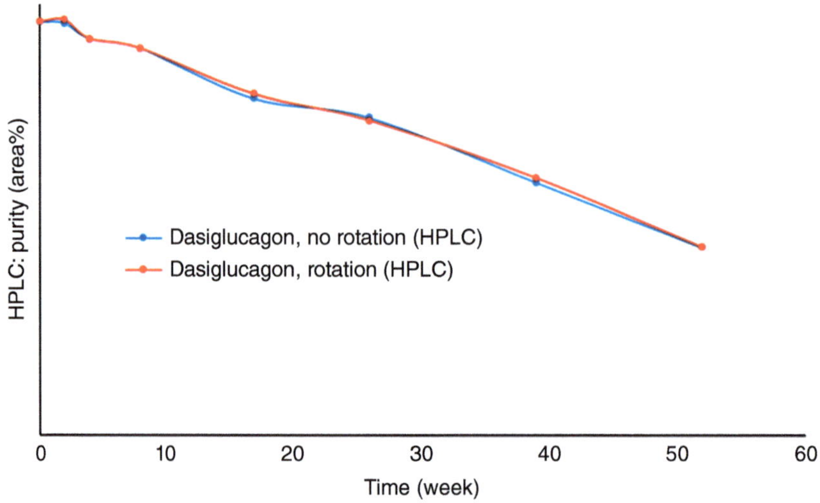

Figure 9.8 Rotation study on 0.6 mg dasiglucagon/0.6 ml, pH 6.5 at room temperature – HPLC purity [area%].

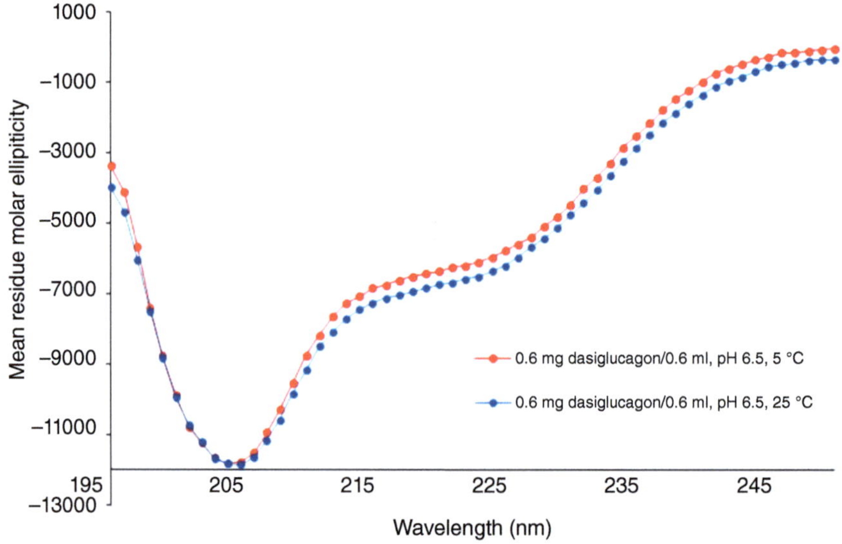

Figure 9.9 Circular dichroism of different drug product batches. 0.6 mg dasiglucagon/0.6 ml, pH 6.5, 25 °C = 0.6 mg dasiglucagon/0.6 ml, pH 6.5 stored 24 months at 5 °C followed by 12 months at 25 °C. 0.6 mg dasiglucagon/0.6 ml, pH 6.5, 5 °C = 0.6 mg dasiglucagon/0.6 ml, pH 6.5 stored 36 months at 5 °C.

Pharmacological Effect of Dasiglucagon in Humans

The pharmacological effect of dasiglucagon in terms of increasing blood glucose was investigated in adults and children aged 6 years and above with type 1 diabetes mellitus. Dasiglucagon at 0.6 mg and glucagon (GlucaGen) at 1.0 mg were administered as a single subcutaneous (SC) injection following a controlled

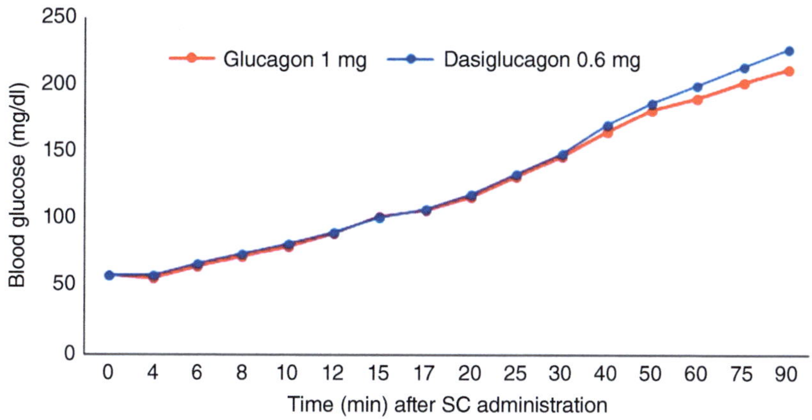

Figure 9.10 Mean plasma glucose (mg/dl) following administration of dasiglucagon at 0.6 mg and glucagon (GlucaGen) at 1.0 mg. Dasiglucagon or glucagon was administered following a controlled induction of hypoglycemia using IV administration of insulin.

induction of hypoglycemia using IV administration of insulin. Administration of dasiglucagon SC was associated with a fast increase in plasma glucose in both adults and children (see Figure 9.10 for blood glucose increase in adults). The increase in blood glucose was comparable to the effect seen following SC administration of reconstituted GlucaGen.

Conclusion

Dasiglucagon was designed as an analog to human glucagon. Five design rounds resulted in 7 out of 14 amino acids in the C-terminal region of the peptide being replaced. These replacements resulted in a peptide with improved physicochemical properties and similar pharmacokinetic and pharmacodynamic properties compared to human glucagon, enabling a "ready-to-use" formulation. Dasiglucagon (Zegalogue®) is currently approved in the United States for the treatment of severe hypoglycemia in adults and children aged six years and above with diabetes.

Amino Acid Abbreviations

Amino acid	3-letter abbreviation	1-letter abbreviation
Alanine	Ala	A
Arginine	Arg	R
Asparagine	Asn	N
Aspartic acid	Asp	D
Cysteine	Cys	C
Glutamine	Gln	Q
Glutamic acid	Glu	E

(Continued)

Amino acid	3-letter abbreviation	1-letter abbreviation
Glycine	Gly	G
Histidine	His	H
Isoleucine	Ile	I
Leucine	Leu	L
Lysine	Lys	K
Methionine	Met	M
Phenylalanine	Phe	F
Proline	Pro	P
Serine	Ser	S
Threonine	Thr	T
Tryptophan	Trp	W
Tyrosine	Tyr	Y
Valine	Val	V

References

1 Banting, F.G., Best, C.H., Collip, J.B. et al. (1922). Pancreatic extracts in the treatment of diabetes mellitus. *Can. Med. Assoc. J.* 12 (3): 141–146. https://www.ncbi.nlm.nih.gov/pubmed/20314060.

2 Kimball, C.P. and Murlin, J.R. (1923). Aqueous extracts of pancreas. III. Some precipitation reactions of insulin. *J. Biol. Chem.* 58: 337–346.

3 Staub, A., Sinn, L., and Behrens, O.K. (1953). Purification and crystallization of hyperglycemic glycogenolytic factor (HGF). *Science* 117 (3049): 628–629. https://doi.org/10.1126/science.117.3049.628.

4 Habegger, K.M., Heppner, K.M., Geary, N. et al. (2010). The metabolic actions of glucagon revisited. *Nat. Rev. Endocrinol.* 6 (12): 689–697. https://doi.org/10.1038/nrendo.2010.187.

5 Ramnanan, C.J., Edgerton, D.S., Kraft, G., and Cherrington, A.D. (2011). Physiologic action of glucagon on liver glucose metabolism. *Diabetes Obes. Metab.* 13 (Suppl 1): 118–125. https://doi.org/10.1111/j.1463-1326.2011.01454.x.

6 Quesada, I., Tuduri, E., Ripoll, C., and Nadal, A. (2008). Physiology of the pancreatic alpha-cell and glucagon secretion: role in glucose homeostasis and diabetes. *J. Endocrinol.* 199 (1): 5–19. https://doi.org/10.1677/JOE-08-0290.

7 Farah, A.E. (1983). Glucagon and the circulation. *Pharmacol. Rev.* 35 (3): 181–217. (In eng).

8 Damm Jorgensen, K., Weis, J.U., and Diamant, B. (1983). Dissociation of the spasmolytic and metabolic effects of glucagon. *Eur. J. Pharmacol.* 90 (4): 315–323. https://www.ncbi.nlm.nih.gov/pubmed/6576908.

9 Lin, T. and Tucci, J.R. (1974). Provocative tests of growth-hormone release. A comparison of results with seven stimuli. *Ann. Intern. Med.* 80 (4): 464–469. https://www.ncbi.nlm.nih.gov/pubmed/4378132.

10 Rahim, A., Toogood, A.A., and Shalet, S.M. (1996). The assessment of growth hormone status in normal young adult males using a variety of provocative agents. *Clin. Endocrinol.* 45 (5): 557–562. https://www.ncbi.nlm.nih.gov/pubmed/8977752.

11 Hirschberg, R.R., Zipser, R.D., Slomowitz, L.A., and Kopple, J.D. (1988). Glucagon and prostaglandins are mediators of amino acid-induced rise in renal hemodynamics. *Kidney Int.* 33 (6): 1147–1155. https://www.ncbi.nlm.nih.gov/pubmed/3404814.

12 Filippi, B.M., Abraham, M.A., Yue, J.T., and Lam, T.K. (2013). Insulin and glucagon signaling in the central nervous system. *Rev. Endocr. Metab. Disord.* 14 (4): 365–375. https://doi.org/10.1007/s11154-013-9258-4.

13 Grodsky, G.M., Bennett, L.L., Smith, D.F., and Schmid, F.G. (1967). Effect of pulse administration of glucose or glucagon on insulin secretion in vitro. *Metabolism* 16 (3): 222–233. https://www.ncbi.nlm.nih.gov/pubmed/6020731.

14 Maruyama, H., Hisatomi, A., Orci, L. et al. (1984). Insulin within islets is a physiologic glucagon release inhibitor. *J. Clin. Invest.* 74 (6): 2296–2299. https://doi.org/10.1172/JCI111658.

15 American Diabetes Association (2019). 6. Glycemic targets: standards of medical care in diabetes-2019. *Diabetes Care* 42 (Suppl 1): S61–S70. https://doi.org/10.2337/dc19-S006.

16 Kedia, N. (2011). Treatment of severe diabetic hypoglycemia with glucagon: an underutilized therapeutic approach. *Diabetes Metab Syndr Obes* 4: 337–346. https://doi.org/10.2147/DMSO.S20633.

17 Abraham, M.B., Jones, T.W., Naranjo, D. et al. (2018). ISPAD clinical practice consensus guidelines 2018: assessment and management of hypoglycemia in children and adolescents with diabetes. *Pediatr. Diabetes* 19 (Suppl 27): 178–192. https://doi.org/10.1111/pedi.12698.

18 Holt, R.I.G., DeVries, J.H., Hess-Fischl, A. et al. (2021). The management of type 1 diabetes in adults. A consensus report by the American Diabetes Association (ADA) and the European Association for the Study of Diabetes (EASD). *Diabetologia* 64 (12): 2609–2652. https://doi.org/10.1007/s00125-021-05568-3.

19 Fabris, C., Farhy, L.S., Anderson, S.M. et al. (2018). Recent exposure to hypoglycemia increases glucose variability following a hyper/hypoglycemic metabolic challenge in T1D. *J. Diabetes Sci. Technol.* 12 (2): 311–317. https://doi.org/10.1177/1932296817729392.

20 Novo Nordisk A/S (2021). GlucaGen HypoKit. SmPC, May 2021, https://www.medicines.org.uk/emc/product/1289/smpc#gref.

21 Eli Lilly and Company (2021). Glucagon for injection. USPI, January 2021, https://www.accessdata.fda.gov/drugsatfda_docs/label/2021/020928s060lbl.pdf.

22 Beaven, G.H., Gratzer, W.B., and Davies, H.G. (1969). Formation and structure of gels and fibrils from glucagon. *Eur. J. Biochem.* 11 (1): 37–42. https://doi.org/10.1111/j.1432-1033.1969.tb00735.x.

23 Joshi, A.B., Rus, E., and Kirsch, L.E. (2000). The degradation pathways of glucagon in acidic solutions. *Int. J. Pharm.* 203 (1–2): 115–125. https://doi.org/10.1016/s0378-5173(00)00438-5.

24 Caputo, N., Castle, J.R., Bergstrom, C.P. et al. (2013). Mechanisms of glucagon degradation at alkaline pH. *Peptides* 45: 40–47. https://doi.org/10.1016/j.peptides.2013.04.005.

25 Bischoff, R. and Kolbe, H.V. (1994). Deamidation of asparagine and glutamine residues in proteins and peptides: structural determinants and analytical methodology. *J. Chromatogr. B Biomed. Appl.* 662 (2): 261–278. https://doi.org/10.1016/0378-4347(94)00203-7.

26 Aswad, D.W., Paranandi, M.V., and Schurter, B.T. (2000). Isoaspartate in peptides and proteins: formation, significance, and analysis. *J. Pharm. Biomed. Anal.* 21 (6): 1129–1136. https://doi.org/10.1016/s0731-7085(99)00230-7.

27 Pedersen, J.S., Dikov, D., and Otzen, D.E. (2006). N- and C-terminal hydrophobic patches are involved in fibrillation of glucagon. *Biochemistry* 45 (48): 14503–14512. https://doi.org/10.1021/bi061228n.

28 Pedersen, J.S., Flink, J.M., Dikov, D., and Otzen, D.E. (2006). Sulfates dramatically stabilize a salt-dependent type of glucagon fibrils. *Biophys. J.* 90 (11): 4181–4194. https://doi.org/10.1529/biophysj.105.070912.

29 Andersen, C.B., Otzen, D., Christiansen, G., and Rischel, C. (2007). Glucagon amyloid-like fibril morphology is selected via morphology-dependent growth inhibition. *Biochemistry* 46 (24): 7314–7324. https://doi.org/10.1021/bi6025374.

30 Pedersen, J.S., Dikov, D., Flink, J.L. et al. (2006). The changing face of glucagon fibrillation: structural polymorphism and conformational imprinting. *J. Mol. Biol.* 355 (3): 501–523. https://doi.org/10.1016/j.jmb.2005.09.100.

31 Oliveira, C.L., Behrens, M.A., Pedersen, J.S. et al. (2009). A SAXS study of glucagon fibrillation. *J. Mol. Biol.* 387 (1): 147–161. https://doi.org/10.1016/j.jmb.2009.01.020.

32 Chabenne, J., Chabenne, M.D., Zhao, Y. et al. (2014). A glucagon analog chemically stabilized for immediate treatment of life-threatening hypoglycemia. *Mol Metab* 3 (3): 293–300. https://doi.org/10.1016/j.molmet.2014.01.006.

33 Rodbell, M., Birnbaumer, L., Pohl, S.L., and Sundby, F. (1971). The reaction of glucagon with its receptor: evidence for discrete regions of activity and binding in the glucagon molecule. *Proc. Natl. Acad. Sci. USA* 68 (5): 909–913. https://doi.org/10.1073/pnas.68.5.909.

34 Spiegel, A.M. and Bitensky, M.W. (1969). Effects of chemical and enzymatic modifications of glucagon on its activation of hepatic adenyl cyclase. *Endocrinology* 85 (4): 638–643. https://doi.org/10.1210/endo-85-4-638.

35 Hilger, D., Kumar, K.K., Hu, H. et al. (2020). Structural insights into differences in G protein activation by family A and family B GPCRs. *Science* 369 (6503): https://doi.org/10.1126/science.aba3373.

36 Qiao, A., Han, S., Li, X. et al. (2020). Structural basis of G(s) and G(i) recognition by the human glucagon receptor. *Science* 367 (6484): 1346–1352. https://doi.org/10.1126/science.aaz5346.

Index

a

A14E B16H B25H 202
agouti-related peptide (AgRP) 215
agouti related-protein (AGRP) 16
Aib (1-aminoisobutyric acid) 272, 274
albenatide 130–131
albiglutide 130–131
alpha-glucosidase inhibitors 147
amino acid peptide amylin 88
amphetamines 159
amylin 87
- brain sites of 91–96
- different molecular forms of 88
- effect on energy homeostasis 89–91
- effects of eating 100–102
- formation in pancreatic islets 102–104
- molecular forms of 99–100
- signaling at the amylin receptor 88–89

amylin-derived fibrillogenic 103–104
amylin-leptin interactions 96–99
- in the AP and NTS 97
- in the VMH (ARC+VMN) 98

amylin receptors 1-3 (AMY1-3) 88
amyloidogenic human IAPP (hIAPP) 102

b

Bardet Biedl Syndrome-6 protein (BBS6) 98
bariatric surgery 224–225
basal insulin drugs 197
basolateral membrane-bound proteins 7
β3-adrenoreceptor agonists 163
β-arrestin 40, 44
BETP 168, 169, 171, 173
biguanides 143, 146–147
bile acid sequestrants 150, 152
Boc5 166
bofanglutide 133–134
boronic acids 205
bovine insulin 198
bupropion + naltrexone (“contrave”) 161

c

cagrilintide 101
calcitonin gene-related peptide (CGRP) 89, 92–93
cardioprotective effects 152
caudal hindbrain neurons 93–94
CB2R expression 162
centrally-acting combinations
- bupropion+naltrexone (“Contrave”) 161
- phentermine+fenfluramine (“Phen-Fen”) 159–160
- phentermine+topiramate (“Qsymia”) 160–161

cholecystokinin (CCK) 1, 2, 5–7
circular dichroism (CD) 280–281
C-terminal amidation 217
cyclic adenosine monophosphate (cAMP) 39, 165

d

danuglipron 173, 176–180
dasiglucagon
- 1st design 268, 269
- 2nd design 268, 270, 271
- 3rd design 270, 272, 273
- 4th design 272, 274–276
- 5th design 274, 277–279
- characterization of
  - circular dichroism (CD) 280–281
  - physical and chemical stability 279
  - rotation study 279–280
- chemical and physical instability 265–267
- design strategy and assays 267–268
- diabetes mellitus 264–265

dasiglucagon (*contd.*)
  glucagon and physiological effects 263–264
  pharmacological effect of 281–282
degludec 201
detemir 200, 201
diboronate insulin conjugates 206
diboronic acids 205
2, 4-dinitrophenol (DNP) 158
dipeptidyl peptidase-4 (DPP-4) inhibitors 4, 12, 37, 150, 217, 226
dopamine-2 agonists 152–153
dorsomedial nucleus of the hypothalamus (DMH) 245
dual amylin calcitonin receptor agonists (DACRAs) 89
dulaglutide 131

e

ecnoglutide 131–132
efpeglenatide 126–127
efsitora alfa 202
11β-Hydroxysteroid dehydrogenase type 1 (11β-HSD1) inhibitors 154
endocrine mode of action 2
endogenous GIP 33
exchange protein directly activated by cAMP 2 (EPAC2) 39
exenatide 124–125
exenatide long-acting release (LAR) 125–129
extended-release (ER) 165
extracellular domain (ECD) 165
extracellular-signal-regulated kinase 1 and 2 (ERK1/2) 39

f

fatty diacid derivatization 227
ferocious appetite 17
Food, Drug and Cosmetic Act (FDCA) 158

g

gastric inhibitory polypeptide 13, 35
genome-wide association studies (GWAS) 50
ghrelin 2, 16–18
ghrelin O-acyl-transferase (GOAT) 4, 16
GIP 13–16
  extrapancreatic physiological effects of
    adipose tissue 49
    body weight 50–51
    bones 52–53
    cardiovascular system 51–52
    central nervous system 53–54
    energy expenditure 51
GIP(1-30)NH_2 36
G protein-coupled receptor kinases (GRKs) 40
G protein-coupled receptors (GPCRs) 37

h

hedonic feeding 1
hedonic processes 1
HEK293 cells 165, 168, 169, 171, 172, 176, 267
high-energy diet (HED) 248
high throughput screen (HTS) 168, 169, 171, 175
homeostatic regulation 1
hormone antagonists 3
HyGlutide 132–133
hypophysiotropic messengers 245
hypothalamic PrRPDMH neurons 252

i

icodec 202, 204, 207
imeglimin 154
immunoglobulin G2 antibody (IgG2) 202
incretin effect 14, 46–48, 121
insulin aspart (B28D) 199
insulin dosing 197
insulin drug design
  glucose-sensitive insulin 198, 204–206
  insulin pumps and cell-based therapy 206
  meal insulin designs and formulations 199
  native insulin 198–199
  once-daily basal insulin designs 199–201
  once-weekly insulin design 201–203
  oral and pulmonary insulin 204
  tissue selective and functionally selective insulin 203–204
insulin glulisine (B3K B29E) 199
insulin pumps and cell-based therapy 206
intellectual property (IP) 270
intracerebroventricular (ICV) injection 12, 218
intravenous glucose tolerance test (IVGTT) model 169

l

lateral dorsal tegmental area (LDTg) 95
LEAP2 18
lipoprotein lipase (LPL) 49
liraglutide 128–129
lixisenatide 126
lorcaserin 161
lotiglipron 173, 176

"low receptor affinity" drug design principle 202
loxenatide 127–128

m
meal insulin designs and formulations 199
meal insulin doses 197
mechanisms of amyloid genesis 102–103
medial prefrontal cortex (mPFC) 95, 96
meglitinides (Glinides) 147–148
melanocortin 4 receptor (MC4R) agonist 91, 163
metformin 146–148, 150, 153, 173, 175, 179, 201
mild hypoglycemia 264
mimicry 2–3
mirabegron 163
mitogen-activated protein kinase (MAPK) 39
2-monoacyl glycerols 7

n
native insulin 197–198, 204
natural polymorphisms 248–249
neuropeptide FF (NPFF) 246
neuropeptide FF receptor 2 (NPFFR2) 243
neuropeptides 2
neuropeptide Y (NPY) 11
  knocking out peptide ligands 218
  primary structure of 216
  receptors and distribution 217–218
  Y1R/Y5R agonism 219–220
  Y1R/Y5R antagonists 220–222
nicotine 155
nisotirostide 227, 230
*N*MeArg^{35} 225–226
NN501 253, 254
noiiglutide 127
norepinephrine–dopamine reuptake inhibitor (NDRI) 161
NPY1-36 215
nucleus accumbens (NAc) 95–96
nucleus of the tractus solitarius (NTS) 245

o
obesity oral agents 154–155
  β3-adrenoreceptor agonists 163
  cannabinoid receptor antagonists 162–163
  centrally-acting combinations 159–161
  dinitrophenol 158
  lorcaserin 161
  melanocortin 4 receptor (MC4R) agonist 163
  nicotine 155
  orlistat 162
  small molecules 164
  thyroxine (T4) 155, 158
obinepitide 227, 230
oligofucosyl/mannosyl insulin derivatives 206
once-daily basal insulin designs 199–201
once-weekly insulin design 201–203
oral and pulmonary insulin 204
orforglipron 176–180
orlistat 162
Otsuka Long-Evans Tokushima Fatty (OLETF) 248
oxyntomodulin 2, 7, 10, 11, 13, 172, 227

p
pancreatic polypeptide (PP) 11
  knocking out peptide ligands 218
  primary structure of 216
  Y4R interaction 222–223
peptide YY (PYY) 2
  bariatric surgery 224–225
  DPPIV 217
  food energy homeostasis 223–224
  GLP-1 or oxyntomodulin 227
  glucose homeostasis regulator 224
  half-life extension of 226–227
  human studies and trials 229–231
  knocking out peptide ligands 218
  obesity and diabetes treatment 231–232
  primary structure of 216
  structure of 216
  Y2R interaction 223
  Y2R-selective 225
Peroxisome Proliferator-Activated Receptor family–PPARγ 148
pharmacological GIPR agonism
  animal studies 54–55
  human studies 55–59
pharmacological GIPR antagonism
  animal studies 60–61
  human studies 61–62
Phentermine+Fenfluramine ("Phen-Fen") 160
Phentermine+Topiramate ("Qsymia") 160
positive allosteric modulators (PAMs) 168, 170
PP-fold peptides 12
Prader-Willi syndrome 17, 222
pramlintide 89, 96, 97, 100, 101
pro-amylin 88, 99–100, 103
proGIP 36, 49
proGIP gene 49
proinsulin 202

prolactin-releasing peptide (PrRP)
 administered systemically 252
 brainstem PrRPNTS neurons 250–251
 central metabolic effects of 246
 discovery of 244
 hypophysiotropic effect 245
 hypothalamic PrRPDMH neurons 252
 natural polymorphisms 248–249
 NPFF signalling 249–250
 pharmacological tool 243–244
 Prlh and *Prlhr* knockout mouse models 248
 prolactin 245
 receptor coupling and distribution 246–248
proopiomelanocortin (POMC) 94, 161, 163
proprotein convertase subtilisin/kexin-1 (PCSK1) 163
protein kinase A (PKA) 39
PrRPNTS neurons 250–251
pulmonary insulin (lung dosed insulin) 204
PYY 11–13

r
Rainbow Diet Pills 159
receptor antagonist, definition 40
rimonabant 163

s
Seemli^er 100
semaglutide 10, 14, 15, 55, 58, 101, 123, 124, 129
single nucleotide polymorphisms (SNPs) 249
small molecule antagonists 3
small molecules glucagon-like peptide 1 receptor (GLP-1R) agonists
 Boc5 166–167
 in clinical development
  danuglipron and lotiglipron 173–176
  danuglipron and orforglipron 180
  orforglipron 176–180
  TTP273 from vTv Therapeutics 173
 ECD 165
 positive allosteric modulators 168–173
sodium-glucose transporter-2 (SGLT2) inhibitors 153
sodium-linked glucose transporter-2 inhibitors (SGLT-2i) 202
sodium N-(8-[2-hydroxybenzoyl] amino) caprylate (SNAC) 129
somatostatin 4, 17, 47, 216, 224
SPPS 219
structure-activity relationships (SAR) 219
sub-postrema (SubP) region 248
sulfonylureas 145–146

t
Tabacco extract 155
taspoglutide 129–130
thiazolidinediones 148–150
thioflavin T (ThT) 279
thyroxine (T4) 155
tirzepatide 10, 14–16, 18, 34, 48, 58–59, 180, 227, 230, 231
tissue selective and functionally selective insulin 203–204
transmembrane (TM) region 165
2, 4, 6-trinitrotoluene (TNT) 158
two-step binding and activation model 37
type 2 diabetes oral agents 141
 alpha-glucosidase inhibitors 147
 amphetamines 159
 biguanides 146–147
 bile acid sequestrants 150–152
 dipeptidyl peptidase-4 (DPP4) inhibitors 150
 dopamine-2 agonists 152
 glimins 154
 meglitinides (glinides) 147–148
 small molecule 154, 164
 sodium-glucose transporter-2 (SGLT2) inhibitors 153
 sulfonylureas 145–146
 thiazolidinediones 148–150
 timeline of history 142

u
utreglutide 132

v
ventral tegmental area (VTA) 95–96
ventrolateral medulla oblongata (VLM) 245
visepegenatide 128

y
Y4R interaction 222–223

z
Zegalogue® 265, 279
ZT002 133